THE EFFECTIVE CLINICIAN

His Methods and Approach to Diagnosis and Care

PHILIP A. TUMULTY, M.D.

Professor of Medicine
The Johns Hopkins University School of Medicine
Baltimore, Maryland

1973

W. B. SAUNDERS COMPANY
Philadelphia · London · Toronto

W. B. Saunders Company: West Washington Square
Philadelphia, Pa. 19105

12 Dyott Street
London, WC1A 1DB

833 Oxford Street
Toronto 18, Ontario

The Effective Clinician   ISBN 0-7216-8915-9

© 1973 by W. B. Saunders Company. Copyright under the International Copyright Union. All rights reserved. This book is protected by copyright. No part of it may be reproduced, stored in a retrieval system, or transmitted in any form or by any means, electronic, mechanical, photocopying, recording, or otherwise, without written permission from the publisher. Made in the United States of America. Press of W. B. Saunders Company. Library of Congress catalog card number 73-77942.

Print No: 9 8 7 6 5 4 3 2 1

DEDICATED
TO MY WIFE,
CLAIRE,
AND TO OUR CHILDREN,
CLAIRE, PHILIP, CATHY, MARY, ALICIA

. . . giving so much, so constantly

Preface

Although many highly effective diagnostic and therapeutic tools are now available, I am convinced that too frequently they are applied to patients' problems in a manner that appreciably lessens their full healing potential for the patient and his family. This in large part results from the fact that the clinician's *approach* to a patient's problem and his *management* of it are sometimes suboptimal. To approach and manage a particular clinical problem most effectively requires the following:

1. Detailed familiarity not only with the patient's specific complaint and his physical status but also with the patient as a person, including knowledge of family and of his life circumstances. This can be realized only if the clinician has acquired great facilty and knowledgeability in *communicating* with his patient, and in examining him, and also in communicating with his *family*, as well. For it is only by means of such communication and physical examination that the basic *clinical evidence* is derived, and this is, after all, the essential stuff behind the clinician's thinking and action.

2. An organized, disciplined, structured method of analyzing the clinical evidence thus derived, so that no specifically treatable possibilities are overlooked in the clinician's diagnostic approach, and consequently in his plan of therapeutic management.

3. Employment of wise principles of management, well tested through broad experience, that emphasize regard for the entire patient and not merely his illness, and even more, regard for the patient as part of a family and a community, not as an isolated being.

4. Securing patient compliance based upon effective communication with the patient (and his family), which aims to accomplish two main objectives: (*a*) *understanding* by the patient of the nature of his problem in terms which are positive and do not generate unnecessary anxiety; and (*b*) *motivation* to do whatever may be necessary for him in order to best meet his problem.

Although dealing with principles, approaches, and methods, this book is by no means a philosophical treatise on the delivery of health care. Rather, it is concerned with their very down-to-earth practical application, and affords a large dose of useful clinical insight and hard information along the way.

Therefore, the subject matter of this book is material dealing with: (1) effective communication between the clinician and his patient, his patient's family, and the chosen consultants; (2) physical examination of the patient at a more sophisticated level than that usually presented in texts concerned with the general principles of physical diagnosis; (3) guidelines for the gathering together and sorting out of all the essential clinical evidence in the most meaningful fashion; (4) the outlining and illustrating of a method of approach to clinical diagnosis based upon an organized, structured method of analysis of the clinical evidence; (5) principles of management of patients and their clinical problems, and suggestions for dealing with their families, as well; (6) the development of a diagnostic and therapeutic plan of management, designed to meet in a total way the patient's problem; and (7) obtaining the patient's compliance and cooperation through inculcation of effective motivation based upon a properly presented understanding on the patient's part of what his problem is really all about. The study and the full understanding of these major steps in the intelligent practice of medicine is the heart of this book.

In addition to general considerations, these matters are discussed in particular relation to some very specific clinical situations that are always especially difficult for the clinician to approach and manage, an analysis of which brings to focus highly useful principles. Finally, the recommended diagnostic approach is illustrated through its application to a wide variety of quite different but frequently encountered clinical problems, which are discussed in some detail.

The list of references following each of these discussions has been chosen largely from articles concerned with the natural course of diseases, or with the fundamentals underlying various methods of diagnosis and management.

It is earnestly hoped that this book will become a source of ideas and information leading to more effective care of the readers' patients, the word "care" being employed in its broadest and deepest connotations.

Because of its broad scope, dealing as it does with practical matters of genuine pertinence to all types of clinical problems, this book is intended for a wide clinical audience—medical students in their clinical years, and interns and residents, as well as practitioners—in fact, for all those who are daily confronted with patients, their families, and the diagnosis and management of their problems.

My years in the practice and teaching of medicine have been happy and valued, years not to be traded. The opportunities for learning have been rich and the types of clinical problems encountered were widely varied. Both the patients and their illnesses covered an exceedingly broad spectrum. Furthermore, those who have taught me have been gifted and challenging and stimulating. So also have been my associates, both on the Junior and Senior

Staffs. I am in debt to many for the clinical opportunities afforded me. To Dr. A. McGehee Harvey I owe the most, for he asked me to join him for two years as his first Chief Resident Physician. Subsequently, for my six most bountiful learning years, we "practiced" together, I acting as his subaltern, making rounds together late in the afternoons, sitting for thought and discussion on the benches in the halls. I enjoyed to the full the refreshment that can only come from contact with brilliance in clinical knowledge and judgment.

Throughout these years, I have been blessed by having a sequence of exceedingly competent as well as attractive secretaries, who have been highly effective right arms and alter egos. None has been more so than Mrs. Joan M. Wood, who helped prepare this manuscript from its very tedious beginnings. I am especially grateful to Mrs. Christine F. Barlow, who assisted in bringing the manuscript to its final form with very great ability and finesse.

Thanks are also owed to the editors of *The New England Journal of Medicine* and *The Johns Hopkins Medical Journal*, who generously allowed me to reprint some material that previously appeared in their much respected journals.

I am grateful to Mr. Jack Hanley of the W. B. Saunders Company for his gentle but expert and experienced editorial hand.

Finally, my warmest thanks are expressed to Mr. Edwin Duncan, Sr., whose generosity enabled me to meet the cost of preparing this manuscript.

PHILIP A. TUMULTY

Leading each chapter of the book are portrait sketches by Mr. Grant Lashbrook of twelve distinguished members of the past and present faculty at The Johns Hopkins University School of Medicine. They were chosen as men whose careers continue to give life to the principles and concepts covered herein. Except for Dr. Osler, this author was taught by all at various stages in his career and to each owes so much.

Contents

Introduction—What is a Clinician and What Does
He Do?............................. 1

Section A—Communication...................... 9

1. Communicating with the Patient—General
   Considerations 11
2. Obtaining the History..................... 17
3. Conducting the "Final" or Summarizing Interview . 29
4. Communicating with the Family 39
5. Communicating as a Consultant.............. 45

Section B—The Performance of the Physical
Examination......................... 49

1. The Physical Examination 51

Section C—Clinical Management................. 99

1. General Considerations in Clinical Management ... 101
2. The Patient with a Functional Disorder 125
3. The Patient with Fever of Unknown Origin (FUO) . 137
4. The Patient with Incurable, Progressive or Fatal
   Illness 171

Section D—Clinical Problem Analysis 187

1. A Systematic Approach to Differential Diagnosis .. 189
2. Problem-Oriented Diagnostic Discussions 201

ix

CONTENTS

- A. A Patient with Hypercalcemia 201
- B. A Patient with Multiple Pulmonary Emboli ... 207
- C. A Patient with Persistent Fever and Malaise after Cardiac Surgery 214
- D. A Patient with Fulminant Pneumococcal Pneumonia 221
- E. A Patient with a Liver Abscess 229
- F. A Patient Suffering Sudden Death 234
- G. A Patient with a Mediastinal Mass 241
- H. A Patient with Obscure Gastrointestinal Hemorrhage 249
- I. A Patient with Chest Pain, Severe Venous In-Flow Block and Coronary Artery Disease ... 258
- J. A Patient with Ascites 268
- K. A Patient with Cryptococcal Meningitis 278
- L. A Patient with the Hamman-Rich Syndrome ... 286
- M. A Patient with Congestive Heart Failure and Aortic Insufficiency 296
- N. A Patient with a Complicated, Chronic, Episodic Polyorgan System Disease 305
- O. A Patient with Amyloidosis 315
- P. A Patient with Chronic Uremia 323
- Q. A Patient with Systemic Lupus and Complications 333
- R. A Patient with Rheumatoid Arthritis and Complications 342
- S. A Patient with a Hemoglobinopathy 351
- T. A Patient with Systemic Lupus Erythematosus (SLE) and Extensive, Profuse Bleeding 362

Index 373

INTRODUCTION

What is a Clinician and What Does He Do?*

Since this course marks your entrance into clinical medicine, it seems appropriate to discuss what a clinician is, and what he does. Sometimes it is easier to describe what something is not than to define what it is, and since a succinct definition of the term "clinician" is not easily conceived, it might be helpful to start with this approach. Thus, a clinician is not someone whose prime function is to diagnose or to cure illness, for in many cases, he is not able to accomplish either of these.

A clinician is more accurately defined as one whose prime function is to manage a sick person with the purpose of alleviating most effectively the total impact of the illness upon that person. Several of the terms used in this definition require development.

MANAGEMENT OF A SICK PERSON

Managing a sick person is entirely different from diagnosing an illness and prescribing therapy for it. A simple example might be offered of a mother, by nature keenly sensitive and perfectionistic, who has three young and perpetually active children and a husband who is preoccupied by his work. She doesn't see much of him, and when she does, they are both tired and the children are boisterous. She visits her physician with complaints of headaches, stiffness and soreness in the back of her neck, persistent fatigability, frequent loose stools with mucus, and a 10-pound weight loss. Her symptoms have reached an intensity that makes it difficult for her to care for her family. After appropriate examination and studies, the final diagnosis is as follows: "anxiety state with tension headaches and a spastic colon." The physician prescribes diazepam (Valium), propantheline (Pro-Banthīne), psyllium muciloloide (Metamucil), and propoxyphene (Darvon). She is told to return in six weeks for follow-up examination.

---

*This article originally appeared in the New England Journal of Medicine, 283:20–24, July, 1970, and is reprinted with permission.

Thus, the physician has correctly diagnosed her condition, and has prescribed appropriate medications—but has he *managed* this sick person? Emphatically not!

Management of this patient would require these additional ingredients: an explanation, in terms highly meaningful to her, of the relation between her symptoms and factors in her personality and home situation; a review of all the elements in her circumstances that might be creating stress; some constructive advice about children's behavior and discipline, and about being a young wife; insistence on an hour's rest period every day after lunch, free of the children; the writing down of a well organized weekly work schedule to bring some order out of household chaos, and insistence upon adherence to it; the suggestion that she employ a day worker every week or two to help with the heavy housecleaning; a conference with the husband to ensure that he understands how to support his wife's position (inquiries about sex adjustments would be apropos at this juncture); efforts to interest the patient in hobbies and activities affording some respite from daily unending household routines; and an admonition to go light on relaxing cocktails and nightcaps during this stressful period, lest dependencies develop.

Clearly, management of a sick person entails much more than diagnosis and the prescribing of medicines, and demands much more of the physician. Also, it gives much more back to the patient.

Management means that the physician comprehends and is sensitive to the total effects of an illness on the total person, the spiritual effects as well as the physical, and the social as well as the economic. With the wisdom born of education and experience, the clinician attempts to prevent or to diminish, or to heal this sum total of effects. Specific forms of therapy are brought to bear directly upon a pathologic process. Management is concerned with the sickened person, and the family, and the community.

Today, even highly sophisticated treatment schedules can be put on tapes, to be printed out at the push of the proper button. Computers are being successfully employed in diagnosis. But the ways of wise management of a sick person can only come out of an understanding spirit, and a sensitive as well as perceptive and educated mind.

A patient given specific therapy has something done to him to aid his recovery. A patient who is well managed is capable of helping *himself* to recovery, for he has been provided with insight and knowledge, hope and security, and the motivation to do whatever may be required.

In incurable illness, treatment of the disease may become a hopeless, vain gesture, and anguished suffering and ultimate death are stark admissions of its failure. However, if the sick person is thoughtfully managed, the effects of incurable illness can be made immeasurably less devastating for both the patient and the family, and triumph can even be had over some of the most mortal effects of fatal illness, which are often far more psychologic than physical.

TOTAL IMPACT OF ILLNESS

In the definition of "clinician," I employed the expression, "alleviating most effectively the total impact of the illness upon that person." Two concepts here require further development.

The impact of sickness upon a person is always multifocal, and the effects highly complex, involving as they do the whole person, with his spiritual, intellectual, emotional, social and economic components.

A pair of kidneys will never come to the physician for diagnosis and treatment. They will be contained within an anxious, fearful, wondering person, asking puzzled questions about an obscure future, weighed down by the responsibilities of a loved family, and with a job to be held, and with bills to be paid. A biochemist or a physiologist can ignore all these secondary factors, and can confine his attention to the kidneys. But the clinician must learn the facts about it all, and comprehend it all, and have a feeling for it all, and develop a plan of management for it all. Otherwise, his approach is superficial.

Finally, sickness rarely affects only the patient. If he is the member of a family, the entire family is inevitably affected, to greater or lesser degrees. Hence, in a peculiar and special sense, *all* clinicians have family practices— even the most erudite and hard to get to see consultants. This magnifies the clinician's responsibility greatly, for his success or failure in managing a patient's problem will be reflected in the welfare of the patient's family members. Few, indeed, shoulder a burden of personal responsibility heavier than the clinician's.

FUNCTION OF A CLINICIAN

So much for what a clinician *is*. How does he function?

First of all, he listens thoughtfully to the patient's complaint. Secondly, he proceeds to gather together all the available clinical evidence pertinent to it, beginning with the history and physical examination. Thirdly, through logical analysis of this clinical evidence, he formulates a reasoned explanation for the cause of the patient's complaint, in the light of his knowledge and past experience. Fourthly, he develops a program of management for the patient, in the terms already discussed.

Clinical evidence is the basic material with which the clinician works. He gathers it from several sources: the history; the physical examination; laboratory studies and special technics (such as x-ray study); and consulting opinions.

The source of the clinical evidence is not the essential point, although experience daily points out the primacy of the history and physical examination. The essential point is that the evidence be both complete and valid, that its total implications be understood, and that it be critically reviewed in relation to other evidence already at hand.

It is foolish to argue that the history is a more important source of clinical evidence than the physical examination, or that the latter is a more valuable source than laboratory or x-ray study. The key evidence in understanding a particular patient's complaint may be disclosed by any of these evidence-gathering technics. A clinician must be equally adept in the employment of all of them. Facts are his concern, no matter how they are harvested, and he must seek them by every means available.

Regard yourselves as indomitable gatherers of clinical evidence. Hunt for it anywhere it might be hidden, in the history or physical examination, in some special test, or in conversation with a family member, or tucked away in some previous medical report, for hidden anywhere it may well be.

Nowadays, in contrast to the past, a diagnosis must often be specifically correct if the patient is to get well, for so many modern forms of therapy have highly specific actions. This scientific advancement compels the clinician to sharpen his clinical skills to the very keenest edge, so that he can extract from a meticulous history and physical examination every particle of pertinent clinical evidence, which he then co-ordinates with evidence gathered by other means. Never before has such a premium been placed upon expertise in the performance of the history and physical examination as the prime steps in the diagnostic process from which all other investigative steps logically proceed.

Once analysis of the clinical evidence has led to a diagnosis, and a plan of management for the patient's problem has been constructed, the physician comes to a highly critical point in his relation with his patient: he must explain to him the nature of his illness and formulate for him the program of management. Unless these matters are handled with clarity and sensitivity, so that the patient understands fully what is wrong and also has the will to marshal his personal resources to co-operate fully, the correctness of the diagnosis and the soundness of the therapy may have no practical meaning whatever for the patient. Ignorance, misconceptions, fears, insecurities, resentments, hopelessness and unanswered queries may block his response.

COMMUNICATION WITH THE PATIENT

This brings us to one of the last but surely one of the most essential considerations of what it is a clinician does—a clinician spends a great amount of his working hours communicating with his patients. What the scalpel is to the surgeon, words are to the clinician. When he uses them effectively, his patients do well. If not, the results may be disastrous.

You are surely aware that physicians are not now as highly esteemed by the general public as formerly. It seems unlikely that the public, so easily impressed by what appears to be scientific, resents the fact that physicians nowadays have become more scientific in their education and methods. Actually, what many patients miss and resent today is their inability to communicate with their physician in a meaningful manner. Patients have questions that they want answered, fears requiring dissipation, misunderstandings that need clarification and abysmal ignorance about themselves that demands enlightenment. Today, many patients with serious health problems leave their physician's offices with less comprehension of what is wrong and what they must do to get well than the average customer understands about his car when he drives it out of the repair shop. "Pay your bill and drive off." "Get these prescriptions filled and come back in two months." And, if the patient feels deprived of adequate communication with his physician, family members often are totally devoid of it.

No wonder the resentments. We clinicians are better educated and more scientific than ever before, but we have a great failing: we sometimes do not communicate effectively with our patients, or with their families. Some of us do not provide the time, or make the effort. Others simply do not know how to talk to sick persons. If this seems exaggerated, it might be recalled that in the entire Marburg Building at Johns Hopkins, there is but one small room suitable for serious family conferences. The general daily practice, therefore, is to discuss critical and frequently shocking issues with relatives while standing in the noisy halls, dodging food trucks and litters. Critical information and advice is given to sick persons and their families buffet style—standing up!

An effective clinician must have a number of skills, and these you must endeavor to make your own. He must be a scientist. He must be knowledgeable about the natural course of common and uncommon diseases. He must be able to harvest clinical evidence from all available sources. He must be a keen analyst of these gathered facts, and through logic proceed to a reasonable conclusion concerning their significance. But, in addition, if these capabilities are to have a practical effect upon the patient, the clinician must have the facility to communicate with him, and his family members.

The wisdom of Thomas Aquinas, the logic of Newman and the clinical genius of Osler will not be effective in making well a patient who does not fully understand why he is sick, or what he must do to get well. A first-rate clinician trains himself to do two things exceedingly well: to talk to his patients, and to listen to them. And he acts similarly with responsible family members.

Through well conceived conversations, the physician hopes to accomplish a number of indispensable purposes, the first being the extraction of all the clinical evidence about the historical development of the patient's illness, followed by the quieting of the patient's anxieties. Here it is essential to realize that all illness in all persons is inevitably productive of varying degrees of fear and anxiety, though they are often well submerged under seeming indifference, bravado or sophistication. These emotions may spring from many causes and assume many forms, but they are always there. If the doctor is powerless to do anything else to aid a patient, he has accomplished a great deal, and has justified his being that patient's physician, if, through his conversation, he strips from an illness ugly, eroding, undermining fears. The fear of cancer is widespread. No less prevalent is the cancer of fear in people who are ill. Its only cure is therapeutic conversation with the physician.

In addition, the clinician must constantly ask patients to undergo diagnostic and therapeutic maneuvers that are costly, or unpleasant or very hard for the patient to accomplish. Recovery from illness often depends on the ability of the patient to exert stern self-discipline over himself. Only full understanding of the problem by the patient can lead to adequate motivation. Only the clinician can bring this about, and only to the degree that he is able and willing to converse with his patient.

Therefore, he has to learn to talk to his patients and—even more important—*like* to talk to his patients. It is his greatest asset as a clinician. The most rewarding study of man *is* man. No one has the privilege of knowing man so intimately, at times of such great personal moment, and under such highly sensitive circumstances, as the physician. He becomes intimately familiar with man as he is born, and as he sickens, and as he dies. Like no one else, he has the opportunity to listen to the laughter and to the cries. Like no other man, he has the opportunity to speak to man, and through his words to guide and to correct him, and to heal him, and to give him solace, to the very edge of eternity.

When the clinician is exceedingly busy, as most clinicians are, there is a widespread tendency to substitute tests for talk, and various therapeutic maneuvers take the place of enlightenment and motivation. One must remember that talk is indeed cheap, but it can be so healing.

Here are some practical guidelines in talking to patients:

Almost all patients, regardless of intellectual capacity, are naïve and simplistic when dealing with their own health problems. One should assume nothing, and start from basic facts, and build upward. A brilliant person is often a dull patient. A less endowed patient is often like a child.

Patients quickly forget what they are told, and are easily confused if told too much at once. Therapeutic conversation should be administered in small but continued dosages, in a preplanned fashion.

Very often, patients will retain only the part of the conversation which agrees with their own ideas, or is pleasant to them. Gentle, firm, persistent reiteration is essential if important concepts are to be acted upon. One must emphasize and re-emphasize, again and again.

Because of anxiety and tension, patients are easily confused and poorly retentive. Therefore, dissipation of anxiety and tension is always the first order of business. Frequently, one accomplishes more with subsequent conversations than with the initial, as rapport develops and first fears fall away. First conferences often merely set the stage for subsequent effective ones. One proceeds in a stepwise manner. If the first are not well handled, not much can be expected later.

Effective conversation with patients must be planned ahead, and cannot be just off the cuff.

Careless or ill planned conversations can be disastrous to the patient. A phrase or word having so little meaning to the clinician that he may not even recall saying it may be seized upon by the patient, and may have a profound effect upon him.

Needless details and technicalities should be avoided. They will not be understood, and may prompt a host of new anxieties.

Above all else, the clinician should be protective of the patient's position, and not of his own. He must be a wise censor, filtering out matters that will either cause needless anxieties or fail to achieve positive motivation. The physician who is impelled to tell the patient or the family (or both) *all* the facts is frequently protecting his own insecurity.

It must be remembered that conversation is therapeutic only to the degree that the patient has confidence in what the clinician says. This, in turn, is directly related to the patient's respect and trust. Most laymen will take clinical abilities for granted, and will not judge the physician in terms of his basic medical skills, which they assume he possesses merely because he is a physician. He will be judged, and then trusted accordingly, solely in terms of the following: the genuineness of his interest; the thoroughness of his approach to the problem; his personal warmth, understanding and compassion; and the degree of clarity with which he gives the patient insight into what is wrong, and what must be done.

DISCUSSION

This brings us back once again to the primacy of the history and physical examination. If they are properly executed, nothing so manifestly demonstrates the qualities of the good physician to his patient as a meticulously accomplished history and physical examination. They set the tone and create the background for future therapeutic relations between the patient and his physician. The patient has the opportunity to see his physician functioning at his best, and he judges him, assaying the qualities of the man and the abilities of the physician.

He becomes willing to entrust himself to this person who gathers so meticulously each relevant fact from the history and who misses no clue during his searching physical examination, each fact, each clue being scientifically scrutinized, and eventually so understandingly interpreted for the patient, whose confidence grows. He already begins to feel better. He knows he has found for himself a superb clinician.

This, as I see it, is the vocation to which you have been called. Understand what it is, and what it requires of you with gleaming clarity. From this first day, immerse yourself in learning its technics and skills. Discipline yourself to accept and meet the burdensome demands that it will continuously make upon you. From now on, you are engaged in the service of the sick. With the knowledge you are acquiring as a scientist, with your clinical art developed through experience, with the warmth of your own spirit and the strength of your own character, with the laying on of your hands, and in response to your words, you can make the sick better, and fill the dying with peace. These are great powers. Always deserve them.

In conclusion, today's young people seek models. Here is an image of a clinician:

He is meticulous in accumulating the historical and physical data from the patient. His questioning of the patient is searching and incisive, like that of a wise barrister. He interprets the clues derived from the physical changes with the precision of an experienced detective. His analysis of the clinical evidence is methodical and disciplined, so that no diagnostic or therapeutic possibility can be overlooked. The reasonableness of his logic makes his conclusions appear inevitable. They are based upon a personal clinical experience of the most sophisticated sort. His special interest is any human illness. His care of the patient does not end with the correct diagnosis. His thoughtful management of the total problems of the sick person makes mere treatment of a disease or a symptom seem woefully inadequate. He is inexhaustibly capable of infusing into his patients insight, self-discipline, optimism and courage. Those he cannot make well, he comforts. Versed in medical science, he also understands human nature and enjoys working with it. Analytical, logical, he is at the same time warm and charming, and although gentle, he is strong in his beliefs and ideals, but never brittle. The things he works with are intellectual capacity, unconfined clinical experience and the perceptive use of his eyes, ears, hands and heart.

SECTION

A

Communication

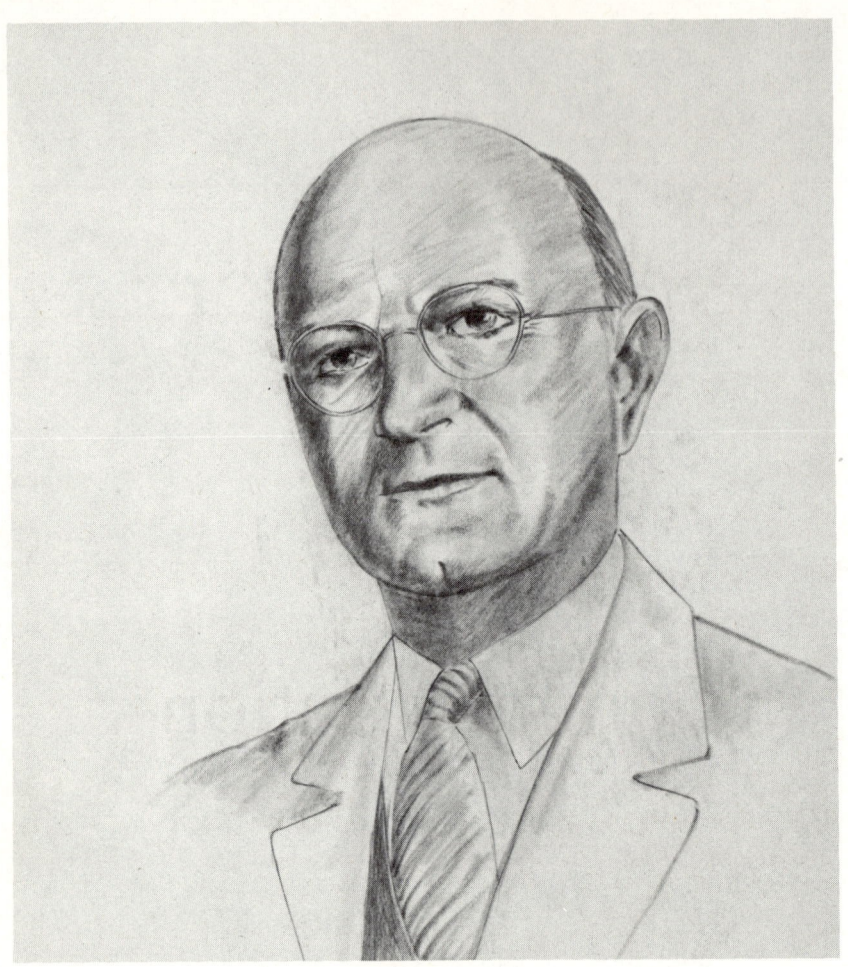

Charles R. Austrian
PROFESSOR OF MEDICINE

All the attributes of a superb clinician were his, and it was a learning experience to observe him examine a patient. He was precise and incisive; not a moment was wasted, yet he was meticulous. The physical inspection of the patient was his grande forte, and his ability to search out and disclose small details, and to draw significant conclusions from them, was startling. His elicitation of the physical findings from the chest was a triumph of ability. He had a real flair, an elegant style, and obviously enjoyed what he was doing. A slight lag of one side of the chest, a retraction, a subtle dullness, rales previously unheard, were given titillating and accurate interpretation. To his far-reaching familiarity with the history and lore of the art of physical diagnosis, he added his own very great perceptive and analytical abilities. He derived much pleasure, and gave even more, by harking back, on summarizing his physical findings, to the observations of the old masters. In discussing the significance of systolic murmurs in the pulmonic area, he would say, "They are the sounds of romance—like romance, they temporarily cause much interest and excitement, but often, ultimately little comes of them."

Having gathered all of the clinical evidence, his eyes would glow with enthusiasm at the challenge their analysis presented. Hedging was not in his nature, and he was bold and forthright in his opinions.

On the wards, he was cheerful and debonair. He guided the young, and gave wise counsel to the older. He left with his patients encouragement, self-confidence, reasoned self-discipline. To those whose health he tended, and to those he taught, Dr. Austrian was a clinician in the tradition of great clinicians.

1

Communicating with the Patient— General Considerations

If a clinician is to communicate with his patients in an effective and meaningful way, it is essential that he appreciate fully the relationships existing between himself and his patients.

Universally, patients are concerned about themselves when they visit their physician, regardless of the nature of the complaint. They inwardly anticipate the worst, although they may cover up with sophistication and braggadocio. Thus, whether the patient is a jovial businessman coming in for his annual check-up, who cheerily assures his physician that "I know I am much healthier than you are," or whether the patient has significant organic disabilities or is going through a period of loneliness and depression, the common theme of the emotional reaction of all, in varying degrees, is apprehension. Whereas many patients are apprehensive lest some organic disorder will be found, others are concerned that *no* organic explanation for their disabling complaints will be discovered and that the physician's conclusion will be that they are "imagining" or "putting on," or are emotionally unstable.

Most patients are naïve and simplistic in medical matters and will give or accept information or advice about their health status uncritically. This applies even to physicians when they become sick, though they are usually thoughtfully analytical about the ills of others. Many patients seek and expect facile answers and easy solutions to medical problems and may be disgruntled if they don't get them.

Most patients trust whatever the physician advises, often unquestioningly. Others are skeptical of anything unless it comes from an "expert," whom they often respect uncritically. A few enjoy challenging the opinions of the physician, basing their arguments upon fragments of medical knowledge.

Some patients have been sensitized to doctors by previous unfortunate experiences or by what they have been told by friends. They suspect that they will be hurried in and out by an overly committed physician who will brush aside their complaints and speed them along once he has "hung a label" on them. They are concerned that they will not be given an adequate opportunity to tell their entire story.

Many patients are worried about their ability to recall all of the facts of their illness, and hence fear that they won't be able to properly relate all of their problems to their physician. This is particularly true of older, anxious patients.

A physician must work around the fact that only a percentage of what he tells the patient will be remembered and that only a fraction of his advice will be acted upon. There are a number of reasons for this. Being anxious and flustered, it is easy for a patient to become distracted, confused and forgetful. Severe illness may dull the memory, as does the aging process. It is natural to block out unpleasant news and to retain only the good. We all pretend not to have heard things we don't like to hear. It is human nature to adhere to advice which is easily followed and to ignore that which requires self-discipline.

Many persons have concealed within themselves areas that are "off limits"—habits, personal problems, ways of reacting and sensitivities that they are unwilling to disclose or will disclose in only a very restricted or distorted fashion.

Some others have very practical reasons for not wanting to speak frankly to their physicians. There may be a variety of motivating factors that control what such patients elect to disclose. Sometimes this results in deliberate manipulation of the facts, but more often it is an inadvertent reaction to a deep desire to have things be different than they actually are.

Many patients feel the need to be reassured and to discuss the same old issues over and over again. The clear has to be made more clear; the explicit more positive; the obvious incontrovertible. In clinical medicine there are few virtues more important than patience!

Many patients are lonely. The want a father confessor, and they will cling to the person who listens with kindness and who gives comfort. They are hungry for attention. Subconsciously, they will invent new reasons to visit their physician.

One must always remember that in many instances illness changes people. It makes the brave timid, sophisticated people naïve, intelligent individuals simplistic, patient persons restive, the easygoing fretful and querulous. In real life, as well as by definition, patients are *not* normal persons! Shortly before his retirement, Dr. Warfield T. Longcope, for many years the very distinguished director of our medical department, told me that it was his experience that sickness *very rarely* brings to flower the very best of human characteristics.

Whereas some patients are very brave, others cringe in terror. All grasp tightly to life, and always some glimmer of hope, no matter how flickering, is essential to the vitality of spirit. It follows that one of the principal functions of a clinician is to give substance to this universal reaching out for hope.

All patients are exceedingly sensitive and suspicious because of inward fears, and they will analyze and re-analyze every word, question, gesture, and even the inflection of the physician's voice and expression upon his face. This is why a considerable number of patients are hurt, and not helped, by clinicians who are careless or thoughtless about these matters. The new physician will be chagrined to observe how often this happens.

A large number of patients become highly dependent. The clinician is the confidante, the port in a storm, the shield, the only one who listens, or who cares, or who understands. What an awesome responsibility to realize that a fellow human regards you as his one and only link to health or to stability. Such dependency may assume highly negative features. The attitude becomes "You, the clinician, must make me well. I lack the necessary maturity and self-discipline and courage, so I turn to you for the laying on of hands, for the working of a miracle." It is altogether human to expect a quick and easy cure.

It is unfortunate that some individuals *are*, in fact, unpleasant and difficult to get along with whether sick or well. Some are their own worst enemies and generate poor interpersonal relationships. A physician may find the personality of a particular patient highly distasteful and grating, but because he *is* the physician he must learn to sublimate his reactions. Once a physician responds with anger and irritation and resentment to such a patient or to the patient's family, his position is weakened, and it may be exceedingly difficult for him to help the patient and to manage his problems thereafter.

A clinician must always keep his cool! His reactions at all times must be controlled and not just "natural." For these and other reasons, instead of hitting back, he must keep in mind that sick persons are not normal, grit his teeth, and turn the other cheek. It is not so easy to do this with members of the patient's family, who are oftentimes more trying than the sick person himself. However, again one must remember that serious illness in one member of a family often psychologically involves the whole family, and hence family reactions may not be normal. From a practical standpoint, to forgive and to forget and to ignore such incidents and attitudes is a must, because to react personally to them will result in distraction, misjudgments, impetuosity and hastiness, all of which breed poor care and sometimes even medicolegal complications.

Very early in his relationship with the patient, the clinician must assay the following points so that intercommunication will be an effective experience both for the patient and himself. What is the personality and character of the patient? How sick is he, both in terms of physical abnormalities and psychological stresses? How intelligent and expressive and sensitive is he? What is his emotional make-up? What are the particular circumstances of the interview and in what kind of a situation does it place the patient? For example, is the patient an executive with many commitments, whose examination report is to be sent back to the company physician? Is the patient the wife of a boorish husband? In the case of a young patient, do the parents want to answer all of the questions? Is the patient an infirm, lonely, elderly person, or an individual who has already been informed that she probably has a very bad disease?

In trying to make these initial evaluations, the importance of observing little details can't be overstated. To an appreciable extent, a clinician must also be a detective. Such significant details include the following: the manner in which the patient greets the physician; his appearance and dress; his deportment toward others in the office or in the hospital; his attitude toward family members and vice versa; if seen at home, the appearance of the home, the behavior of the children, and so forth. Is the bedside table littered with bottles of medicine? Little things tell a lot, and nothing is to be overlooked.

One must realize that effective conversation with a patient is not something which a physician stumbles upon. It must be learned and studied and planned and experienced. To be effective, conversation must be a dialogue, and not a monologue by either the physician or the patient. The conversation period is a time of giving and receiving, and if the physician doesn't give of himself, he will not get back anything that has value or meaning. If he is impatient or seems harassed, or if he is short-tempered or cuts the patient off, the patient cannot be expected to respond well. Effective conversation with patients is tiring. It demands much of the clinician. It can't be accomplished in a hurry. Time is its essential ingredient, and hence the physician must not overschedule himself to the degree that a meaningful dialogue with his patients is impossible.

At the first meeting, the patient will be immediately responsive to the attitude and appearance of his physician. Very early he will start forming his conception of the physician, which he may never alter. Therefore, from the very start it is essential that the physician's image be one of intellectual capacity, understanding, reasonableness, reassurance, compassion and patience. Ideally he should seem to have a blithe spirit and a warm sense of humor. He must be meticulous. He must appear to have adequate time no matter how rushed. Most importantly, it must be evident that he is interested in people and that he *likes* people.

The physician should demonstrate these qualities to the patient in a variety of simple and practical ways. For example, even though he may be planning only a very short visit with the patient, he should sit down comfortably in a chair in a relaxed manner; he should not stand, or lean on the side of the bed. The conversation should be carried out in a quiet area in an atmosphere conducive to friendly, intimate interchange. The physician should make sure that the patient is comfortable throughout the conversation by adjusting the bed or the chair, seeing to it that the light is not shining in the patient's eyes, and so forth. These are small gestures, but they will be noted by the patient as indicants of the genuineness of the physician's interest.

Whereas the clinician must lead the patient in conversation, he should not seem to dominate it or to push too hard. It should never appear that he is prying into sensitive areas or trying to force open doors that have been closed for a long time. Obviously, one has to establish understanding and confidence and friendship before one can begin to delve into keenly personal areas. One rarely reads an entire book at one sitting, but rather chapter by chapter. So should one become acquainted with the vagaries of the patient's life, and his reactions to them. As confidence and familiarity increase, the plot will begin to thicken.

Finally, it must be remembered that, for a variety of reasons, a patient may be loath to discuss his problems unless in private. Parents or an overbearing husband or wife overhearing the conversation may inhibit the patient. Therefore, there is great value in insisting upon first interviewing the patient alone, and only later bringing relatives into the picture, accepting the fact that some relatives may resent this approach.

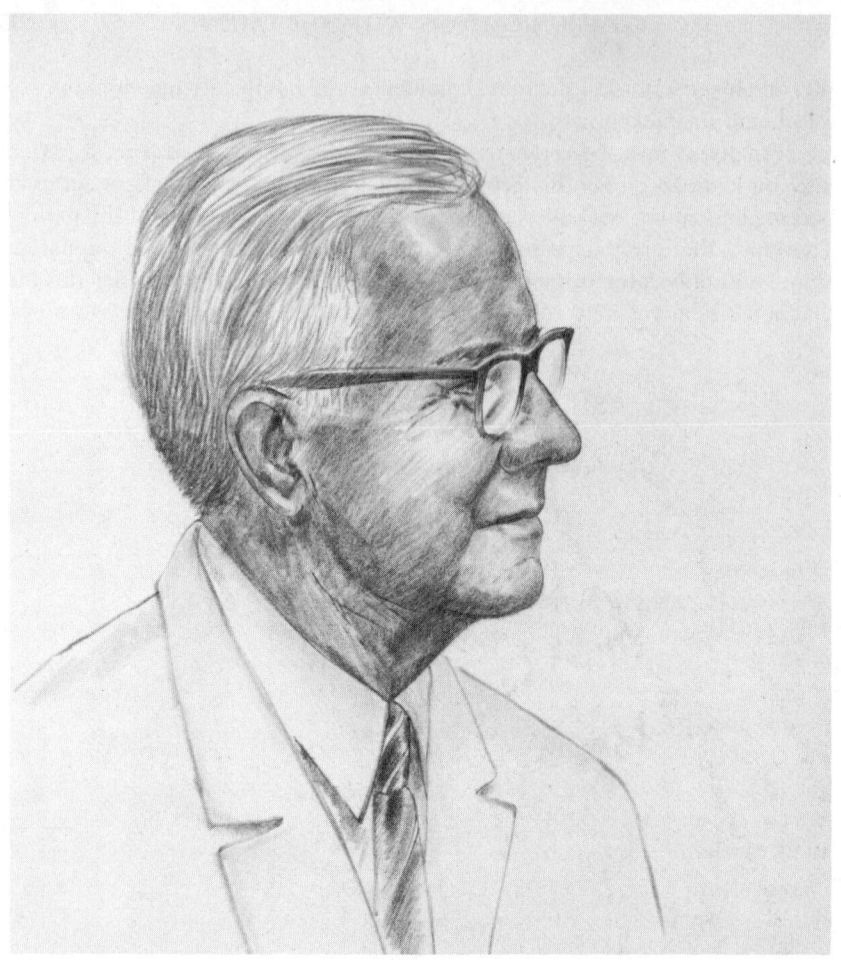

Alfred Blalock
PROFESSOR OF SURGERY

Few physicians have had their accomplishments so honored as did Dr. Blalock as he advanced to a foremost position in surgery in the United States. Few have received recognition more modestly.

By nature a shy person, his manner was characterized by dignity, charm, and warmth. A quick, puckish sense of humor made him a delightful companion who loved to be with people, especially young people. They always found him easily approachable and understanding, despite his high stature. His interest in people and ready comprehension of their problems, coupled with wise judgment, drew many to seek his counsel, especially his students and subordinates.

Because of these personal qualities, and his skills and achievements, he attracted persons of unusual abilities to his House Staff. A most impressive relationship, almost like father and sons, developed between him and the men he schooled. It produced a closely knit, intensely loyal group of men, many of whom have become heads of departments or professors of surgery, and continue as "The Blalock School of Surgery."

Nothing could have pleased him more, for the ideas and the techniques which he brilliantly initiated could not have been fully exploited in the life span of just one man, and he had the wisdom and the foresight to pass on to his young associates the inspiration, the devotion, the skills, and the energies to ensure that his contributions would be enduring. They are!

2

Obtaining the History

One hears it said that the day is approaching when the "routine" medical history will be obtained by a computer or by a physician's assistant. It is difficult to understand how this might be accomplished successfully, for there should never be anything routine or automated about securing a clinical history. The history is the first step, and often the most important, in the process of making a differential diagnosis. As the patient relates his story, he drops clues as to what might be wrong, clues that the physician should closely pursue with discerning questions designed to produce even more clues. The more expert the physician is in the complex analysis of differential diagnosis, the more meaningful will be the history he obtains, for it is his knowledge and experience that converts the patient's statements into clues. A history taken in a "routine" fashion indicates that the physician has no clear-cut concept as to what might be wrong with the patient. The way a patient appears and reacts when he is questioned, what he emphasizes, his attitude, the particular words he chooses, these are small, but essential factors that may lead to what is truly happening. Taking a meaningful clinical history is similar to playing a game of chess. The patient makes a statement and, based upon its content and mode of expression, the physician asks a counterquestion. One answer stimulates yet another question until the clinician is convinced that he understands precisely all of the circumstances of the patient's illness.

As previously emphasized, all patients are apprehensive. Being questioned by a physician is often a new and unusual experience, and although desiring to be helpful, patients are not sure of their role or of the procedure to be followed. Some try to relate everything, others seem reluctant to reveal anything. Some describe their symptoms in vivid detail, others are vapid and monosyllabic. Some are intelligent and sensitive, others dull and unresponsive. Some have already reached fixed conclusions as to what ails them and slant what they say accordingly, for personal, financial or other reasons. Many, rather than give a specific account of the manner in which the illness has developed and affected them, relate in a circuitous way the general circumstances *surrounding* their illness. Everything is told to the clinician except what he really wants to know, that is, precisely how the illness has evolved and exactly how the patient has been affected by it.

Perhaps the majority of patients have unclear or mistaken concepts as to what constitutes excellence in medical care. They often equate the performance of numerous laboratory tests with quality care. This conviction may be so firm that the patient becomes restive and churlish when a detailed history is taken; he is impatient to proceed to the really important part of his medical care—the testing!

Hence, before interviewing a patient, the clinician should thoughtfully review any available background material, such as the patient's previous clinical records, information from other hospitals, or data from his visits to other physicians. Such information will allow the clinician to be more direct in his questioning, confining the patient's answers to areas more likely to contain useful information.

Since patients are often neophytes at history-giving, it is wise to precede the actual questioning by a brief explanation of the methodology of history-taking that you plan to follow. Doing this will secure better cooperation and understanding from the patient, relax some of his tensions, and ultimately save time. The points to stress are these:

First, you want the patient to give a brief yet inclusive summary of the general nature of his problem; in other words, why has he come to you? Such a statement gives the examiner an overall view of the general nature of the patient's problem, which will later help to steer the questioning into pertinent areas. He will not be flying totally blind.

Second, you want to hear about any sicknesses in other family members, because some disorders run in families or may be passed from one family member to another.

Third, you need a succinct but complete review of the patient's health status, from the earliest he can recall to the present.

Fourth and last, you want the patient to describe in detail, step by step, starting from the very first symptom until the latest, how his present illness has evolved and affected his health status.

This explanation to the patient of the methodology of history-giving should be concluded by emphasizing the following points:

1. The patient should not worry about inability to recall exact dates or circumstances, for approximations or educated guesses are satisfactory.

2. He should not be hurried or rushed: obtaining all the significant facts is time well spent.

3. He should understand that pertinent items you are anxious to have him describe are *not* so much the general circumstances in which the illness has evolved, but rather the total impact and effect the illness has had upon his general health, which should be related in a step-by-step manner.

There are times when it is distinctly advantageous to secure the history of the present illness *before* commencing the system review; at other times just the reverse is true.

Early discussion of the present illness is wise (a) when the patient is very acutely ill, uncomfortable, agitated, fretful, uncooperative or at all obtunded as a result of his condition; (b) if the patient is unusually verbose, rambling or overdetailed in his recounting, or if he has multiple minor complaints; (c) finally, if the physician is very fatigued.

There are several advantages to preceding the discussion of the present illness by the system review. Some disorders, for example systemic lupus, may unfold episodically over a period of sometimes many years, recurrently involving one and then another organ system. Therefore events in the past history may give new meaning to present occurrences. Thus, for example, a young woman who enters with an acute pericardial effusion, initially regarded as being probably of viral, tuberculous or idiopathic origin, undergoes a system review which discloses past episodes of arthritis, unexplained anemia, and a transient skin rash. This places an entirely different interpretation upon the most likely etiology of the presenting disorder, namely, systemic lupus erythematosus.

Also, as a patient relates his health story from the very beginning, the observer obtains not only a meaningful evaluation of the patient's general health status but also an estimation of the kind of person with whom he is dealing. This will make subsequent evaluation and interpretation of the data of the present illness much more meaningful. Thus, a 58 year old patient who arrives complaining of severe weakness and fatigue, in a somewhat vague manner, but whose entire system review contains few or no complaints, is more likely to have a serious organic cause for his present nonspecific complaints than a patient whose recounting of the past is packed with a host of minor complaints. The state of a patient's past health is obviously a helpful background against which to judge events of the present. Little bits of information included in a review of the past history may significantly contribute to the accuracy of the interpretation of the present happenings. In other words, it's best to start a story at the very beginning.

SPECIAL POINTS REGARDING THE PRESENT ILLNESS

Make certain that the patient starts the story of his illness with Chapter 1, and not Chapter 2 or 3. Many patients do omit the earliest chapters, and often begin with some dramatic or (to them) significant event, skipping over the prior, more subtle, insidious events. It is a must to insist that the patient start at the very beginning and that he describe even the most banal initial events, for knowing these, and interpreting them properly, will lead the clinician to a proper appreciation of what followed. Thus, a patient starting the description of his illness with a vivid account of a sudden left-sided stroke may fail to mention that for two months he has been cranky and irritable, has lost 10 pounds, has had mild night sweats and vague, transient joint pains. These facts, if presented to the clinician, would have led to the suspicion that the "stroke" was not a primary event, but an embolic occurrence secondary to bacterial endocarditis.

Therefore, it is good practice to explain to the patient how important each little detail can be and that you want to be told all of them from the very beginning. A good technique is to ask the following questions: "When is the last time you felt *entirely* and *completely* well? When did you first begin to feel not quite up to par? What was the very first suggestion you had that your health status was *not entirely* normal?" Once the clinician feels certain that he has pushed the patient back to the very beginning, he should then say, "Now tell me what happened after that, step by step, in great detail."

Often the patient may skip over details, describing only what he thinks are the major points. Not at all uncommonly, however, the real clues are in the seemingly unimportant details. Such "inconsequential" circumstances as the fact that the patient has been on a picnic, or that the pet bird was sick, or that the patient coughed very heavily before he "passed out," may be the keys to understanding the whole story. It is wise to advise the patient with a statement similar to the following: "You start telling me *everything* you can recall—*I'll* decide what is significant. Don't you be the censor."

Many patients are not able to accurately and fully verbalize their symptoms. To many, a pain is a pain, and dizziness is dizziness. They cannot furnish the physician a *description* of the little details or employ the colorful, definitive adjectives which commonly are the payoff in differential diagnosis. In these instances, it is essential to stress to the patient the importance of such little details and to give him adequate time and assistance to supply them as well as he can. The physician must suggest suitable differentiating adjectives and ask questions specifically designed to stimulate verbalization.

Many times the patient may feel too sick to give a detailed history at a single interview, or may be too elderly or under too much psychological stress, and may become exhausted upon extensive questioning. The excitement of being examined for the first time may fluster the patient, causing him to become forgetful. This will be particularly true if the physician pushes the patient too hard with his questions in an effort to save time. Therefore, there are occasions when the initial interview should be devoted only to securing an overall understanding of the patient's problem, the essential details being sought at the subsequent interview.

Many patients insist upon clinging to seemingly "silly" explanations of things that have happened to them. Here a word of warning is needed because occasionally such explanations prove to be not so silly, and, if objectively pursued and analyzed, may lead to the right answer. Whereas the physician has to filter out and assess the value of information given to him, he must be careful not to select only those data that fit his prejudgment of the case. Each fact presented to him must be screened and analyzed before it is discarded.

Ask the patient to express in some objectively measurable way any physical changes that lend themselves to quantification. For instance, dyspnea should be expressed in terms of level blocks walked or steps climbed before shortness of breath is felt; diarrhea in the number of stools per day; weight loss in pounds per unit of time, and so forth.

The physician should challenge, rather than accept, every diagnosis that the patient claims was made in the past by other physicians. An episode of so-called "pneumonia" may not have been pneumonia at all, but rather a pulmonary embolism. A "gallstone attack" may lend itself to much different interpretation when the details are known. To blindly accept such proffered diagnoses as factual may be to start off with some very wrong assumptions, which, if challenged, occasionally reveal some excellent clues as to what has really transpired.

Take nothing for granted. If a patient has been seen by another physician or has been previously hospitalized, call or write for an abstract of all of the clinical information relative to that episode. Don't accept the patient's explanations of what happened, which may well be inaccurate. If possible, obtain and re-examine all old x-rays and—very important—all pertinent biopsy material. This is the only way you can be sure that the evidence upon which you are building your analysis will be valid.

Many patients are confused and forgetful, as already emphasized, and hence the physician should repeatedly review the history with his patient. Unfortunately, some physicians conclude that they have obtained *the* history simply because they have systematically interviewed the patient initially. However, it is not uncommon for the pertinent facts to be revealed only after several interviews. Not until the physician is satisfied that he has the fullest comprehension of the entire course of the patient's illness should he stop requestioning the patient. Facts that the patient can't recall today may be recalled tomorrow, and these may be the key points. Also, as clinical evidence is accumulated from laboratory and other sources, new leads open up.

After the patient has satisfactorily answered all questions pertaining to the present illness, it may be very helpful to ask him, "What have been *your* thoughts as to the cause of all of your troubles?" The answer to this somewhat disarming question is often very revealing, and it may give insight into the patient's perceptiveness, motivations, and apprehensions.

Finally, the pen should be put down, and the patient should be asked, in a way which implies that there is still plenty of time available, "Now, is there anything else you would like to tell me about yourself or your illness before I start examining you?" Such a question may bring out hitherto hidden anxieties or a description of one of the "silly" symptoms which are every now and then the key clue.

The taking of the history should be a quiet yet animated dialogue between physician and patient. This atmosphere is destroyed if the physician is constantly writing his notes as the patient answers the questions put to him. History taking is a conversation—not a dictation!

PAIN AS A SYMPTOM

The clinician should employ a planned approach to an analysis of the symptom of pain, no matter where its point of origin.

Pain as a symptom merits very special consideration since it is frequently the only or the predominant clinical manifestation of a wide variety of different types of disease processes. The physician must become expert at analyzing the patient's description of his pain if he hopes to discover its etiology.

Patients often have had such limited personal experience with pain that they give misleading or totally inadequate information about it. As a matter of fact, they may be so unfamiliar with pain as "pain" that they deny that they have it if asked simply, "Do you have pain?" For example, the patient with a peptic ulcer may not recognize the hungry, tight feelings he gets in his epigastrium in mid-mornings and afternoons as "pain." Nor may the patient with angina pectoris appreciate as true "pain" the constriction he gets in his chest when he becomes excited. These and other conditions have been often overlooked by physicians who do not realize that, whereas patients are amateurs in dealing with pain, clinicians must be experts in its analysis.

The symptom of pain should always be methodically analyzed under the following headings:
1. Location.
2. Radiation.
3. Character.
4. What causes it, or increases its intensity?
5. What makes it go away, or decreases its intensity?
6. Associated phenomena.
7. Time relationships.

Let us consider each of these in turn:

1. Location. It is basic to have the patient locate exactly the point of origin of his discomfort. He may sometimes confuse the area of *radiation* of his pain with its point of *origin*, and hence mislead the physician. It is best to take the patient's index finger and tell him to point with it to the area from which the discomfort seems to stem. It should be noted that functional illness is sometimes characterized by the patient's inability to do this.

2. Radiation. It is equally important to have the patient trace out with his finger the pattern of radiation of his distress. It must be re-emphasized that oftentimes the point of origin of the pain is totally "silent," and the area of radiation may be mistaken for the point of actual origin, leading to diagnostic errors. Thus, angina pectoris may present to the patient solely as a "peculiar sensation" he gets in the left hand when he hurries to the bus, or a peptic ulcer may be mistaken for an orthopedic condition because the patient's total complaint is of back pain at night.

3. Character. As already indicated, patients are frequently unfamiliar with pain as an experience in life, and their concept of what the word pain connotes may be very limited. To some it may simply mean the sensation they had when they closed a finger in the car door or burned themselves cooking. Many patients are not aware that they are experiencing what the physician technically speaks of as pain. Also, some patients, out of fear or shame, will deliberately avoid admitting that they are bothered by pain. They may so distort their symptoms that establishment of a diagnosis may be difficult, if not impossible. This kind of personal reaction is the basis for the old adage, "The toothache disappeared as soon as I got in the dentist's chair."

Therefore, it is wise to avoid use of the more narrow expressions, such as "Do you have pain?", and to employ broader expressions such as "distress," "discomfort," or "uncomfortable" or "unpleasant." The physician must aid the patient in verbalizing his sensations by suggesting to him a variety of descriptive phrases, such as toothachy, burning, knifelike, tight, constricting, tearing, heavy, gnawing, eating, cramping, and so forth.

Much information of diagnostic value can be derived from a patient's accurate description of what his discomfort feels like to him. For example, the presence of a true colicky pain generally means that one is dealing with spasm of a smooth muscle viscus, such as ureter, gallbladder or gut. Special questioning may be required to bring out the fact that the patient is, in fact, having true colic. "Does it grab and let go intermittently? Is it like the sensation you have when you need urgently to move your bowels, but can't?" A superficial, uncomfortable, burning sensation is typical of nerve root irritation. Persistent, deep, boring, I-can-never-get-away-from-it kinds of discomfort, particularly if worse at night, are characteristic of new growths. Gnawing, burning, eating, hungry, tight-fisted sensations are common in peptic ulceration. Bloating, distending, dyspeptic feelings are the marks of gallbladder trouble. Tight, constricted, pressing, pushing, heavy sensations are characteristic of coronary insufficiency. A tearing may be described by the patient with dissecting aneurysm. Obviously, an accurate, full description of his discomfort is of great diagnostic value.

4. What Causes It, or Increases Its Intensity? It is essential to extract from the patient a detailed description of the exact setting in which his pain occurs. A general description will not suffice. The particulars of the story are frequently the keys. *Precisely what* was the patient doing when he got the pain? What were the *specific circumstances* surrounding the occurrence of the pain? What factors, has experience shown, seem to precipitate or increase the pain? Is it affected by emotions, activity, coughing, breathing, or eating? This is the kind of information that must be gotten. If the pain is episodic, ask the patient to describe a typical spell in the greatest detail, from start to finish.

Lack of clear-cut answers to this kind of probing questioning is sometimes an indication of functional illness, although one has to be circumspect in this area, since some important organic diseases may be characterized initially by a very vague, hard-to-put-into-words kind of discomfort, and one can make serious misjudgments.

5. What Makes It Go Away, or Decreases Its Intensity? Again, one must insist upon a complete listing of all the factors which seem to diminish the discomfort. These factors generally should be suggested to the patient by the physician, so that no important categories are omitted.

Experience teaches one not to discount *any* of the factors that the patient claims play a role in his discomfort, even though they may sound inconsequential or even bizarre. The diagnosis may be contained in the very peculiarity of the patient's story. It is usually prudent to accept the patient's story on its face value; it is often an error to censor the patient's account to better accommodate one's thinking.

In order to evaluate accurately the character of a patient's pain and related changes, it is essential that the observer be familiar with whatever medications the patient has been receiving, for several reasons. Drugs may ameliorate or alter the key symptoms or manifestations of an illness. Morphine, for example, may profoundly change the pain and muscle spasm associated with a ruptured appendix. Drugs may induce symptoms or changes that have nothing whatever to do with the underlying disease process, but that are by-products of the drug itself, and may mislead and confuse both patient and physician. For example, the development of acute polyarthritis as a manifestation of penicillin sensitivity, the drug having been given for treatment of tonsillitis, may suggest rheumatic fever.

Dependency upon drugs of various sorts may significantly color the patient's description of his symptoms and make the differential diagnosis of chronic or recurrent discomfort particularly difficult. Patients who have become drug dependent are often extremely sensitive about their predicament and make great efforts to conceal it. It is wise to appreciate this and to proceed slowly and delicately until a warm rapport has been established. Abruptness may rob the physician of his only chance to help the patient. It is good practice to ask, in a casual way, "What different kinds of drugs have you found necessary to take in order to control your discomfort?"

Finally, it is obvious that many drugs affect patients' ability to give accurate information, either by blunting their sensibilities, clouding their reactivity, or inducing depression or euphoria.

6. Associated Phenomena. In this cateogry are included all of the physical alterations associated with the patient's pain, such as anxiety, dyspnea, sweating, nausea or vomiting. Again, the physician must insist upon an unabridged listing, and he must act as the prompter.

7. Time Relationships. The average duration of an episode of discomfort is of obvious significance, as is the frequency of recurrence. It is helpful to try to determine whether there is any pattern of recurrence, seasonal or otherwise. The tendency for peptic ulceration to worsen in the spring and fall is well recognized; peptic ulcer is also one of a very few conditions that cause chronic, recurrent abdominal discomfort at night. Nocturnal worsening of skeletal pain is frequently observed in metastatic carcinoma, and repeated episodes of chest discomfort at night would bring to mind the possibility of angina decubitus or hiatus hernia. Here, too, should be included questions relating to any environmental factors, at home or on the job.

I have found it very helpful to always ask the question, "Have you *ever* had pain at all similar to this one before?" Patients have a way of describing an episode of pain as though it is a unique experience, misleading the physician into thinking that he is confronted by some acute and newly formed process, only to later discover that this illness was actually one of several similar episodes dating back many years. The knowledge that an episode of pain is part of a *recurrent* process vitally affects one's thinking about the nature of the process; hence the need to pursue this point with forcefulness.

PERSONAL AND SOCIAL HISTORY

One learns much about the patient by observing his dress, deportment and attitude, the manner in which he tells his story, how he responds to the challenge of being questioned, and so forth. At the initial interview, it is both poor taste and bad judgment to attempt to intrude upon the patient's private life; to open doors that have been kept tightly closed for a long time. Later, with finesse and tact on the part of the physician, these doors will begin to open spontaneously, one by one.

Initially, therefore, questions should be general and not probe too deeply. But answers to the following questions can be very revealing:

1. How far did you go with your education? Why did you stop?
2. How long have you been married? In general, has your marriage been a satisfying one?
3. Have you had any children? If not, why? Are they healthy? Do you enjoy them? Have they done well in school? Any particular problems with them?
4. What type of employment do you have? Is it enjoyable? What other types of work have you been in? How long have you been with your present company?
5. Were you ever in the Armed Forces? For how long? Where did you serve? Were you ever sick while in the service? What kind of illness?
6. Do you have any special hobbies or interests? Do you give much time to them?
7. Do you have any particular habits, such as smoking or use of alcohol? How much do you smoke or drink?
8. Have you ever traveled? Where?
9. In general, has life been good to you? Have you had more than your share of personal and business problems?

Recording the History

Clinicians are exceedingly busy persons and any method of recording clinical information must take this into consideration. The recording must be brief and succinct, with no wasted words. At the same time, the history is both a scientific and legal document, and hence must be complete, factual, and detailed whenever a full understanding of the disease process demands particulars.

Since it is a legal document, and as such is subject to perusal by a variety of interested persons, it is open to challenge. What is said must be a fair as well as correct presentation of the facts. Thus, there is real potential danger for both the patient and the physician if the clinical chart contains such statements as "the patient is an alcoholic," "the patient is emotionally unstable," or "the patient is exaggerating his complaints and demanding drugs," unless the stated facts substantiate such declarations. "Would this statement hold up in court?" is a good question to ask oneself when making a report, and it is a wise habit to regard each history as a document that someday might be challenged by a group of one's peers.

For insurance purposes the clinical chart must document the precise role the physician has played in caring for the patient and fully justify the fees that have been charged. This justification must be not only quantitative but qualitative as well.

Obviously there is no place whatsoever in such a document for humor, or sarcasm, or invective, or exaggeration, or for unfounded statements, sniping at one's confreres, or expressing off-handed suspicions.

If an organ or structure is normal, simply say so! The only negatives that should be noted and described are those in which the presence of normality or the absence of abnormality has a special impact upon the diagnostic possibilities. For example, the absence of clubbing in a patient suspected of having subacute bacterial endocarditis should be specifically stated.

The use of various abbreviations and symbols should be assiduously avoided. Reading charts containing multiple abbreviations and symbols is sometimes like trying to grasp a local dialect, and requires an interpreter who speaks the local jargon. Often, such notes are meaningful only to the person who wrote them.

Anything that lends itself to measurement should be quantified. The statement should not be "the patient continues to lose weight," but rather "the patient lost three pounds in the past two days."

The patient's present illness should be described in chronological sequence, each paragraph being a description of another major step in the evolution of the illness. The paragraphs should begin with a phrase indicating the time sequence, which is underlined, as in the following example:

10 days ago—The patient had a mild upper respiratory tract infection, but continued working.

4 days ago—His cough became worse and productive of thick sputum.
2 days ago—He had a shaking chill and complained of pain in his right chest on breathing.
Yesterday—He had a high fever and additional chills.
Today—He was brought into the Emergency Room in shock.

It is a small, but essential point: *All* notes must be *signed and dated.*

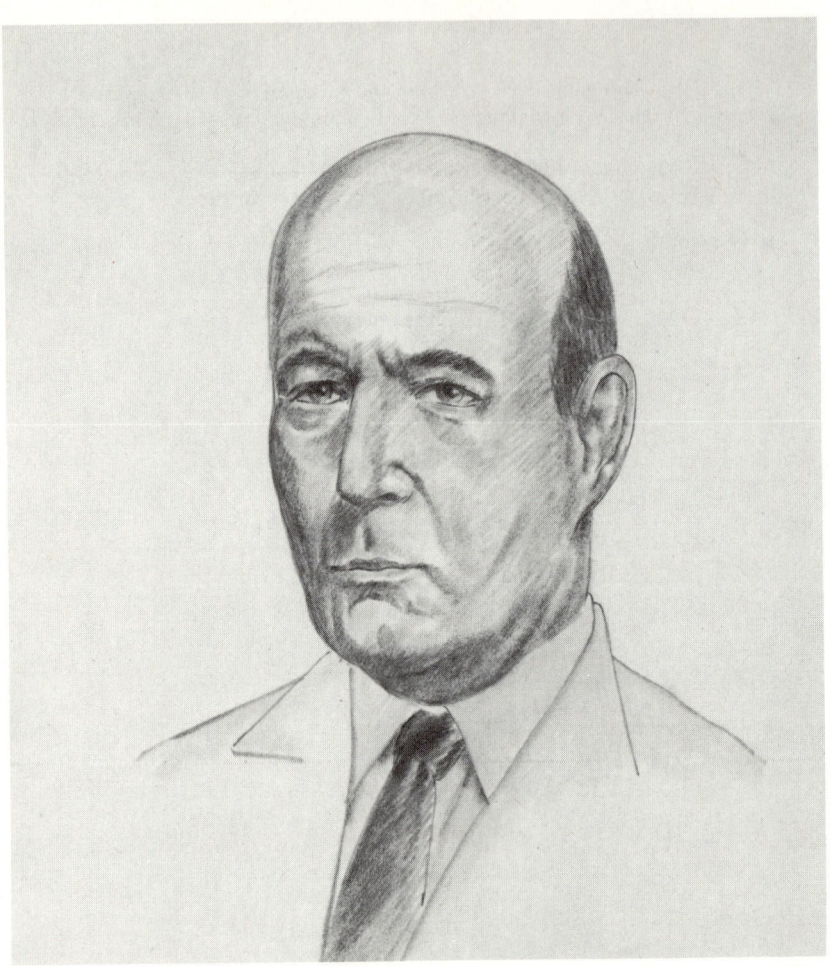

Frank R. Ford
PROFESSOR OF NEUROLOGY

Frank Ford rates very high in any listing of the truly great clinicians who have contributed to the Johns Hopkins Medical School and Hospital. It is beyond challenge that he corrected more mistaken diagnoses than any other clinician during his half-century of service. He was affectionately known as "the Judge" by colleagues in almost every department of the hospital. His contributions to neurology have been many and significant, but we will only mention one. His textbook, Diseases of the Nervous System in Infancy, Childhood and Adolescence, is an internationally recognized reference. It encompasses much more than diseases of the young, and for many of us it has been the neurological bible.

Mild and quiet, his subtle humor was delightful. His ability to listen thoroughly before assessing any problem or situation was of a degree that is rarely encountered. Little scraps of notes taken at the bedside were assembled into a succinct yet comprehensive consultation which often put to shame more labored recordings and less incisive thinking, for it was made baldly evident what the problem really was and illuminated the answer as well. Often, Dr. Ford would include pertinent references to the literature.

Dr. Ford's teaching was at the bedside and in the clinic, not from the podium. There the force of his impact upon students and staff was very great, for his warm, dryly witty personality, combined with vast experience, his ability to get to the point quickly through brilliant analysis, and his blunt honesty made of him a model worth striving to emulate, the very image of a physician one would richly like to be. What he has done for many students and colleagues within the Johns Hopkins Hospital and throughout the world may rarely be equalled, but cannot be surpassed.

3

Conducting the "Final" or Summarizing Interview

By the expression "final interview" is meant the conference that the clinician has with his patient (and sometimes members of the family) after the history, physical examination and diagnostic studies have been completed, and during which the physician discusses the results of these studies, the diagnosis they indicate, and the plan of management to be followed. The expression "final interview" is really a misnomer because, therapeutically speaking, far from being the *final* interview, such conferences are actually the beginning of a long-term relationship between the patient and his physician. An exception would be those instances where the patient is being seen in consultation and is to be returned immediately to the care of the referring physician. In any event, this conference marks the transition of the patient from the stage of investigation to the stage of management of his problem. It is critical that such a conference be handled in an optimum fashion, for bungling may mean that the therapeutic program is defeated before it begins, and the healing relationship between patient and physician may be irreparably damaged.

Unfortunately, young physicians are taught little or nothing about the structuring of these conferences and the finesse required in conducting them. Often, it is a case of hit or miss, and of learning by one's errors, of which, unhappily, many are made. Whereas the success of such conferences obviously depends upon the knowledge, wisdom, experience, tact and compassion of the individual physician as well as on his ability to communicate, there are some general principles and guidelines for the conducting of such conferences that are helpful to follow. Let us consider them.

As already indicated, a patient must be motivated to accomplish what must be done to overcome his health problem. Such motivation must sometimes be very strong, for often a physician must ask of the patient sacrifices and self-discipline of major proportions if he is to get well. The patient may have to change long-established habits, undergo suffering, accept distasteful

29

forms of therapy, and even see and acknowledge in himself destructive qualities which he has long hidden. Often, although the spirit required for recovery is generally willing, the flesh is weak, and it will respond only to impelling motivation.

But without understanding, motivation of a human being cannot be brought about at all, or at the least only transiently, or half-heartedly. Therefore, the twofold purpose of such a final conference is first to bring about understanding within the patient as to the basic nature of his problem, and second, to motivate him so that he can and will continue to do whatever is necessary to overcome, or at least to modify, his medical problem.

In addition, as we have repeatedly stressed, fears and anxieties are a part of every health problem, and hence the allaying of these and the consequent instillation of self-confidence is an essential goal of such conferences, for understanding and motivation are not likely to have positive results unless a patient has confidence that his efforts have the potentiality of bearing fruit.

STRUCTURING A FINAL INTERVIEW

Such conferences are not likely to be effective if a physician simply sits down with the patient and starts talking without prior consideration of what goals he specifically wants to achieve. To be effective, such a conference must be planned beforehand, step by step. We have already discussed the general principles of communication with patients. In no other relationship with the patient is it so imperative that these principles be well applied as during these conferences, for they can be either the beginning or the end of the physician's opportunity to help the patient.

It is well to begin such a conference by stating that you have studied the patient's problem very carefully and have reviewed thoughtfully all of the clinical evidence gathered through the various studies just completed. The accuracy of this statement will be appreciated at once by the patient, who will recall how carefully his history was reviewed, and how meticulously he was examined. Hence, your relationship is off to a good beginning.

Next, tell the patient that it is your desire to review all of this clinical data with him in terms he will understand, explaining what was done, why it was done, what the results were, and the conclusions to be drawn from them. Thereafter, you will outline a program of management. Finally, you will give him an opportunity to ask any questions he desires. If the format of the conference is thus explained to the patient, he won't be frequently interrupting the physician, and the discussion can continue in an orderly fashion.

The discussion of the patient's problem should begin with a recapitulation of his major complaints. Whereas this should be a brief summary, it should be detailed enough to reassure the patient that you have correctly understood his reasons for coming to see you. If he gets the impression at this stage of the conference that you have not comprehended the basic reasons why he came to see you, the remainder of the conference can be a fiasco.

This summarization should be followed by a brief account of what was found on physical examination. Here, it is imperative not to employ expressions that will frighten the patient. Descriptive terms may need to be modified, and at times, some findings actually omitted. For example, a patient with hepatomegaly should be told that he has "mild" or "moderate" enlargement of the liver, and not that his liver is "huge." Rather than describing heart murmurs one can say, "There is some evidence that rheumatic fever has mildly affected the functioning of one of the valves of your heart." Findings which are not pertinent to your explanation shouldn't be mentioned at all, and never should the patient be made unnecessarily anxious.

Next, the information obtained from the various special studies should be explained in detail and in terms the patient will understand: "You are not anemic. The different kinds of white blood cells are normal. The urine is clear. The electrical tracing of your heart is normal, and so on." It is wise psychology to outline *all* of the studies and not just the pertinent ones, so that the patient will appreciate the wide scope of the studies that were accomplished. The following are to be assiduously avoided:
1. The use of technical expressions.
2. The reporting of results that are highly equivocal.
3. The relating of data that is unnecessarily anxiety-producing.
4. The description of results that are not pertinent to the patient's problem and that may be a seed for future concern, such as, "Your chest film shows an old scar" or "Your T waves are slightly inverted" or "Your cholesterol level is just a little high." These abnormalities, although quickly dismissed by the physician, are likely to be retained for a long time by the patient, producing unnecessary tension. Subsequent assurances by the physician that "These changes don't really mean anything" may fall upon deaf and distracted ears.

In the next step, the meaning of all of this clinical evidence in terms of the patient's complaints should be synthesized in simple, understandable terms: "What does all of this information add up to and how does it pertain to these disabling headaches you have been having?" This final diagnosis should be formulated in plain, easily understood terms, unequivocally, concisely, and in a manner so as not to generate undue fears.

Obviously, it is not nearly enough to simply tell the patient the name of the disorder he is thought to have. Understanding will only be instilled in the patient when the basic nature of the process is made clear to him. This must be done in such a way that he is left with a reasonable explanation of the development of the process, how it has produced the disabilities he has experienced, and how it can be beneficially affected by the treatment program you are about to outline.

At this juncture, it is important to reflect upon the impact that the diagnosis you are presenting to the patient may have upon him. One must be prepared to soften its impact, if it is a negative one, as gently and understandingly as one can. This will require pre-thinking and pre-planning. Having already formulated a conception of the patient's character, his sensitivities and reactions, and being aware of the circumstances in which the patient finds himself, the clinician must attempt to set the stage for a maximally positive response to the information he is giving the patient. To be avoided are statements leading to the development of fear or panic or depression within the patient, or of hopelessness, or of a feeling of being overwhelmed or that he is "in over his head." The patient's fears of chronic invalidism or of impossible goals to be achieved should likewise be assuaged by the clinician. To accomplish this, the truth will sometimes need to be molded and even some of the facts may be withheld.

In presenting an explanation of the diagnosis, the use of simple diagrams or photographs may be very useful, to "save one thousand words." There are several booklets published containing useful material for this purpose. In describing the pathogenesis and treatment of a duodenal ulcer, for example, a simple drawing of the stomach and duodenum can be exceedingly helpful. Not infrequently, patients have asked, "Could I take that drawing home?"

In presenting the explanation of the diagnosis the clinician has reached, the following should be stressed, as applicable:

1. The common occurrence of the condition.

2. The fact that many patients with the same condition handle it exceedingly well.

3. The condition need not be feared; it will not be progressive and crippling in the future.

4. It is not "catching" or inherited.

5. There are varying degrees of involvement of the condition; the patient's appears not to be advanced or extensive.

6. The patient may have many misconceptions about the condition, some of them leading to gloomy conclusions, and these you desire to dispel, for many patients who are affected by it handle it very well indeed. This approach is essential in dealing with disorders such as systemic lupus erythematosus, where the general reaction is oftentimes one of dread and hopelessness. In such instances it is wise to employ a direct assault upon these fears and to say something like the following: "I realize there have been articles in some women's magazines portraying this condition as a progressive and destructive one, and perhaps such misconceptions are in your mind. If so, dismiss them, for in many, many instances this is not correct, and numbers of patients who have the condition lead normal, long and productive and happy lives. There is no reason why you shouldn't also be one of these!"

7. In dealing with chronic conditions such as renal, cardiac and hepatic disorders, it is helpful to point out that these organs characteristically possess large functional reserves and have great ability to accept and make adjustments to injury, as well as having very impressive healing powers. It is comforting to the nephritic patient to be told, "After all, a person can be well even if he has less than one entire kidney."

8. In chronic disorders, it is well to stress the considerable impact that treatment will have in "making the disorder behave itself." Although it is correct that the condition can't be gotten rid of completely, it can be brought under control. Although there may be some downs and ups in the future, there will be more ups than downs as time goes on and as the plan of management begins to have its full effect. This may take some time, however. Also, let the patient know that impressive accomplishments in research are occurring in this field, of which you are and shall continue to be fully aware.

There are, however, several groups of patients who should be dealt with in a very firm, explicit and direct fashion, with no softening compromises. These include alcoholics, diabetics, and the significantly overweight. With such patients, the facts should be laid on the line in an "either/or" fashion. To suggest that there are easy ways to solve these types of problems, and that one can make a choice and drift half-heartedly along, is to invite eventual failure. Such patients must accept the reality of what they are told and act forcefully upon it or they will not prosper. They must not be allowed to refer their failures to the inadequacies of others. Their fate is truly in their own hands.

In thus formulating the diagnosis, the physician must be ever conscious of the potentially heavy impact of his message upon the patient. He may be telling an executive with many commitments that he has coronary artery disease and must "take it easy," or a young mother with four children that she has to "get plenty of rest and quiet," or a recently married couple that they must not have children. Surely the imparting of such information and advice calls for great understanding and infinite tact and finesse.

Oftentimes psychological blows that have to be delivered can be softened by avoiding finality and inevitability, by leaving the door a little ajar instead of slamming it tightly shut. In other words, leaving room for hope, by saying things like "You can't do that right now but perhaps in a few months or so you will be able to," or "As time goes on and you progressively improve, you will be able to do that."

A physician is at a distinct disadvantage when his best diagnostic efforts have failed to bring him to a satisfying conclusion regarding the nature of the patient's complaints. (This problem as it relates to functional illness is discussed in Section C, Chapter 2.) In this circumstance, he has several alternative moves. If his judgment is that the patient may well have some kind of obscure organic disorder and that it may have serious potentialities or is likely to be rapidly progressive, then, especially if specific forms of beneficial therapy are available, the wise and proper alternative is to tell the patient frankly about one's concerns and to insist upon further investigation, employing consultative help and perhaps hospitalization. If adequate consultative help is not available locally, the patient must of course be referred to an area where the necessary facilities *are* available. The patient should be advised where to go, and his arrangements should be facilitated as much as possible.

On the other hand, if in the physician's judgment of the clinical evidence this is *not* a disorder which is likely to progress if not specifically treated, he may explain to the patient and the family that the present evidence does not allow a specific diagnosis to be made ("We can't put a name on the baby just yet") at this particular juncture. He should inform them that the evidence gathered does indicate that there is no progressive, potentially serious condition present, and certainly none which requires immediate, specific therapy, and hence the wise course to follow is one of continued watchful observation, which will be carefully carried out. In the meantime, the physician will outline a simple program of therapy that will make the patient symptomatically better. It should be pointed out to the patient that it is not at all unusual for a patient to have complaints for which a ready answer is not available. Many such complaints vanish as mysteriously as they have come. The studies have shown that there is no evidence of present injury to any of the organ systems, and that the patient's general health status remains good. The essential and wise thing to do under the circumstances is not to force a diagnosis when the answer is not evident, but rather to follow a conservative program of support and periodic re-examination, retaining an open mind as to the basis of the patient's complaints. The large majority of patients will respond positively to such frankness and to obviously honest and wise counselling, and will be grateful that they weren't given some off-hand explanation. They will recognize in their physician qualities they respect, and will therefore get support from what this obviously wise and honest person tells them. They will be willing to work together with him in future re-evaluations of their complaints.

Suggestions regarding the method of conducting a final interview with patients having functional illness and progressive fatal disorders are discussed in Section C, Chapters 2 and 4.

OUTLINING THE PROGRAM OF MANAGEMENT

The presentation of the program of management to the patient must be accomplished in such a way that the patient understands both *what* he is to do, and *why* he is to do it. Each step in the program must be explained in a detailed and explicit fashion that leaves no room for equivocation or misunderstanding. The program must be broad in scope and not be a mere recitation of medications to be taken. It must include little items as well as major issues. It must be a program that the patient can live by in terms of his financial and psychological resources. Since patients during such conferences are usually anxious and easily confused and forgetful, any detailed instructions relating to medications, diets, and the like should be written down in such detail that it would be difficult for the patient to make an error. Many patients at the conclusion of such conferences are beset by doubts that they will be able to "do the right thing" after arriving home. Such perplexity may lead to discouragement and then to laxness followed by discontinuance. If a form of treatment is important enough to prescribe, it is important enough to outline in writing for the patient in an unmistakable fashion. Simply handing the patient a set of prescriptions is not nearly enough.

In outlining the program of management for the patient, the following items are important:

1. The patient shouldn't be given too much advice at once for he is easily confused and will forget much of what he is told. At the first conference the general features of the program should be outlined and the most important items stressed in detail. At subsequent conferences the basic features should again be reviewed and more details stressed. In other words, the patient is indoctrinated regarding the program in a stepwise fashion, adequate opportunities for reinforcement of its details being afforded.

2. It is a mistake to demand too much of the patient. Asking for the impossible will result in discouragement and withdrawal. One should be moderate and willing to compromise wisely, suiting the program to the character and situation of the particular patient.

3. It is thoughtless and deleterious to make recommendations that are beyond the patient's means, for to do so will only increase the patient's tensions. To insist with someone who can't leave his job that a "move to a very dry, hot climate" would be helpful for his asthma, or to tell a young mother with four youngsters that she "must get 2.5 hours of complete rest" each noon, is unrealistic and does not help the patient.

4. The patient should never be pushed into making major decisions that he is reluctant to make (unless it is critical that he do so, as for an emergency appendectomy). After explaining his reasons for the recommendations he has made and answering the patient's questions, the clinician should push no further but say, "This is what I would do if I were you, knowing what I do about your condition. But take time to think it over. Don't decide now. See how things go for a while and then let's discuss the matter again."

5. The patient and, if included in the conference, his family, should be afforded adequate time to ask questions. The physician must anticipate the following and other types of reactions to what he has had to say, and he should note such reactions in his summarization of the problem and its management:

   a. Antagonism;
   b. Incredulousness;
   c. Fear, or even panic;
   d. Quotations from statements made by other physicians or gleaned from magazines or other sources;
   e. Determined debate and rebuttal ("If what you say about my headaches is true, doctor, how do you explain this. . . ?");
   f. Displeasure and disenchantment with previous medical care obtained elsewhere ("Why didn't Dr. X tell me what you have said?").

These attitudes and responses have to be handled in a variety of ways, depending upon their specific presentation, and only general principles can be outlined.

Whatever the patient's response, and however bitter or unpleasant or out of place it may be, the clinician must, at all costs, "not lose his cool." He must meet unreasonableness with sensibleness, irateness with equanimity, and immature behavior with wisdom. To retaliate by following the patient's bad example is to court disaster and chance disruption of any positive relationships with the patient and his family. One has to stand one's guard with calm reasonableness and stick to the facts as one has judged them to be: "I have tried to present the nature of your problem to you as clearly as I know how, and I have told you the way in which I believe it can best be handled. I can appreciate that it is difficult for you to understand this explanation and how hard it can be to follow the advice I have given. However, I have come to my best conclusions. Under these circumstances, perhaps we should get Dr. X to see you and obtain his viewpoints. I'll be delighted to arrange this consultation for you. If he has a better solution for your problem than I, we will certainly pursue it. My only desire is to help you get well."

In explaining the failure of other physicians to have reached the correct diagnosis in the past, it should be pointed out that one cannot judge the past by the present. If often takes time for changes to occur to the point where a correct diagnosis is possible. In medicine the answers to problems are sometimes not clearly evident any more than they are in other fields. There are no easy answers to hard problems. Often things are not black and white but rather are matters of experience, judgment, and opinion. The physician does his best to draw the correct conclusion from the clinical data at hand at the time he studies the patient. Obviously the data changes as the patient's illness progresses. You, the clinician, are giving your best judgments based upon presently available information. You presume this is what the patient's other physicians have done as well. The patient is free to accept or reject your advice or, if he desires, you will be happy to invite other opinions.

Whatever is said, say it in an affable, understanding, and generous fashion, once more realizing that sick people don't react like healthy ones, nor do their families!

At the conclusion of the "final" interview, the patient should be given the requisite prescriptions. Be certain they contain unambiguous directions. As already stressed, so many patients arrive home only to puzzle over what they are *really* supposed to do. Handing the patient several prescription blanks won't do. It only requires a minute or two to prepare a brief outline listing in a coordinated manner what the patient is to do. This is a must of good patient management. Always have the druggist put the name of the prescribed drug and dosage instructions on the bottle. This will forestall the patient calling to ask, "How long shall I take the blue capsules with the red stripes on them?" Finally, if the drugs are expensive or must be taken for a long period of time, advise the patient where he can obtain them most economically.

Also, because many patients are totally mystified by things medical, may tend to develop excuses for not following the advice given them, or delay

CONDUCTING THE "FINAL" OR SUMMARIZING INTERVIEW

its application, the clinician must be highly specific and precise in his directions, and take pains to see to it that it is made as easy as possible for the patient to do what he has been told. Most patients like to have a program spelled out specifically and precisely. Thus, it is not enough to say "gargle with salt water," or "raise the head of your bed at night," or "get more rest and relaxation, and exercise every day." General advice must be particularized. If a patient needs a reduction diet, make an appointment for the patient to have a conference with a dietician on a particular day. If a patient is to wear a supporting girdle, tell her specifically where she can get it, and supply the necessary details to make certain the correct girdle is purchased.

Not only will this kind of detailed planning and explanation bring about greater patient compliance, but it will further convince the patient that his problem is, indeed, in sound, effective, considerate hands. He will feel a responsibility both to himself and to his physician to carry out the advice given him.

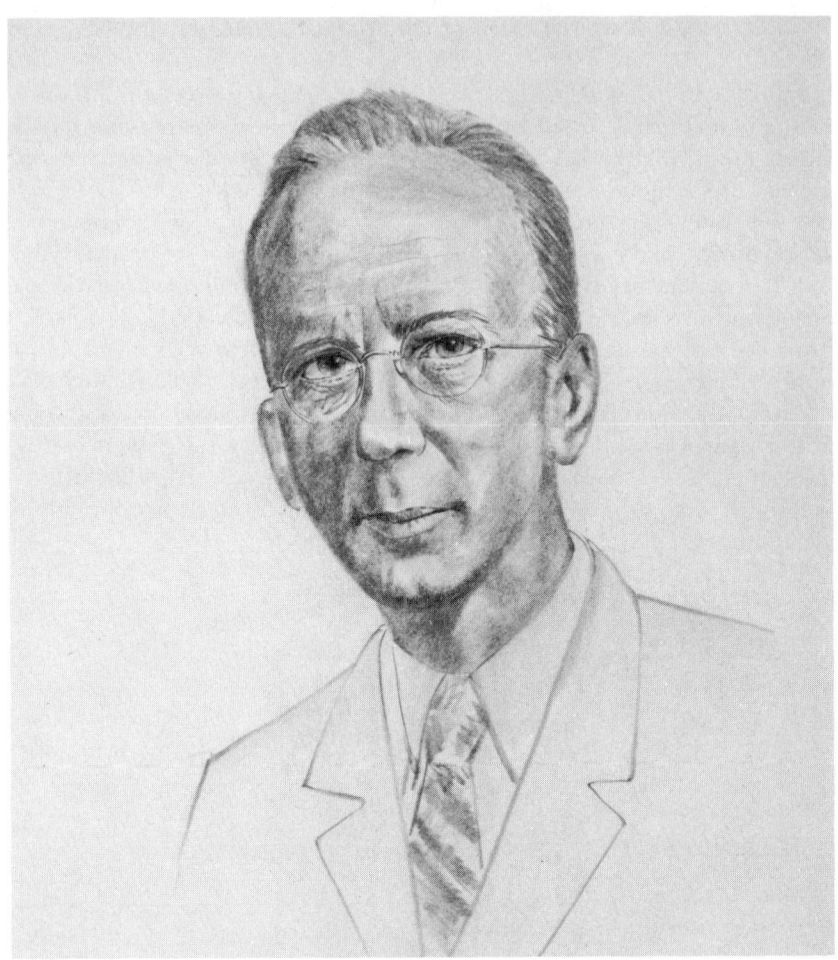

Louis Hamman
PROFESSOR OF MEDICINE

Dr. Hamman is well remembered for many reasons. To his students, he was the model clinician. Meticulous in accumulating the historical and physical data from the patient, his questioning was searching and incisive, like that of a wise barrister, and he interpreted the clues in the physical changes with the precision of an experienced detective. His analysis of the clinical evidence was severely methodical, so that no diagnostic or therapeutic possibility might be overlooked. The reasonableness of his logic made his conclusions appear inevitable. They were sometimes brilliant, always sound, and usually correct. They were based upon a wide personal clinical experience of the most sophisticated sort, for his special interest was any human illness.

His care of the patient did not end with the correct diagnosis. His planned, thoughtful management of the problems of the sick individual made mere treatment of a disease or a symptom seem woefully inadequate. He was inexhaustibly capable of infusing into his patients insight, self-discipline, optimism, and courage. Those he could not make well, he comforted. Versed in medical science, he also understood human nature, and enjoyed working with it. Analytical and logical, he was at the same time warm and charming. Although gentle, he was strong in his beliefs and ideals, but never brittle.

The tools he worked with were intellectual capacity, unconfined clinical experience, and the perceptive use of his eyes, ears, hands, and heart. His harvest was great good; his legacy to us was inspiration.

4

Communicating with the Family

Regrettably, patients' families are often very badly neglected by physicians. They may be actively avoided altogether or their questions may be cut short. This is very unfortunate for a number of reasons, such as the following:

1. Every sickness in a member of a family is a family sickness. If the husband is sick the wife shares in it, and vice versa. If the children are ill, the mother and the father are participants. Children are often profoundly affected by sickness in their parents.

2. To get well, the patient will certainly need the support and understanding of the entire family. It may be necessary for the family to make various sacrifices in order to help the patient, and obviously this requires comprehension of the reasons for their sacrifices.

3. Not uncommonly, family members have information about the patient and the development of his illness that may be crucial. They may have noticed things that the patient has consciously or subconsciously ignored, such as changes in personality, mental capacity, bodily appearance, increase in his use of various drugs, including alcohol, and so forth.

4. The cooperation of the family in carrying out the program of management can be just as essential as the cooperation of the patient. If the family does not like the attitude of the physician, both he and the patient are in for an uphill fight! An exceedingly clever but inexperienced clinician may wipe out the advantages of a brilliant diagnosis and a sound plan of management for his patient simply by not bothering to bring the family into the problem in a thoughtful manner, for it is often the family that will have the strongest influence on the patient. It is wise to make an ally of the family from the very start.

In general, at the very onset, it is a wise idea to talk with the responsible family members together with the patient, giving them a preliminary summary of what is thought and what is being planned. It is unwise to talk behind a patient's back. This may breed anxiety. One leak from a member of the family may wash out the confidence that the patient has developed in his physician. Also, families not infrequently distort or misinterpret what is told to them, and their misstatements may confuse the patient. If it is necessary to have an interview with the family away from the patient, either outline to the patient beforehand exactly what you intend to tell the family or, as soon as the family conference is completed, outline to the patient precisely what you did say to the family. It is utterly destructive to patient-physician-family relationships if either the patient or the family begins to suspect they are being two-timed.

Beware of confiding "secrets" to the family. Most members of the family won't be able to keep them. In a large family, select a responsible member and deal directly with him if there are confidential matters. It is very unwise to give different opinions to various members of the family. They will check and double check with each other and become very suspicious and apprehensive if everything doesn't jibe satisfactorily.

Any explanation to the family should be simple and straightforward. It should not contain too many details, which will probably not be retained and may only cause confusion or misinterpretation. In discussing serious illness be honest and frank, but keep some glimmer of hope burning as long as it is reasonable to do so. (See Section C, Chapter 4.) Even though what you have to say may contain some bad news, try to give it a positive slant, for the patient needs the family support and it is difficult to supply this when news is bleak and hope is slender.

By the same token, the family must be made honestly aware of the general progress of the patient's disease and of the critical areas that lie ahead, For example, it is an unfortunate mistake to give the impression that a complicated operation is a relatively minor one, or to imply that a particular type of treatment will no doubt produce improvement beyond real expectations. Be modest, conservative, and realistic in what is said, but at the same time always try to suggest some hope if the facts of the patient's illness will permit any at all.

In dealing with the family, always put the patient's welfare ahead of your own. Unfortunately, some physicians are so preoccupied by the fear that time will prove them wrong, thereby incurring family disapproval, that they design their conversations with the family not with the goal of maximally supporting the patient, but rather with the aim of strengthening their own position and buttressing themselves against the possibility of future criticism. Hence, they will unload upon the family every concern, every doubt, every unhappy eventuality that the patient's illness could possibly contain. This protective device of "telling it to the family before it happens" undermines the family's morale and is inevitably transmitted to the patient. A clinician must be ready to defend the position he has taken in meeting each of his patient's problems. He must not make the family the whipping-boy of his own insecurities. If the family has consistently been dealt with compassionately, if a reasonable understanding of what is wrong with the patient has been communicated to them, and if they comprehend what it is you are trying to do for the patient, the likelihood of such unfortunate consequences as law suits, refusal of autopsies, and so forth, will be negligible.

On the other hand, unfortunately there *are* some patients and families who are seeking an opportunity to entrap the physician in order to create a basis for legal claims. Although such instances are few, they are common enough for a physician to be constantly wary. His conduct must always be such that he would be willing at any time to have his actions reviewed by a group of his peers. His attitude toward the patient must always be strictly professional, and he should never do or say anything that is not a regular or usual part of routine medical practice in his environment. I recall a young house officer who had an exceedingly nervous female patient with a cardiac neurosis in the hospital. While the physician was making his evening rounds, the patient encountered him in the hall and complained of intense precordial distress and palpitations. Because of her concern he volunteered to listen to her heart. Since the two ward examining rooms were filled at the time, he suggested that she step into the nurses' cloakroom for a brief examination. The patient later accused the physician of fondling her. His position was made difficult by the fact that the circumstances of his examination were unusual. This episode clearly shows why special precautions should be taken when the patient or family appears to be emotionally unstable, or when one is dealing with a coquettish female or a homosexual. A witness should be present when such individuals are examined or when any sensitive subjects are discussed.

One of the best protections for a physician is the notes placed by him in the clinical chart. They should of course always be complete, but if trouble seems to be brewing, the physician should take great pains to see to it that his relationships with the patient and the family are documented in particular detail. This is especially true when some unfortunate incident occurs, such as the giving of a wrong drug dosage. Regardless of the nature of the incident, there should be a frank, honest, and complete description of it in the patient's clinical chart, including an account of what was done to correct the error once it was recognized and a detailed description of the patient's physical state before and after the incident. Any indication of a "cover-up" can be legally mortal for the physician.

Another protection is to ask the family to select a consultant to see the patient and if they are reluctant, to insist that they do so. The consultant's opinions and recommendations must also be recorded in the chart.

If critical decisions have to be made under such trying circumstances, the pros and cons should be discussed with the patient or the family or both in the presence of a witness, and concurrence obtained before action is taken. The key questions to be asked (and the answers to be recorded in detail in the chart) are these: (1) "Have I made the entire problem clear to you?"; (2) "Do you understand everything I have said or are there more questions?"; and (3) "Should we proceed, or would you like other opinions?"

Some patients or their families will want favors done for them dealing with insurance matters and so forth. Such requests must be turned aside with pleasant but firm amiability. Although granting them may create the impression of "he's a great fellow," this is a short-term gain, for one favor inevitably leads to another, and clearly, in the long run, the image of the physician as a person of unassailable integrity will be smudged.

Although it is obviously beneficial for the physician to get close to the patient and his family, and to establish warm and friendly relationships, it is important not to get *too close* or overly familiar. The physician must remain just a little apart, on a slightly different plane, or he will not be able to effectively lead and direct either the patient or the family. The physician should never appear to be lounging in the room when he visits the patient or family professionally, nor should he smoke, or tell jokes that could be misinterpreted in any way, or use slang, or have cocktails with them. He must maintain an air of dignity. People will not entrust their most serious problems, indeed their very lives, to someone they do not respect and admire. Therefore *look* the part of a clinician and *act* the part of a clinician—constantly.

Above all else, relatives want to feel that everything possible is being done for their loved one. It is exceedingly destructive for them to even suspect that their relative might have avoided disability or death if the family had only acted differently in some way. The conclusion that a mistake was made can be devastating. Sometimes guilt feelings enter into this reaction. For these and other reasons, relatives may sometimes be overzealous and overinquisitive; they may push suggestions and offer information that is not helpful. They may become very demanding. The physician will have to be extremely patient in dealing with such reactions. He must try to understand the motivations behind the relatives' attitudes and be tolerant of them. As already indicated, family support of the clinician is frequently essential to the welfare of the patient and to the success of the clinician's efforts. It may have to be bought at a high price of tolerance and patience.

The best attitude toward the family is one of patient cooperation, but there are times when it is necessary for the physician to be firm with relatives for the patient's sake. The physician must not let the family's emotional reactions overly influence the patient and his management. When one senses that this is beginning to happen, the family should be brought together with the physician, and the matter should be dealt with in a forthright manner. The medical problems should be explained to the family so that they are fully understood, and then the physician must insist upon the family's cooperation in enabling him to manage the patient as he believes best. Rarely, it may be necessary to turn the patient over to some other physician. If one senses that the patient is being adversely affected by his family's reactions, it may be helpful to explain to him that you know that he appreciates how families sometimes react to sickness and therefore, that he should not get upset, because together you can handle the disturbing situation with tact and diplomacy.

Calling in a consultant is a must when the family gets sticky. Supply the family two or three names and let them choose whom they want.

Above all, as already emphasized, a clinician should never "lose his cool" when dealing with families. Anger, sarcasm, bitter words will always come home to roost. Honesty, fairness, reasonableness, understanding, patience, communication—these are the effective responses to such trying situations.

Letting a family know that you are always readily available to them should they need you for support or questioning is an effective way of desensitizing an overly anxious group. Inaccessibility will only markedly increase their restiveness. The simple statement, "I know just what it is like to have someone very sick in the family, so if you become concerned or have questions, simply call me, and besides, I'll be in every day to see you and to answer your question after I have examined the patient" will often quiet troubled waters. Tell them the approximate time you expect to see the patient so they can prepare for your visit. A liberal application of the Golden Rule is necessary when dealing with reactive families.

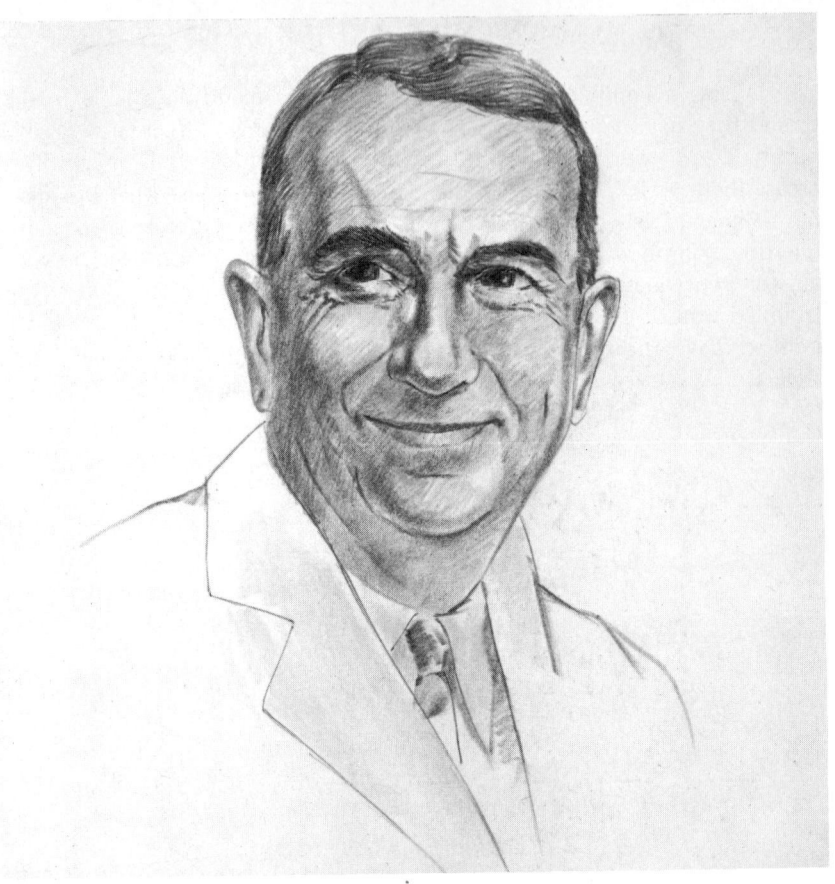

A. McGehee Harvey
PROFESSOR OF MEDICINE

Through the years, the characteristics we have most observed and felt are a gentle moderateness touched with a little shyness, strength and forthrightness, tireless perfectionism, unyielding tenacity, brilliance in the clarity and reasonableness of his analysis of any problem, farseeing and progressive, albeit conservatively so.

He is a member of a small hierarchy of academicians seemingly no longer to be encountered, who had talents and were able to make significant contributions in such diverse fields as research, clinical teaching, and administration. And so he built a great Department of Medicine, well balanced in both research contributions and clinical productiveness. Many will have read some or all of his papers and books. His Staff, year after year attracting brilliant and highly competent young physicians, is a perennial "hats off!" salute to a matchless clinician. With his guidance and example, the department has continued to adhere to Oslerian principles and methods in its approach to patients' problems, and in its support of complete personal involvement and responsibility in patient care.

Having had uniquely broad clinical experience, his analysis of clinical problems is methodically reasoned, developed with infinite logic and based upon meticulously gathered clinical evidence. He is able to make a very obscure answer to a clinical problem seem strikingly obvious, not by employing special technical maneuvers, but by disclosing some historical or physical fact not previously appreciated, or by highlighting in his analysis features hitherto not regarded as pivotal.

Undemonstrative, he teaches quietly, soundly, reasonably, and thoroughly, demonstrating to the students what a disciplined mind, in possession of accurate clinical evidence and reasoning methodically can accomplish for the care of sick persons.

Succeeding to Osler's chair, he has enriched and embellished the clinical tradition which his predecessor left behind. As his students, which all of us continue to be, we have learned and grown and come to be something better medically than we would have been without the setting and atmosphere he helped to create.

5

Communicating as a Consultant

Obviously, the role of a consultant is to help the patient by aiding his primary physician and is not to supplant him or to override him or to push him aside. Unfortunately, some consultants, by a variety of missteps, make it even more difficult for the primary physician to play his essential role in the care of his patient. One of the most common of these is giving information directly to the patient or his family, or making suggestions to them regarding diagnosis and treatment, without first touching base with the primary physician. Such actions may put the primary physician in a disadvantageous position because he may not have considered these particular suggestions previously and may not agree with them after further deliberation, or he may already have considered and discarded them for his own very good reasons. Because these are the consultant's opinions, and, therefore, presumably the "expert's," it may be difficult to erase them from the patient's and his family's minds if they are not followed. Therefore, doubts may be planted and confusion may begin to grow. The primary physician may start to lose control of his own patient's management.

Unfortunately, but thankfully infrequently, some consultants are overzealous in their desire to appear to always have the right answer and to seem clever, and they may talk to the patient or family in a demeaning or condescending manner with regard to the actions of the primary physician. They may use such expressions as "I don't understand how he could possibly have told you that!" or "You mean you have been on prednisone all this time?"

The consultant should be ever mindful of the difficult problems encountered in the everyday practice of medicine, and he should therefore make a deliberate effort to buttress the position of the primary physician. If the consultant concludes that the primary physician is in error, the matter should be discussed with him directly. It is exceedingly wrong to sacrifice the equanimity of the sick person and his worried family because of bungled relationships between the consultant and the primary physician.

Therefore, after completing his examination, the consultant should simply state to the patient and to his family that he will thoroughly discuss the problem with the responsible physician at once, that he has carefully reviewed the clinical evidence to date, and that he will make every effort, working together with the primary physician, to speed the patient's recovery. Under no circumstances, at this time, should the consultant give to the patient or his family *any* information of a specific nature relating to diagnosis, treatment or prognosis, *unless* he is directly requested to do so by the primary physician. Certainly the consultant should always try to say something that will help to comfort the patient and the family, and that will also support the position of the responsible physician, but his remarks should be confined strictly to these areas. If the patient has a complicated illness, it should be pointed out that although it may take time to achieve the correct answer, the patient is meanwhile in excellent hands; the problem is being studied carefully and thoroughly. The consultant should point out that he will continue to serve the patient and Dr. Blank in any helpful way. He should make it clear that he is only the consultant and that he will not in any way be supplanting Dr. Blank. He should make it evident that Dr. Blank will call him when *he* needs him.

If, after examining the patient, the consultant is backed into a corner by members of the family, who insist upon getting an opinion from him, it is always possible to gracefully put them off by saying something to the effect that the x-rays or other laboratory information must be critically studied, and that it is essential to review certain aspects of the problem with Dr. Blank before forming an opinion. The consultant should always suggest that another consultant be brought into the problem if he concludes that the matter is not in his special field of knowledge. Obviously, the welfare of the patient demands that the available physician with the most experience be the one selected to guide the patient's management.

Before he visits the patient, it is imperative that the consultant personally review in detail *all* of the clinical evidence that has been accumulated. He should read the clinical chart in its entirety. He should study the x-rays himself, and not simply accept on face value the reports pasted in the chart. He should question the patient in detail and examine him meticulously, taking nothing for granted. He should start his analysis of the problem from the beginning and challenge *all* of the historical and physical data already accumulated, forming his own personal judgment about each item. His should be a fresh and brand-new look, and not simply an overview of old material already assembled. He should trust no one's judgment but his own and rely only upon that clinical data which he has evaluated himself.

To be avoided assiduously for the sake of good patient care are what might be called "quickie" consultations. By these are meant off-hand, in-the-hall or around-the-luncheon-table kinds of consultations, in which the consultant is merely presented with a brief synopsis of the case as the primary physician sizes it up. Such off-hand consultations may lull the primary physician into unwarranted feelings of security. An opinion that isn't solid shouldn't be offered at all. A consultant's opinion should be based upon the most meticulous examination of *all* of the clinical evidence, not just part of it, and in particular, not upon a synopsis obtained from a second party. The consultant should not use any secondhand data. He must get all of the facts for himself.

Immediately after seeing the patient, the consultant should always write a note. If his opinion needs to be expressed in a long note to be dictated in his office or over the hospital Dictaphone, the consultant should nevertheless at least write a short summarizing note in the chart. The more detailed note can be added to the chart later. A telephone call to the primary physician as soon as the consultant has seen the patient is also highly desirable. It is both rude and ineffective for a consultant to see a patient and then not let the responsible physician know his conclusions for 24 or 48 hours, as unfortunately occasionally happens.

In summary, as soon as a patient is seen in consultation, the opinion of the consultant must be stated briefly in the chart and communicated rapidly by some means to the responsible physician. Nothing makes the primary physician look more inadequate in the eyes of the family and the patient than the discovery that the primary physician does not know the conclusions of the consultant whom *he* selected to see the patient.

If, after examining the patient, a conference with the family and the consultant is requested by the primary physician, and if the consultant disagrees with the responsible physician, he should clearly be exceedingly tactful and diplomatic in expressing his conclusions: "As Dr. Blank has explained to you, he believes that your trouble is most likely due to gallbladder disease. I can certainly appreciate his reasons for coming to this conclusion. However, having the advantage that I have had of looking back at the course of events in your illness and studying how it unfolded, it seems to me more likely that this is not gallbladder disease but rather hepatitis."

At this juncture, the family may question why the consultant doesn't agree with the primary physician. It is wise to point out that medical problems are oftentimes not clearly black or white, and determination of the exact nature of an illness is many times not an open and shut case. One and one doesn't always quickly add up to two. Nor are medical problems, once defined, always easily solved. After study of the clinical evidence, different opinions may be drawn from it by different clinicians. Frequently these are matters of opinion and judgment and experience. The clinician's responsibility is to make every effort to meticulously study the clinical evidence and to develop the most reasonable plan of management. You, the consultant, and the primary physician are now attempting to do exactly this, in a cooperative way.

During such a conference, the most essential items are these:

1. To give the patient and the family ample opportunity to ask any questions that they might want to ask.

2. To support the patient by trying to strengthen his confidence in his primary physician and to avoid any remark or attitude that might lessen it.

3. To present only as much specific information and advice to the patient has the primary physician has agreed that he wants you to give.

One of the most difficult situations is that in which the consultant has come to the inescapable conclusion that the patient is being mishandled by the primary physician. In this unfortunate situation, the consultant should first make every effort to see to it that the primary physician understands the seriousness of the problem and the deleterious effects of his decisions upon the patient. If, after ample dialogue, the responsible physician will still not alter his position, the consultant should firmly suggest that other opinions be brought in to try to resolve the dilemma. A note put into the clinical chart by the consultant clearly stating the points of disagreement between himself and the primary physician may be very effective in this regard.

If these approaches are of no avail and the responsible physician persists in a program which the consultant thinks is harmful, then the consultant should explain to the patient or the family or both that it is necessary for him to withdraw from the matter because he can no longer be helpful to them in view of the differences in judgment, and he should suggest that they seek yet another opinion. In employing this approach, however, it should be made clear to the patient and family that the matter is one of failure to agree; they should *not* be told by the consultant that he is necessarily right and the other physician is wrong. It should again be stressed that medical problems are like all other problems; there is room for disagreement.

It is obviously extremely wrong to just "go along." The consultant is serving the patient, and has a grave responsibility to him as well as to the primary physician. *He* brought you, the consultant, into this relationship with the patient, and it is not enough simply to excuse yourself if you think the patient is being poorly handled. Of course, the primary physician should be informed of what the consultant intends to do. As already stressed, a properly composed note in the patient's chart is generally the only stimulus needed to get the primary physician to request additional consultative help, which is the only proper answer to this kind of unfortunate impasse.

SECTION

B

The Performance of the Physical Examination

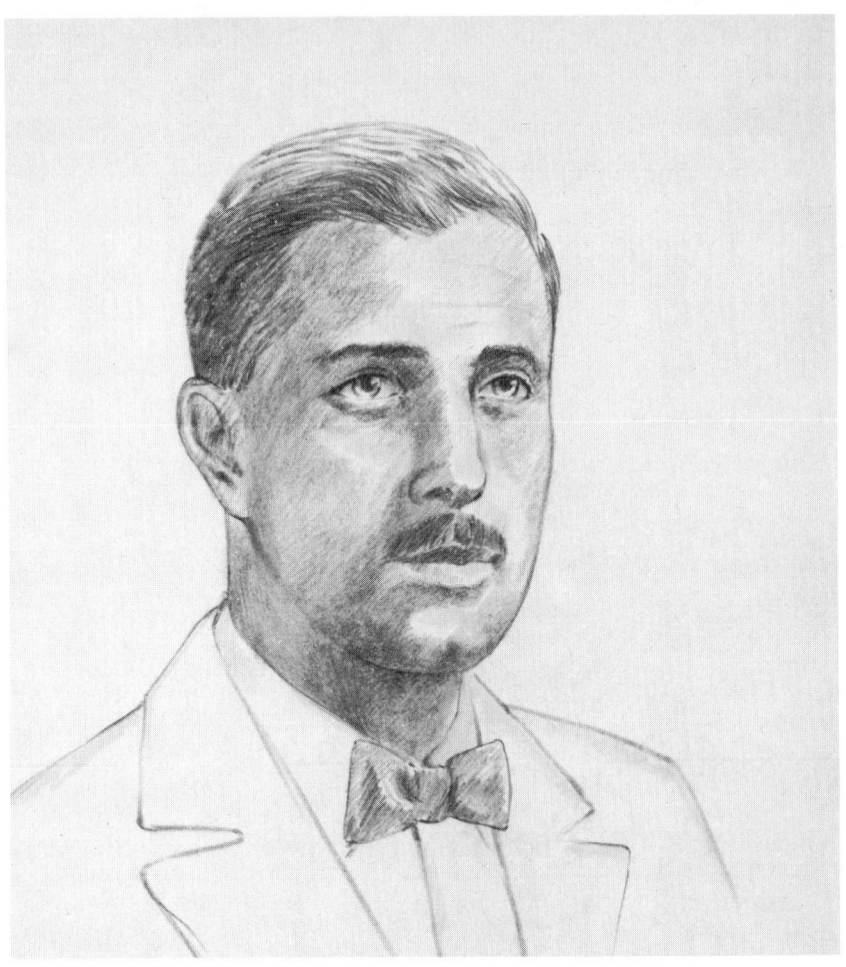

Joseph L. Lilienthal, Jr.
PROFESSOR OF ENVIRONMENTAL MEDICINE

The passage of time distills our memories, leaving behind the most vivid. A gay and charming spirit, blooming with humor, brilliant, dynamic, tireless, a compendium of knowledge of all sorts of subjects, fiercely loyal to causes strongly held—these recollections of Joe come to us now most readily.

It was a delight to meet him in the corridor or at luncheon, for to be with him was to learn and to enjoy. He had strong convictions, and he was always ready to take up cudgels against injustice, intolerance, and chicanery in any form. He could wither with a few words stupidity, pretense, or posturing. He was equally and superbly talented as an investigator, clinician, teacher, and administrator. To be his intern when he was an Assistant Resident was a memorable and rich experience, but not an easy one, for he insisted upon excellence and could be stern when less was given. Trying to keep pace with his fertile, imaginative mind was just the right exercise for young associates, bewildered—but also vastly stimulated—by the extent of his knowledge. Because of his balanced judgment, he seemed assured of his bearings even when dealing with clinical problems not previously encountered. Working for Joe was hard, because he worked hard, but there were episodes of exhilarating humor, and his praise was generous and sincere.

His achievements in science and academic medicine were important ones, and he became one of the most distinguished members of this faculty. Although death came early to Joe, he has left us a rich harvest.

The Physical Examination

INTRODUCTION

This section is not intended to be a restatement of basic material readily available in textbooks of physical diagnosis. It assumes such an introduction and endeavors to make observations which will increase the yield of clinical information derived from the use of the basic techniques of physical diagnosis. Throughout this discussion, the potential diagnostic value of little and sometimes seemingly unimportant details will be repeatedly stressed, for such details are oftentimes the revealing clues. The physician must not just look, but *see,* and not just see, but *analyze,* and not just analyze but *interpret*—not just *some* of the data but *all* of it.

GENERAL OBSERVATIONS

General observation of the patient is often the most revealing part of the entire physical examination although, unfortunately, it is often neglected. While many young clinicians are very proficient in their examination of specific organ systems, it is my impression that some overlook many highly rewarding clues because of their lack of proficiency in general observation of their patients. Either the obvious appears so obvious that its telltale diagnostic implications are overlooked or else it is not known how to derive significant meaning from the less obvious. Recently, with a junior colleague, I saw an elderly white female admitted with severe congestive heart failure. My colleague recited the cardiac findings in precise detail, concluding that "The patient probably has degenerative myocardial disease." But he failed to notice on general observation that the patient was quick and jerky in her movements; she had an unusually "bright eye"; her hair was stringy and hanging down "because I can't keep it up"; the frontalis fossae were quite prominent; and she complained of weakness of the muscles of her shoulder girdle—all, of course, classic manifestations of hyperthyroidism, which proved to be the actual cause of the congestive failure. My young colleague's proficiency in examining the patient's cardiovascular mechanism did not pay off because he had failed to make the meaningful and necessary general observations. Therefore, each physical examination should start with an all-encompassing view of the patient, with special attention to the following elements:

The General Setting. The clinician must be a detective, for small details reveal a great deal; for example, the appearance of the patient and her surroundings—are they neat and bright or tasteless and depressing? Are the shades pulled down and is the room dark? Is the patient, supposedly in great pain, nicely groomed? In introducing her husband, does the patient say, "I'm glad you met my husband today. He's constantly so busy you probably won't ever have a chance to meet him again!"?

The Attitude of Those in Attendance. Are they overly concerned or indifferent? Does the illness seem to be bothering them more than the patient? Do they insist upon answering most of the questions for the patient? Does one sense concealed antagonisms? Frequently, illness affects all members of the family—not just the patient.

The Character of the Patient's Response. Is he animated and responsive or dull and clouded? Is there any indication of blunting of the sensorium or of difficulty with mentation?

The Patient's Personality. What sort of a person does the patient seem to be on first encounter? Is his emotional make-up simply constructed or complicated, is he outgoing or introverted, sensitive or insensitive? Are there any outstanding peculiarities in his appearance, actions, or traits of character? Such an initial impression may have to be completely revised later, but it is basic in attempting to form a working evaluation of the patient's way of reacting, since it will critically affect one's interpretation of the symptoms and signs as they are elicited. Thus, the evaluation of abdominal tenderness in a sensitive individual who tells her story tearfully and flinches each time she is approached is necessarily different from that of a stolid, rugged individual with the same condition. The observations already made regarding the patient's surroundings, attitude of attendants, dress, speech, and so forth, will help in early appreciation of the patient's personality.

General Appearances. Does the patient seem to be having any particular type of distress, such as pain or dyspnea? Does he appear to be ill? Has he lost weight? It is wise to correlate such evidences with the general observations already outlined. Does he have a tic or stutter? Does he move about or walk oddly? Is he restless and agitated?

The physical position which the patient assumes may have diagnostic significance. The patient with true vertigo wants to lie flat and motionless, and to be undisturbed. Pleurisy may cause the patient to splint his affected chest. Frequently the patient with pericarditis prefers to sit very erect, leaning forward. The patient with carcinoma of the pancreas may be very loath to lie flat on his back, preferring a rolled up or fetal attitude. Irritation of the psoas muscle by an inflammatory process such as appendicitis may result in flexion of the affected thigh. An inflammatory process in the hip joint may favor flexion and internal rotation of the thigh. An acute myocardial infarction may cause the patient to become exceedingly restless, tossing and turning in an agitated manner, even insisting upon getting up and walking about. A patient with a pulmonary embolus may be found sitting up, markedly anxious.

General Body Structure. Here there is no need for a highly technical categorization. In ordinary terms, is the patient tall or short, thin or obese, athletic or asthenic? Note the general body structure at the start, since it will have significance in your interpretation of the heart size and the palpability of organs such as the liver and kidneys. Obviously, any special peculiarities of body structure, whether congenital or acquired, are to be sought and interpreted. Some examples are pigeon breast, pectus excavatum, tower skull, kyphosis, long tapering hands and feet, and so on.

Vital Signs. An elevation of temperature is always a significant finding which requires explanation. Oral temperatures may be highly deceptive, and rectal determinations should be required if there is any question of the validity of the recordings. I have seen the real cause of a serious illness overlooked because of apparent absence of fever, only because oral temperatures were misleading. Factitious fevers are not uncommon, and the manner of their production may be difficult to detect. If there are any suspicions, it is a good plan to have the observer simultaneously take an oral and rectal temperature at a time other than the routine. The buttocks should be left exposed so that the thermometer can be observed constantly while the pulse rate is being counted. The observer must make certain to get back the same thermometer given to the patient, for some patients will make stealthy substitutions. Another technique, if a temperature elevation is under suspicion, is to take the temperature of the patient's urine immediately after voiding. It should match the body temperature. Even with such precautions I have encountered instances in which the factitious nature of a fever could not be definitely established, even though suspected for a long time. Factitious fevers occur most commonly in members of the medical or paramedical profession, or their family members.

The only abnormality indicating the presence of such serious conditions as pneumonia, pulmonary embolism or congestive heart failure may be an increased respiratory rate. Respiratory rates of 18 or 20 breaths per minute are sometimes recorded on hospital charts without the true rate having actually been counted. Therefore one must be sure that the reported rate is valid before attempting to interpret it. In addition to increased rate, alterations in the quality of breathing have important diagnostic meaning and must be observed.

Likewise, changes in the rate or quality of the peripheral arterial pulses may be the only indication of major physiological dysfunction, as in acute gastrointestinal hemorrhage or a pulmonary embolus. The golfing businessman who says he had a little precordial tightness on the 18th hole but now feels fine, and on examination is found to have an excessively rapid or irregular pulse, is a candidate for further investigation.

Few clinical observations are more carelessly performed than the determination of systemic blood pressure. Patients are not infrequently given erroneous and worrisome information about their health as a result of improper interpretation of a blood pressure determination, which may also lead to unnecessary use of potentially harmful drugs. A blood pressure reading can be significantly influenced by the structure of the patient's arm and by his emotional reactions. Large, fat arms may give pressure readings which are too high, whereas thin arms may give values which are too low. Although it is widely appreciated that emotional tension induces moderate elevation of the systolic blood pressure, the marked degree to which this elevation sometimes occurs is not so well recognized, nor is the fact that the diastolic pressure may also be very much increased. Thus elevations in the range of 180/115 or higher are not at all uncommon in a highly reactive person. Tact and repeated observations on the part of the physician usually overcome some of the emotional over-reaction and lead to a more accurate approximation of the patient's true pressure. The use of a wide cuff, or over-wrapping a standard cuff with some material to prevent bulging-out and overinflation of the pneumatic bag, is necessary when dealing with an excessively large arm.

PARTICULAR OBSERVATIONS

In examining the patient it is essential that he be stripped and examined completely, if possible in a bright, direct light. All areas must be inspected. A British clinician once defined an American patient as "a person having a front but no back," reflecting the fact that so often we examine the patient's front assiduously, but so infrequently is he completely stripped and turned over. For example, the illness of a young man with fever, rash, and toxicity was considered to be a diagnostic mystery until a more careful physical examination disclosed a tick buried in the pudendal hair. Dentures must be removed in the search for mucosal lesions, and nail polish must come off.

The particular items mentioned in the following sections are by no means intended to be a complete listing or compendium of the various types of changes which can or should be noted on physical examination. Rather, they are simply examples of the kind of useful information which can be gathered if the observer looks with ingenuity. It is hoped that by outlining some of these more evident clues, the observor will be stimulated to discipline himself to keep constantly searching for others.

Coloration

Unless the patient is observed in a bright, direct light it may be extremely difficult to detect even major degrees of pallor, cyanosis and icterus. A decision regarding the presence or degree of pallor or cyanosis should be made only after the palms of the hands, the nail beds, the conjunctivae, and the mucous membranes of the mouth and tongue have been sequentially and comparatively investigated. It should be recalled that at least 5 gm. of unsaturated hemoglobin are required for the production of clinically detectable cyanosis. Therefore, a patient with severe anemia may never be cyanotic while a patient with polycythemia may readily appear very blue. Cyanosis of the tongue indicates an extremely low degree of oxygen saturation. Icterus should be sought for not only in the eyes and skin but under the tongue as well. The skin and mucous membranes may remain icteric even after the eyes have cleared. While it is common to refer to "scleral" icterus, it is actually icterus of the conjunctivae which is seen. Icterus should not be confused with discoloration due to atabrine, which does not stain the conjunctivae, nor with carotenemia, which has a distinctive pinkish yellow tinge. There is an appreciable time lag between a fall in serum bilirubin levels and disappearance of the pigmentation from the tissues. Pruritus of the skin may begin before icterus is discernible, and start to subside before there is appreciable fading of the skin pigmentation, particularly in patients who have been chronically jaundiced. Chronic severe jaundice leads to dark bronze pigmentation of the skin (sometimes suggestive of hemochromatosis) as well as to yellow discoloration.

Increased or decreased pigmentation of the skin, or a mixture of the two, are common accompaniments of a wide variety of local as well as systemic disorders. The earliest change in several important systemic diseases may be such altered pigmentation, as in scleroderma or thyroid dysfunction. The distribution of such changes, whether localized or generalized, and whether the mucous membranes are involved as well, may be important from a diagnostic standpoint. A characteristic feature of Addison's disease is a deposit of pigment about old scars and abrasions as well as in the buccal mucosa. In scleroderma, altered pigmentation is frequently first observed over the extremities, the face or the neckline area. The finding of small pigmented spots on the lips is characteristic of the Peutz-Jeghers syndrome. A number of factors, including local vascular changes such as venous stasis or lymphedema, or exposure to physical or chemical trauma, as from the wearing of a tight girdle or chronic scratching, may result in abnormal pigmentation—hence the need for making a detailed analysis of the setting in which the altered pigmentation is discovered before drawing any conclusions regarding its etiology.

One should examine the texture of the skin with care, by viewing and stroking, and by folding and creasing the skin and subcutaneous tissues. Often, recent alteration in its texture is more significant than the observation that the skin is smooth or rough, or dry or moist, for such changes in texture may indicate underlying systemic disease. For example, in hyperthyroidism the skin may become very fine and silky. This can be misleading in the Negro, in whom smooth skin is a racial characteristic. It is important to test the elasticity of the skin. Decreased elasticity is a typical feature of the Ehlers-Danlos syndrome. A loss of normal skin turgor may indicate a serious degree of dehydration or electrolyte depletion.

Increased thickening of the skin or its adherence to subcutaneous tissues or both, which may be very local or quite generalized, are prominent features of a wide variety of disorders which will require clinical differentiation, sometimes quite difficult to make. These include scleroderma, scleredema, myxedema, myxedema circumscripta, acropachy, sclerodactyly, chronic venous stasis, lymph stasis (when congenital, Milroy's disease), amyloidosis, sarcoidosis, chronic or recurrent cellulitis (erysipelas), tumor infiltration, and massive hemorrhage into the subcutaneous tissues as in bleeding disorders.

Hair

The color of the hair may give a meaningful hint as to the nature of the patient's underlying disorder. A youngster with painful joints and a fever and red hair may well have rheumatic fever. Premature greying of the hair in a blue-eyed individual is a characteristic of pernicious anemia. Occasionally there have appeared on the market hair dyes which have been hepatotoxic or have induced thrombocytopenia. The general appearance of the hair may tell a story. Thus, an otherwise fastidious female with unkempt hair is probably significantly ill, physically or psychologically.

Loss of hair, either local or generalized, may be associated with a host of organic and functional conditions, and hence the finding of alopecia is of little specific diagnostic help. Conditions as disparate as anxiety and disseminated tumor may lead to focal or generalized loss of hair. Whereas in the past change in the texture of the hair has been emphasized as being a characteristic feature of abnormalities of thyroid function, in our own experience a much more typical story of thyroid abnormality is the patient's complaint that he or she can no longer get their hair to stay fixed: "I fix my hair and within a short period of time it is down around my neck again. My hairdresser has given up."

The distribution of body hair is well known to be of clinical significance. However, one must be cautious in interpreting the meaning of excessive quantities of hair on the face and other portions of the body since this may be a familial characteristic. Correct interpretation of this physical alteration is dependent on a careful family history.

Scars and Tattoos

The presence of scars, operative or otherwise; sites of needle injections; sinus tracts; or puncture wounds, produced by the bite of an insect or animal or induced by some other trauma, can be of diagnostic pertinence. For example, the patient with recurrent hypoglycemia may be inducing hypoglycemic episodes by injecting himself with insulin. A healed sinus track in the region of lymph nodes raises the question of old, healed tuberculous lymphadenitis or of other granulomatous or suppurative infection. The prick of a rose thorn may lead to the indolent lymphagitis of sporotrichosis. Tattoo marks are often seen in individuals who are emotionally unstable, such as chronic alcoholics, or in those having similar personality disorders. Viral hepatitis can be acquired by tattoo.

Edema

Two of the main determinants of localization of edema are tissue pressure and the force of gravity. Since the tissue pressure about the eyes is low, one of the earliest sites of generalized edema formation is the periorbital region. Because of the effect of gravity, collection of edema in the recumbent patient should be first sought in the buttocks and presacral area, and *not* in the lower extremities. It is important to recall that a number of additional factors may be involved in edema formation, including changes in serum proteins, alterations in fluid and electrolyte balance, diuretic factors, vascular permeability, anemia, anorexia, inflammatory changes, hypersensitivity, arteritis, lymph stasis, and mechanical obstruction to lymphatic or venous return. Hence, one's analysis of the presence of edema in a particular patient must include the necessary observations to exclude or include the role of each of these factors. For example, the discovery of the wearing of a very tight panty girdle may shed important light on the finding of edema of the lower extremities in a fat lady with incompetent veins.

Vascular Lesions

There are a large number of vascular lesions which may signal the nature of an underlying systemic disorder. While such lesions may be numerous, far more often they are sparse and only detectable upon the most careful survey. A case in point is a patient who presented with repeated gastrointestinal hemorrhage of unexplained origin and was ultimately discovered to have a single Osler-Weber-Rendu lesion high in his nasopharynx.

Vascular spiders are usually seen on the flush areas of the body. Contrary to common belief, they may appear and disappear quite suddenly. Whereas generally regarded as an accompaniment of hepatic impairment, which is progressive, these lesions may appear as a badly damaged liver begins to regenerate or, on the other hand, they may actually fade as the injury continues to advance, because of an altered balance in estrogen–androgen metabolism.

Telangiectases, sometimes large, are a common, very early feature of scleroderma, and may be seen both in the skin or in the mucous membranes. They may exactly simulate those of Osler-Weber-Rendu disease. Of interest was a patient who presented with congestive heart failure, thought originally to be due to idiopathic or degenerative myocarditis, but which eventually proved to be due to scleroderma of the myocardium. The telltale clue was one large telangiectatic lesion under the patient's tongue, others in the buccal mucous membranes, and a few scattered over his extremities. Vascular lesions like those seen in Osler-Weber-Rendu disease are also sometimes seen in systemic lupus erythematosus.

The distribution of purpura should be noted carefully, for it may have diagnostic meaning. Thus, purpura appearing at the base of hair follicles, and about the eyes and the neck, is quite characteristic of amyloidosis. It may be a very early change in this disorder. In Waldenström's hyperglobulinemic purpura, the lesions are confined almost entirely to the lower extremities. Perifollicular hemorrhages are also typical of scurvy, whereas small ecchymoses may be an indication of a variety of disorders associated with a bleeding tendency, including Cushing's syndrome and steroid therapy. It should be emphasized that easy bruising is not an unusual phenomenon in many healthy women, particularly in association with their menstrual cycle.

Subungual splinter hemorrhages and petechiae are seen not only in blood stream infections such as bacterial endocarditis but in other disease states as well, including trauma, fat emboli, tumor emboli (myxoma of the left auricle), acute rheumatic fever, all of the various forms of arteritis, and marantic endocarditis. The soles of the feet are a common site for petechial lesions, as is the area about the ankles. The lesions may appear and disappear rapidly; hence, frequent examination of the patient is essential for their detection. A common cause of "splinter hemorrhages" under the nails *is* splinters, or some other form of trauma. Erythematous spots or hivelike lesions following trauma or pressure are typical of urticaria pigmentosa.

Skin Eruptions

Disorders of the internal organs often manifest through alterations in the integument. Such changes are frequently the earliest or the only manifestations of serious, progressive internal disease. Therefore, it is essential to first closely examine the skin and mucosal surfaces before proceeding to a study of the deeper structures. In analyzing any changes in the integument, it is well to remember that one and the same internal disease may be capable of producing a large number of totally nonspecific alterations of the mucocutaneous structures; conversely, a particular kind of change in the skin or mucous membranes may be associated with a wide variety of entirely different systemic diseases. Thus, long before any other changes are evident, a lymphoma may be associated with pruritus of the skin, altered pigmentation, urticaria, purpura, or a papular eruption, all of these being nonspecific. On the other hand, a specific dermatologic lesion like erythema nodosum may be associated with any one of the so-called "immune" disorders, new growths, drug reactions, sarcoid, granulomatous infections, and enterocolitis, among others. I recall a businessman who felt well but for the complaint of a nonspecific, pruritic papular eruption on his forehead of several months' duration. Not until 18 months later was it discovered that this nondescript, "unimpressive" eruption was the initial manifestation of a hidden lymphoma from which the patient ultimately succumbed.

Since even the most subtle alterations may be of great diagnostic significance, it is urgent to examine the entire integument in a bright direct light as well as in a cross light. Unless the entire body is checked, the skin has not been properly examined. Changes of diagnostic importance may appear and fade very rapidly—hence the necessity for frequent re-examination. I recall a 45 year old male patient who stated that he had had a shaking chill and fever every third day for six weeks, during which hivelike lesions would transiently appear over his lower extremities. In the intervals he felt well. Such an occurrence is not uncommon in recurrent meningococcemia. An episode was observed, and subsequent blood cultures were positive for the meningococcus.

Deposits, Infiltrates, and Nodules

Deposits and infiltrates in the integument may tell an important story. Xanthomatous deposits about the eyes, for example, are frequently seen in individuals with a high serum cholesterol. When seen in a young person they may be an indication of premature vascular degeneration. They may be associated with early arcus senilis, which Dr. Osler called "old man's spectacles." These shouldn't be worn by a young person! When they are, they may be an indication of premature aging of his vessels. However, for reasons still unclear, they are common in apparently healthy young Negroes. Cholesterol deposits, particularly around tendon sheaths, occur in biliary cirrhosis and with primary familial hypercholesterolemia. The significance of uric acid deposits is well known. Calcium deposits may appear in a number of circumstances in addition to states associated with hypercalcemia, such as hyperparathyroidism. Calcium salts will deposit in any area where there is dead tissue, chronic inflammation, or inadequate blood supply. Thus, calcification may occur in old hematomas or in infarcted tissues. Calcification of the skin, subcutaneous tissues and muscles may be prominent features of scleroderma and dermatomyositis, as well as benign or malignant primary or secondary tumors of the soft tissues, or chronic granulomatous infections.

Granulomatous processes, including those due to sarcoid and fungus infections, may appear as very small scattered areas of infiltration or in confined patches. These changes may be very hard to discern unless viewed in a cross light. Systemic fungus infections, including Cryptococcus, may form small, nondescript nodules which characteristically appear about the face or within the oropharyngeal cavity, although they may occur anywhere in the integument. There may be only a single or very few such nodular lesions. They are easily disregarded as being cutaneous papillomas of no importance. At the Walter Reed Hospital I once saw a sergeant who presented with a six-month history of headaches, weight loss, personality deterioration and finally a patch of pneumonitis in the left upper lobe. Just above the labial fold on the left was a small, isolated, pigmented protuberant nodule, direct smears of which on biopsy showed the cytococcus; this same organism was later obtained from the patient's spinal fluid and lung.

Malignant tumors of a variety of sorts, and especially carcinoma of the lung, may first become evident by small, focal metastases to the skin and subcutaneous tissues of the face or other areas of the body. I recall a businessman who, while shaving, nicked a small papilloma which had recently appeared on his face. His physician had the wisdom to make a biopsy of this lesion. It was a metastatic squamous cell carcinoma of the lung. Only months later was small nodule observed in a chest film. Thus, whenever the presence of a malignant tumor is suspected, it is worthwhile to check the entire integument for the presence of a single or perhaps several subcutaneous lumps, biopsy of which might give a specific answer. The navel is of particular importance in this regard, for a number of intra-abdominal tumors, including carcinoma of the gut and the pancreas as well as of the ovary, may metastasize to the umbilicus long before they go elsewhere. This is a lesion easily examined by biopsy.

The presence of rheumatoid nodules along tendon sheaths is best disclosed by flexing the joints so that tension is put upon the tendons. The observer then rakes his examining fingers along the stretched tendons. It is not well recognized that rheumatoid nodules may become very enlarged, so that they can be mistaken for cysts when seen about a joint, particularly behind the knees, simulating Baker's cysts. These nodules may also appear behind the ears and in the scalp and be mistaken for lymph nodes and other mass lesions. Whereas typical of rheumatoid disease, they may occur in other disorders of this spectrum, including systemic lupus erythematosus. Pulsating nodules along blood vessels are seen in polyarteritis nodosa as well as in giant cell arteritis, but only infrequently. A characteristic clinical feature of giant cell arteritis is the appearance of so-called "phantom" spots in various areas of the scalp. These are small, tender, painful areas, sometimes nodular, which alternately appear and vanish. Very rarely they break down, becoming gangrenous. Frequently it is impossible to distinguish between subcutaneous lipoma, fibroma, or neurofibroma on clinical grounds, and biopsy is required. The identification of a neurofibroma may be important since it is infrequently associated with a pheochromocytoma or hypoglycemia, or with tumors involving the brain or spinal cord, or those presenting as mediastinal or intra-abdominal masses. Such lesions may be associated with a cafe au lait spot on the skin.

The Subcutaneous Fat

Weight loss and its degree are highly significant clinical observations. Marked wasting of subcutaneous fat and muscle is oftentimes made obvious by deepening of the frontalis fossae. The degree of wasting of the soft tissues may be readily estimated by picking up and palpating with the fingers a fold of skin, particularly about the margins of the thoracic cage.

Whereas a fat trunk and slim extremities are characteristic of Cushing's syndrome, this is not an uncommon finding in females as well as males who eat excessively, and it may also be a familial trait. Unusual and excessive deposition of fat, e.g., in the buttocks, thighs, or breasts, may also be a familial trait. Although deposition of fat at the base of the neck, the so-called "dowager's hump," is typical of Cushing's syndrome, less frequently there is pronounced deposition of fat in the supraclavicular fossae, the patient assuming a Kewpie doll appearance. This has also been noted in a patient with myxedema. Only recently has it become well recognized that similar deposits of fat may occur within the mediastinum, exactly mimicking the appearance of a solid or vascular tumor. Such deposits may be small or very large. I am acquainted with a patient who was on steroids in moderate dosage for a year because of rheumatoid arthritis. He presented with a huge mass extending outward from the mediastinum. He was operated upon with the conviction that he had some sort of a malignant new growth, but only fatty deposits were found. Such fatty deposits regress when steroid administration is halted or upon control of the Cushing's disease.

Tender, painful inflammatory and sometimes necrotic nodules in the panniculus adiposus are hallmarks of Weber-Christian disease. The lesions vary from 0.5 to more than 10 cm. in diameter. An oily liquid may be extruded from them. Characteristically, healing is associated with scarring and atrophy leading to small depressions in the skin, which sets these lesions apart from other types of disorders affecting fatty tissues. Similar lesions are infrequently observed in various diseases of the pancreas, including pancreatitis and pancreatic carcinoma. These kinds of lesions may be confused with lipomatosis, cellulitis, adiposis dolorosa (Dercum's disease), erythema nodosum, erythema induratum, sarcoid, and insulin atrophy.

The Muscles

Myositis of a nonspecific sort may be an early, and sometimes the only, indication of the presence of a large number of systemic diseases of widely varying etiology, some very common, others unusual, including the "autoimmune" disorders such as scleroderma, rheumatoid arthritis, hypersensitivity angiitis, polyarteritis, giant cell arteritis, and systemic lupus, as well as sarcoidosis, generalized granulomatous infections such as tuberculosis and histoplasmosis, the dysproteinemic states such as Waldenström's disease, and unusual conditions like Whipple's disease. Similar changes may herald the presence of any malignant new growth, such as bronchogenic carcinoma or carcinoma of the pancreas or stomach, as well as various types of lymphomas and leukemia. Hyperthyroidism, particularly in the older male, may be mistaken for a primary muscle disorder because of pronounced shoulder and pelvic girdle weakness and atrophy even in the absence of most of the usual signs of thyroidism, including significant enlargement of the thyroid gland. In all of these diverse conditions the symptoms and signs may be, for a significant period of time, primarily muscular in nature, and unless the observer is alert to this important relationship, the true nature of the patient's illness can be misinterpreted. Widespread myositis may be present without any physical changes in the muscles other than weakness or atrophy, alterations such as local tenderness, heat, or swelling more often that not being absent. There may be marked discrepancy between the clinical and histologic appearances of the muscles, apparently healthy-looking muscles being quite abnormal when examined histologically, and vice versa. In all these disorders, the shoulder girdle and hip and thigh muscles frequently demonstrate the earliest and most pronounced change. Hence, very early complaints made by these patients include difficulty combing the hair, shaving, raising the arms above the head, going up stairs and getting out of a chair or car. As truncal muscles become involved, generally at a later date, the patients complain of trouble turning over in bed and in sitting upright.

In this same group of systemic disorders which cause prominent and sometimes diagnostically confusing muscle changes, arthralgia and arthritis may be prominent features, and simulate rheumatoid or other forms of primary joint disorders. Peripheral neuropathy may be yet another accompaniment. A wide variety of skin eruptions may also appear, some nonspecific in character and others simulating the kind of vascular alterations once regarded as "specific" for so-called "idiopathic dermatomyositis," Now we realize that the clinical picture of dermatomyositis secondary to a new growth may precisely simulate that of the idiopathic variety. Hence the correct diagnosis depends upon excluding some background disorder, frequently latent.

It is very helpful from the standpoint of clinical diagnosis to regard the concomitance of myositis, peripheral neuritis, arthritis, arthralgia, and a variety of nonspecific skin eruptions as a clinical complex observed in a group of disorders of widely varying etiology, but all having the common denominator of some type of immune hyperreactivity. Included in this group are drug reactions, sarcoidosis, granulomatous infections, chronic focal infections (such as subacute bacterial endocarditis), any kind of new growth (including lymphoma, myeloma and leukemia), the dysproteinemic states, enterocolitis, Whipple's disease and Mediterranean fever. These represent a group of disorders in which clinical differentiation may be most difficult, for, like Mike and Ike, initially they may look alike. Early in their course, acting predominately through immune mechanisms, the alterations they produce are exactly similar, with the most prominent early changes very often being in skin, muscles, joints, and peripheral nerves.

The Extremities

So much of diagnostic value can be learned from the extremities that it is a wise habit to always inspect them in detail before starting to examine the chest and abdomen.

First, note their general structure. In acromegaly the fingers are broad, and thick and pudgy, and the ends appear blunted, producing a "spadelike" appearance. By contrast, the fingers in pituitary insufficiency may be long and slender. Long, slender fingers and palms, and also feet, with hyperextensibility of the digits, are also present in Marfan's syndrome (arachnodactyly) and in sickle cell anemia, pulmonary stenosis and the Ehlers-Danlos syndrome. Sausage-shaped fingers may be a result of granulomatous dactylitis owing to tuberculosis or syphilis. Spindle-like deformity is observed in a variety of circumstances, including the "collagen" disorders, osteoarthritis, psoriasis, and sarcoidosis. In the rheumatoid family of disorders the proximal phalangeal and metacarpophalangeal joints are first and principally affected, whereas in osteoarthritis and psoriasis it is the distal phalanges that are most often involved. A single broadened and flattened distal phalanx is sometimes seen in sarcoidosis. Shortened fourth and fifth metacarpals occur in pseudohypoparathyroidism and in pseudo-pseudohypoparathyroidism. Malposition and abduction of the fifth finger is a part of Turner's syndrome.

Polydactyly and syndactyly occur in association with a wide variety of congenital cardiovascular abnormalities, as does arachnodactyly and hyperextensibility of the digits. A few instances in which a pheochromocytoma was associated with neurofibromatosis and arachnodactyly have been described. High arching of the feet is seen in some congenital degenerative disorders of the neuromuscular system, such as Huntington's chorea, and at times the cardiac muscle shares in these changes, leading to congestive heart failure.

The palms of the hands are warm, moist, and velvety in many patients with hyperthyroidism. This is in contrast to the moist but cold palms of the patient with neurasthenia and tension, or the dry, thickened palms of the patient with hypothyroidism. Whereas palmar erythema is seen in 5 to 10 percent of normal persons, it is also observed in a wide variety of disorders, including hepatic cirrhosis, pregnancy, hyperestrogenism, mitral insufficiency, polycythemia, inflammatory rheumatism, tuberculosis (acroerythrosis), nutritional deficiency, and arsenic poisoning. Blue palmar creases are seen in generalized purpura, and pale silvery or white creases in significant anemia. Dark brown or black creases may be a feature of Addison's disease.

Dupuytren's contractures are noted in a variety of circumstances and their recognition may be very important. They are seen in normal persons, particularly those in the older age group and in those who have performed hard work with their hands. There is a familial incidence. It is not uncommonly reported to occur in association with diabetes mellitus, epilepsy, cirrhosis, Raynaud's syndrome, scalenus anticus or other "cervical outlet" syndromes, syringomyelia, and after a myocardial infarction. Significantly, it is rather frequently associated with premature vascular degeneration in younger persons, and can be the tip-off to the presence of coronary artery disease in the young individual. Thus, if a male aged 40 complains of "indigestion" after a heavy game of golf, and a Dupuytren's contracture is seen, premature coronary artery disease could well be present. In its earliest stage, a Dupuytren's contracture is noted as an indurated dimpling of soft tissues, usually at the base of the fourth and fifth fingers when the hands are hyperextended and the tendons are put on stretch. Dupuytren's contractures are also seen on the soles of the feet. They most often occur in the right extremity first. They may be associated with Peyronie's disease of the penis.

Acropachy is an interesting alteration sometimes seen in association with states of altered thyroid (or more accurately, thyro-pituitary) function. At times it occurs with "malignant" exophthalmos or with myxedema circumscripta, and may have a common etiologic background. Both the hands and feet may become involved. The fingers and toes become thickened and broadened as a result of subperiosteal new bone formation, with thickening and adherence of the surrounding soft tissues. Similar changes involving remarkable thickening and distortion of the face and scalp are seen in an unusual condition called pachydermoperiostosis (primary hypertrophic osteoarthropathy).

Clubbing of the fingers and toes is an early sign of a host of congenital and acquired conditions implicating the heart and lungs as well as other organs. The most common causes of clubbing are pulmonary emphysema, bronchogenic carcinoma and congenital heart disease with right to left shunting. The former conditions are frequently associated with long bone periostitis (hypertrophic osteoarthropathy) but are rarely seen with congenital heart disease. Clubbing also occurs in such diverse disorders as ulcerative colitis, regional enteritis, sprue, intestinal infections such as amebiasis and tuberculosis, cirrhosis of the liver, myxedema, polycythemia, and hyperparathyroidism. Periostitic changes involving the hands and feet are often an early indication of the presence of an intrathoracic new growth, such as bronchogenic carcinoma. In fact, they may be the only manifestation, even radiographs of the chest being clear. The symptoms and signs resulting therefrom can be easily mistaken for the changes of rheumatoid arthritis. Joint pains, either "rheumatoid" or nonspecific in character, so often herald the presence of some latent new growth that the clinician must keep this possibility foremost in his consideration when following the course of patients past 40 who present initially with such complaints.

In examining an affected joint, one should make a careful analysis to determine whether one is dealing with a true arthritis or actually a periostitis. This can be done by carefully manipulating the joint and applying pressure over the periosteum of the bones just proximal to the joint proper to see if there is point tenderness. Periostitis is not one of the usual forms of uncomplicated arthritis and hence its detection is important.

A number of significant vascular lesions may be seen on the extremities, including those of the Peutz-Jegher's syndrome and those of familial hemorrhagic telangiectasia (Osler's disease). A 25 year old male was recently admitted with epileptic convulsions. The diagnosis of a congenital cerebrovascular anomaly was suggested by the finding of a small vascular plexus on the palm of one hand, and a cerebral arteriogram showed a large arteriovenous tumor in the right temporal area. Petechial spots have a predilection for the hands and feet, as already emphasized. Osler's nodes and Janeway lesions are characteristic of bacterial endocarditis. Osler's nodes are pea-sized, tender nodules occurring in the palms or on the sides of the digits. The Janeway lesions are small, reddish-purple, erythematous or hemorrhagic patches, somewhat nodular and sometimes tender, found on the skin of the palms or digits. All of these lesions result from a focal arteritis, and all occur on the feet as well as on the hands.

Examination of the skin of the extremities can be very helpful in the early diagnosis of "collagen-vascular" disease. In scleroderma, for instance, one of the initial alterations is a change in the pigmentation of the skin, with areas of hyperpigmentation and vitiligo. The skin becomes thickened, waxy and adherent, the normal creases disappearing. In systemic lupus erythematosus and dermatomyositis, a useful physical sign is the appearance of an erythematous lacelike eruption over the joints and at the base of the fingernails. Pulsating nodules resulting from aneurysmal dilatations of small arteries are typical of polyarteritis nodosa as well as of giant cell arteritis, but do not often occur. Deposits of calcium, sometimes ulcerated and extruding calcium salts, are seen in advancing scleroderma. Raynaud's phenomenon may be a part of the natural course of all of the "auto-immune" disorders and may precede all other manifestations of these disorders by years. This is particularly true of scleroderma. When chronic and severe, atrophy of the fat pads of the digits may occur, their tips characteristically becoming tissue-paper thin, and tender, pinpoint, moonlike craters developing. Actual necrosis of the finger tips may follow. Severe and prolonged Raynaud's syndrome or arterial insufficiency of any cause may lead to sclerosis and atrophy of the fingers or toes, resulting in sclerodactyly or acrosclerosis. The end states can be confused with scleroderma, which is but one of several agencies for these alterations.

Observation of changes in the fingernails can reveal much that is valuable. Splinter hemorrhages have already been discussed. Nails that are bitten or deformed by picking indicate a nervous, reactive personality. Ridges or transverse white lines across the nails occur in nutritional disorders and in a very wide spectrum of systemic diseases too broad for such signs to be diagnostically helpful. Brittleness of the nails has similar implications, as does the presence of white spots or striations. The so-called Hippocratic or "watch glass" nails are indicative of chronic respiratory and circulatory disorders, especially pulmonary tuberculosis, and also cirrhosis of the liver. "Spoon nails," concave on the outer surface, are seen in several circumstances in addition to hypochromic anemias, including endocrinopathies, trauma, dermatoses, syphilis, and nutritional deficiencies. In Wilson's disease abnormal deposition of copper may occur in the nail moons, producing an azure coloration. This change has also been produced by the ingestion of phenolphthalein.

Lymph Nodes

The answer to an obscure problem may be found in the discovery of a single enlarged lymph node in the neck, reflecting disease originating within the thoracic or abdominal cavities. Hence, thorough search behind the ears, in the cervical triangles, and particularly above and below the clavicles and at the insertion of the sternocleidomastoid muscles, may pay dividends. In feeling for axillary nodes, elevate the patient's arms over his head to bring the superficial nodes to the surface. The deep variety are best felt by having the arms held close to the side, the examiner gently inserting his fingers as high as possible into the axilla and methodically combing downward. Enlargement of an epitrochlear lymph node is frequently of significance, but spotty enlargment of the inguinal or axillary nodes is often merely the result of some long-healed local infection. Although emphasis has been placed on the value of the consistency of lymph nodes in differential diagnosis, we have often been misled by overemphasizing whether or not glands are tender or not tender, matted together or distinct. Sometimes nodes involved by neoplasm or infection are tender and sometimes not; sometimes they are matted together and sometimes they are quite distinct. In my experience diagnostic value of the consistency of lymph nodes is limited.

In searching for the cause of localized lymph node enlargement, as in the neck for example, look for old scars that might represent a sinus tract healed from infection due to tuberculosis; a fungus; or some suppurative disorder. Always check carefully the areas draining to a particular group of enlarged lymph nodes for evidence of local inflammatory or malignant processes.

The Parotid Glands

It is sometimes difficult to discern parotid gland enlargement. It is best identified by the appearance of a small tongue-like projection of parotid tissue extending below and behind the ear, just above the temporomandibular joint. Failure to feel this projection should raise the suspicion that a mass in the region of the parotid may be due to some other cause, perhaps a lymph node. A history of episodic, recurrent swelling of the parotid glands, usually suggesting a benign rather than a malignant condition, nevertheless sometimes occurs in malignancy. Involvement of the contiguous facial nerve generally indicates a new growth, but has been observed in sarcoidosis. Enlargement of the parotid glands sometimes occurs in various types of diffuse liver disease and after the administration of drugs, such as the iodides. The area of Stensen's duct should be palpated to help rule out a calculus as the cause of parotid enlargement, and examination of some material extruded from the duct after palpation of the gland may help confirm the diagnosis of infection.

Head and Face

Abnormalities in the gross contour of the head and face, such as the tower skull of patients with sickle cell anemia, the round face in Cushing's disease, and the thickening of the features in myxedema and acromegaly are well recognized. Deepening of the frontalis fossae is an indication of marked wasting of muscle and soft tissue, as might be associated with a malignant new growth or a chronic infection such as tuberculosis. It is, moreover, a frequent indicant of the presence of hyperthyroidism.

In scleroderma, the normal facial markings may be obliterated, the nose and ears becoming sharp and pointed, and the vermilion borders of the lips markedly narrowed, resulting in a smirking expression. Owing to lack of wrinkles, the patient with scleroderma may actually look younger than his or her stated age. A smirking expression is also seen in patients with myasthenia gravis, and when associated with drooping eyelids or gaping mouth is almost diagnostic.

The scalp should be carefully palpated for nodules and percussed for areas of tenderness. Occasionally a tumor metastasis or a rheumatoid nodule may be located in the scalp. A persistently tender area over the cranium may suggest a brain abscess or a localized osteomyelitis. Reddened, thickened, or tender temporal arteries, or the presence of tender "phantom spots," mentioned previously, suggest cranial arteritis.

Examination of the head should always include careful auscultation of the skull. A soft bruit may lead to the discovery of a vascular anomaly or tumor. Similar bruits may be heard in the presence of very severe anemia and are normal findings in youngsters under 5 years of age. The importance of bruits over the carotid vessels in pointing to the possible cause of various neurological manifestations is well recognized.

The Eyes

It is very difficult to estimate clinically the degree of exophthalmos that may be present. This can be accomplished accurately only with the use of an exophthalmometer. However, one can estimate the degree of exophthalmos to a reasonable degree clinically by studying the relationships of the margins of the lids to certain landmarks. When the normal individual looks straight ahead, the lower lid usually just touches the lower border of the iris, or there may be a very small rim of sclera visible. The upper lid generally drifts approximately halfway between the upper border of the pupil and the rim of the sclera. In the presence of exophthalmos, one may find depression of the lower lid or elevation of the upper lid beyond these usual positions, or both lids may be retracted. Apparent exophthalmos is a racial characteristic of many Negroes, particularly Negro males. If exophthalmos is present, one should check for pulsation of the orbit, indicative of some vascular abnormalities, and one should also estimate, by gently pressing upon the orbit, the degree to which the exophthalmos is compressible. In severe degrees of "malignant" or progressive exophthalmos, there is oftentimes very firm and noncompressible exophthalmos. One should auscultate the orbits for a bruit, which might indicate hyperthyroidism, a vascular tumor, or an aneurysm. Increased pigmentation of the lids and periorbital tissues is another indicant of "malignant" hyperthyroidism. Likewise, periorbital edema, conjunctivitis, and chemosis of the lids are often important accompaniments. Other causes of edema about the eyes, with or without the presence of exophthalmos, are blockage of the superior vena cava, pseudotumor of the orbit, venous sinus thrombosis, severe emphysema, intraorbital tumors, amyloid deposits, sarcoidosis, cellulitis, and angioneurotic edema. I have also observed edema in a few patients given large dosages of prednisone.

Reiter's disease, some drug reactions, systemic lupus, spirochetal infections such as Weil's disease, brucellosis, Stevens-Johnson syndrome, temporal arteritis, trichinosis, and keratoconjunctivitis blennorrhagia are all characterized by their ability to produce brilliant conjunctivitis and edema.

Alterations in the uveal tract may reflect a very large number of systemic disorders, including tuberculosis, sarcoidosis, ulcerative colitis, regional enteritis, and the various so-called auto-immune diseases, to mention but a few. Sarcoid may also involve the conjunctiva, and this is readily available for biopsy.

Scleritis and episcleritis may also occur secondary to a large number of general disturbances, among them polyarteritis nodosa and other forms of arteritis.

When dealing with a patient with a fever of undetermined origin, examination of the eyes should receive special attention, since important clues as to the origin of the fever may be present there, as emphasized in Section C, Chapter 3, dealing with the patient with FUO.

In examining the fundi, it is imperative that a systematic pattern of examination be followed and that the pupils be dilated if necessary. One should first examine the nerve head and then study the branches of each fundic vessel all the way to the periphery in a clockwise fashion; otherwise, telltale information, not infrequently confined to a very small area of the fundus or fundic vessel, may be overlooked.

Recognition of papilledema is not difficult, but there is an unfortunate and dangerous impression in many minds that an appreciable degree of papilledema is a more or less universal accompaniment of increased intracranial pressure. Actually, many patients with very marked degrees of intracranial pressure may show little or no papilledema, or it may occur only very late. The importance of distinguishing papilledema from optic neuritis should be clear. Conditions other than increased intracranial pressure, such as severe emphysema and pseudotumor cerebri, may, of course, also be responsible for papilledema.

Attention should be paid to the degree of tortuosity of the fundic arteries and veins, for a characteristic feature of several systemic disorders, including sickle cell anemia and other congenital anemias as well as polycythemia and macroglobulinemia, is increased tortuosity ("corkscrew") of the fundic vessels. Excessive width and fullness of the fundic veins is observed in increased intracranial pressure, and also in plethoric states and conditions associated with sludged blood, such as Waldenstrom's macroglobulinema. The latter is also accompanied by "boxcars" in the vessels, and exudates and hemorrhages.

Whereas the degree of arteriosclerotic alteration in the fundic vessels oftentimes accurately reflects vascular degeneration occurring elsewhere, including the coronary, cerebral, and renal vessels, it should be pointed out that not at all infrequently there may be very impressive degenerative changes in the fundic vessels with little or no evidence of vascular degeneration in other organ systems. On the other hand, one may have a marked degree of coronary or other localized sclerosis in the presence of fundic vessels that look amazingly youthful.

Sometimes one sees tiny round flecks within the fundic arteries that look like brightly shining copper plaques or like the yellow lights on a Christmas tree. These represent cholesterol plaques or, less often, cholesterol emboli.

One should look very carefully for the presence of cytoid bodies in the fundus. These are small, round or irregularly shaped, white or dirty white patches which have been called by the British "cotton wool spots," since they sometimes resemble pledgets of cotton stuck on top of the retina. They are generally located centrally adjacent to the fundic arteries. In the older literature these were called hard exudates, but they are not really exudates but rather very small areas of anemic degeneration in the nerve fiber layer of the retina. The presence of cytoid bodies has genuine diagnostic significance. They are seen generally in the following situations: (1) a marked degree of increased intracranial pressure; (2) profound degrees of anemia; (3) blood stream infections, such as bacterial endocarditis; (4) states of marked vascular degeneration, such as that associated with diabetic retinopathy; and (5) various types of arteritis, in particular, polyarteritis and systemic lupus. Their significance lies in the fact that through simple clinical observations or the history, one can usually rather readily eliminate the presence of increased intracranial pressure, severe anemia, blood stream infection or diabetes, and, in the absence of these conditions, the likelihood of some type of vasculitis becomes a good one.

Although Roth spots are frequently regarded as being a pathognomonic manifestation of bacterial endocarditis, this is not so, since they may be seen in any of a variety of conditions that may result in focal vascular damage.

The Nasopharynx

It is well recognized that the specific cause of acute pharyngitis or tonsillitis is impossible to determine on clinical examination alone. The final distinction requires cultures and other special studies. When the course of such an inflammatory process is atypical, prolonged or unresponsive to usual nonspecific methods of treatment, one should consider less common etiologies such as syphilis, gonococcal infection, leukemia, lymphomata, tuberculosis, histoplasmosis, and Bacteroides infection. The latter organism may produce a retropharyngeal cellulitis or abscess and become associated with a gram-negative sepsis. In this day of altered mores, syphilitic and gonococcal infections have to be kept very much in mind, unfortunately.

It requires emphasis that chronic sinusitis is perhaps as often the result of chronic bronchopulmonary infection as it is the cause of it, although many mistakenly regard upper respiratory tract infections as always being the initial change.

A frequently observed clinical syndrome is very persistent and recurrent paroxysms of severe, hacking, nonproductive cough, worsened when the patient lies down and often interfering with sleep. The coughing is secondary to sinus infection with postnasal discharge, and often appears 7 to 10 days after "the flu" or "a head cold" went away. A nasal voice, or tenderness over the sinuses and a postnasal discharge may suggest the right answer.

Lips and Oral Cavity

Persistent herpetic lesions on the mouth and buccal mucosa often accompany chronic emotional and physical fatigue or an altered immune response associated with new growths, collagen vascular diseases, myeloma, and so forth. Herpes simplex characteristically occurs with pneumococcal lobar pneumonia and meningococcal infections, among others. The Coxsackie viruses and sometimes other enteroviruses may present with small, punctuate, hemorrhagic lesions on the buccal mucosa and oropharynx. Ulcerative lesions may occur in systemic fungus infections, including histoplasmosis, and should be carefully searched for when such systemic infections are suspected. Syphilis and tuberculosis may produce similar changes.

Leukemia may first be detected by the finding of boggy overgrowth of the gums, often with bleeding or secondary infection. Such changes were once thought to be characteristic of monocytic leukemia but are now recognized as being also associated with other forms of leukemia, as well as with Dilantin administration, Wegener's granulomatosis, macroglobulinemic states, and amyloidosis.

A dirty mouth due to poor oral hygiene, with infection of the teeth and gums and heavy dental scaling, may be the source of chronic bronchopulmonary infections, including lung abscess. It may also be the locus for the development of bacterial endocarditis.

Malocclusion of the teeth is a common cause of obscure and occasionally very severe pain in the temporomandibular joints radiating to the sides of the face. Another major cause of pain in the jaws and face occurring upon strenuous chewing is temporal arteritis. Such pain may be the earliest and only clinical manifestation of this sometimes destructive disorder. If malocclusion and temporomandibular arthritis of rheumatoid or other etiology can be excluded, this complaint is pathognomonic of temporal arteritis.

Examination of the tongue is now frequently ignored, although our predecessors often relied heavily upon it to make astute diagnoses. The size of the tongue should be noted since very large tongues (macroglossia) may be found in amyloidosis, acromegaly, myxedema, or Mongolian idiocy. The general appearance of the tongue gives a clue to the patient's state of hydration and even the chronicity of his illness. A very smooth, atrophic tongue is found in pernicious anemia and other vitamin deficiency states. Ulcerations of the tongue may occur in syphilis, tuberculosis, carcinoma, or giant cell arteritis. The tongue should be carefully observed for evidence of motor weakness and atrophy, and for fasciculations, which may occur in conditions such as amyotrophic lateral sclerosis.

The Neck

The conformation of the neck should be noted. Older individuals with short, stocky necks, and those with "dowager hump" are particularly subject to osteoarthritis and the so-called "outlet syndrome," characterized by aching, numbness, and tingling in the shoulders, arms, and hands. Observation of the posture of the patient as he sits in the chair is important, as even moderate degrees of malposture involving the neck and shoulders may lead to chronic fatigue, aching, soreness, and stiffness, as well as tingling, sometimes simulating the distress of coronary insufficiency, particularly in the anxious person. The possibility of a cervical rib should be excluded and the mobility of the neck and the presence of joint crepitus should also be checked. It is important to note whether sharp rotation of the neck induces dizziness or other indications of cerebral ischemia, which may result from impingement of vertebral spurs upon the vertebral arteries.

In palpating the thyroid gland, it is essential to employ both an anterior and a posterior approach, for some glands are more readily palpable from one direction than from the other. Each examiner should develop his own routine for palpating the thyroid; one which he uses regularly and with which he feels comfortable and assured. Generally one can secure a much more accurate idea of the size and consistency of the thyroid using the posterior approach, in which one palpates from behind the patient as he sips water. The sipping of water is essential. It is sometimes difficult to distinguish so-called "diffuse enlargement" of the thyroid gland from the nodular variety.

One should not overestimate one's ability to clinically evaluate the size, consistency, or tenderness of the thyroid gland. The distinction between a cyst into which there has been recent bleeding and a solid tumor is often impossible on clinical examination. Hashimoto's struma is now being recognized more frequently. It may occur in hyperthyroidism, hypothyroidism, or euthyroidism. Only histologic examination allows one to firmly establish its presence. In considering the likelihood of the presence of Hashimoto's thyroiditis one should check for lacrimal, parotid, and salivary gland enlargement, together with dryness of the eyes, nose, and mouth, for features of Sjögren's syndrome are at times associated with Hashimoto's struma.

When listening for a bruit over the thyroid gland, as may be heard in hyperthyroidism, one must be careful to exclude both a venous hum in the jugular veins and a systolic bruit in the carotid vessels. The venous hum is easily excluded by compression of the venous channels above the thyroid gland. Carotid bruits are usually propagated up the neck well beyond the thyroid. Diffuse tenderness of the thyroid gland may indicate an acute inflammatory process whereas local tenderness is associated with hemorrhage into nodules, a rapidly growing tumor, or a diffusely overactive gland.

It is important to recall that a variety of malignant tumors occasionally metastasize to the region of the thyroid gland, where they may be mistaken for thyroid or parathyroid tissue. There was a case of a young woman who presented with weakness, weight loss, and hypercalcemia. A mass was felt in the region of the thyroid gland. She was thought to have a parathyroid adenoma but at operation a metastatic hypernephroma was discovered. Lymphomata may also appear to originate within the thyroid gland.

The Trachea

While investigating deviations of the trachea, one should be sure to check for a tracheal tug. This should be done both when the patient is recumbent and when he is sitting erect, as some tugs are better felt in the one position than in the other. In addition to being associated with aneurysms, tracheal tugs may be produced by solid tumors that are contiguous to pulsating arteries.

The Chest

It is unfortunate that examiners so often take only a cursory glance at the conformation and movements of the thoracic cage before beginning to percuss and auscultate. The experienced clinician observes the chest in a methodical way.

First he acquires an appreciation of the general conformation of the chest. He realizes that without this, correct interpretation of the significance of the physical signs that will become apparent later is impossible. Second, he analyzes the mobility of the chest. Movements of the chest are to be viewed not only anteriorly but also posteriorly (if the patient can sit erect), for a lag in movement not visible anteriorly may be easily seen when viewed from behind. Detection of a lag in the inspiratory takeoff of one side of the chest, or decreased expansion of one side, may help to localize the disease process. Are movements full and free, or limited? Are they painful or are they abruptly halted by pain? Are they associated with coughing or wheezing? As the patient breathes, do the interspaces retract, indicating generalized or local bronchial obstruction? The observer should not only closely watch the chest movements but he should also spread his fingers along the lower costal margins and actually *feel* the movements of the chest, comparing one side with the other. In addition, he should place the flat of his hand over the various portions of the anterior and posterior chest in order to detect any localized vibrations, pulsations, or impulses that might indicate the presence of a bronchial obstruction, tumor mass, or vascular abnormality.

It is worthwhile to ask the patient if he has been aware of any localized noises in his chest when he lies down at night in a quiet room. Patients with bronchial obstruction, especially that resulting from new growths, may notice such focal wheezing. Similarly, patients may locate the site of origin of a hemoptysis by indicating where they feel a "warm, trickling sensation" in their chest.

If, because of the abrupt onset of chest pain or shortness of breath, a patient is suspected of having an acute condition such as pleurisy, pneumonia, or an infarct, always check carefully to exclude a fractured rib. Ribs may fracture with surprising ease, even in young, healthy individuals, after a paroxysm of coughing, sneezing or yawning, or after sudden exertion such as fly casting or swinging a golf club. This is even more true of older individuals and of those who have osteoporosis. Repeatedly I have seen fractured ribs overlooked and mistaken for some much more serious condition. Fractured ribs are easily overlooked in x-rays of the chest, which compounds the problem.

In addition to searching for rib point tenderness, one should also test for muscle tenderness in these same circumstances, because acute myositis due to Coxsackie or other virus infections may exactly mimic coronary occlusion, pneumonia, pleurisy, pericarditis, or pulmonary infarction. This is not at all an unusual occurrence. In particular, one should examine the cervical muscles, the shoulder girdle muscles, and the muscles inserting about the borders of the diaphragm, for these are the groups most commonly affected by the Coxsackie and other viruses. (See Section C, Chapter 3.)

Before lightly percussing the chest, it is helpful to slap the anterior and posterior chest with the tips of the fingers, using a gentle, smart tap. Often this maneuver will make immediately evident major abnormalities in the resonance of the chest, which will subsequently help to guide the examiner in performing more refined clinical observations.

Failure of one of the diaphragms to move as well as the other, or the elevation or depression of one or both diaphragms, may give critical information. Acquire the habit of always marking the levels of the diaphragms with a skin pencil. The only physical manifestation of a subdiaphragmatic abscess may be elevation or poor movement of the affected leaf of the diaphragm. The same may be true of other inflammatory or neoplastic processes affecting the upper or lower surfaces of the diaphragm. It is not so well recognized that inflammatory or other processes involving the upper lung fields as well may cause decreased mobility of the diaphragm on the affected side.

Any inflammatory process that causes irritation of either surface of the diaphragm, whether it be tumor, infection, or of other etiology, may produce reflex discomfort and tenderness to pressure of the upper border of the corresponding trapezius muscle. A subdiaphragmatic or splenic abscess, a spreading pancreatic carcinoma, or a liver abscess, among other conditions, may be suggested by the discovery of increased sensitivity to gentle squeezing of the upper border of the trapezius muscle on the affected side. In interpreting this physical sign, one should realize that it is also induced by myocardial ischemia, and hence may be a helpful indication of occult myocardial infarction. In such instances the tenderness is usually more marked, or only present, on the left side.

In auscultating, the observer should breathe quietly through his mouth and not through his nostrils. Also, he should learn to concentrate his attention upon *particular* phases of the respiratory cycle and not just listen in a general sort of way.

The elicitation of post-tussic rales is an essential component of one's examination of the chest, for there are some highly important conditions associated with no physical abnormalities in the chest other than the fine crackling rales that appear only after the patient sharply inspires following a brisk cough. In early tuberculosis, in viral pneumonias, and in a variety of interstitial pneumonias, there may be no dullness or change in quality of the breath sounds whatsoever, and unless post-tussic rales are elicited, the chest may be mistakenly regarded as normal.

One must remember that wheezes and rales require the passage of air through the small and large bronchial tubes. Patients with severe obstructive pulmonary disease may be regarded as improving because their wheezes and rales are waning, when actually they are nearing an acute stage of marked respiratory failure. The point is that they are moving such a small quantity of air through the bronchial tree that no rales or wheezes can be produced. It is critical to be aware of this situation, as it means that urgent measures are required or death may ensue.

Inspiration made noisy by wheezes, rattles, and crowing sounds must not be mistaken for asthma. Such inspiratory sounds indicate a large airway obstruction, such as that resulting from laryngospasm, hematoma in the neck, or a foreign body, and their presence demands immediate efforts to localize and correct the obstruction.

Sometimes patients who complain of shortness of breath and "asthma" are regarded as having a functional disorder because examination of the chest performed while the patient is sitting and breathing quietly reveals nothing remarkable. The patient's complaints seem exaggerated. However, if the patient is exercised, and forced to exhale very, very deeply, one can hear distinct wheezing, and the real nature of the patient's problem becomes evident.

One must appreciate the very fleeting nature of many pleural friction rubs. Repeated examinations of the chest are required if these significant sounds are to be discovered.

The physician should be fully aware of the limitations of physical examination of the chest. At times it is impossible to distinguish massive atelectasis from consolidation or from compression of the lung by fluid. The wise physician combines a meticulous physical examination with x-rays of the chest when indicated, and does not push his clinical self-confidence too far. In this regard, the frequency with which pneumothorax—even of massive proportions—is overlooked is worthy of mention. A patient may be in acute respiratory distress from a massive pneumothorax and yet show few or none of the characteristic physical abnormalities. A chest film is mandatory.

Gross assessment of the patient's breathing capacity is extremely helpful both in diagnosis and follow-up, yet it is frequently ignored. In patients with various types of neuromuscular disorders, such as myasthenia gravis, it is a necessity. The patient's cough will become feeble long before other signs of ventilatory embarrassment become evident. Inability to blow out a lighted match is an indication of advanced difficulty. Bulging of the intercostal muscles with coughing indicates weakening of these muscles. Provided the patient is not obese, one can gauge the strength of contraction of the intercostal muscles. Anxiety, tachycardia, and the patient's need to use accessory respiratory muscles are other indications of serious trouble with exchange. The breathing capacity of patients with emphysema can be assessed and followed by evaluating the ease with which the patient can rapidly expire a forced volume of air.

The Mediastinum

One of the most elusive differential diagnoses to make accurately by clinical means is determining the nature of a mass presenting in the mediastinum. There may be no clinical features whatsoever which can help to determine whether such a mass is a vascular tumor or a solid one. Tracheal tugs, compression of the bronchi, pulsations of the chest wall, the demonstration of intrinsic expansion of the mass, and bruits heard over the mass are all changes which may be common to both solid and vascular tumors. Perhaps the most helpful clinical distinction is observation of an appreciable difference between the volume of the arterial pulses and the level of the blood pressure in the two upper extremities. This phenomenon occurs often with aneurysms but very rarely with solid tumors.

The Sternum

Tenderness of the sternum to light palpation may be a useful sign, suggesting some myeloproliferative disorder or a metastatic tumor. However, patients with any chronic, debilitating disease may develop generalized hyperesthesia, and hence may demonstrate tenderness upon sternal compression; this should be kept in mind when evaluating this response.

Superior Vena Cava

Obstruction of the superior vena cava is most commonly caused by new growths, predominantly malignant in nature, by aneurysms of the aorta, or by chronic mediastinitis due to tuberculosis or other granulomatous infections, such as histoplasmosis. Less common causes are thrombosis associated with sepsis, leukemia, polycythemia vera, and an arteritis.

The characteristic signs are edema of the head, neck, and arms, a peculiar "ruddy cyanosis" of the face and neck, and the development of widespread collaterals which may extend down the lateral aspects of the trunk to the femoral veins. Papilledema, with exudates and hemorrhages, and distention of the fundic veins, may be present, and sometimes the patient appears dull and obtunded. Rarely, convulsive seizures are observed and the patient may complain of marked vertigo, especially when bending over. Hoarseness may result from laryngeal edema. There may be considerable dyspnea, particularly on exertion. Disturbances of vision and hearing, worsened by stooping, and conjunctivitis and periorbital edema may be the earliest signs and complaints.

The Heart and Circulation

As already noted, inexperienced clinicians, when confronted by a patient with suspected cardiovascular disease, often turn immediately to auscultation of the heart or to some technical examination such as an electrocardiogram, disregarding the fact that *prior general observation of the patient* is essential for correct interpretation of more technically acquired information. Important clues to cardiovascular problems are often found in areas of the body quite remote from the heart itself, as is obvious from the preceding discussions.

Accurate assessment of the gross functional capacity of the heart to determine whether or not there is congestive failure can be accomplished, for most practical purposes, by simple clinical methods. Rarely should one have to call a cardiologist to "see if the patient has heart failure." If the patient, lying comfortably flat on the examining table, has no venous congestion (as is indicated by flat neck veins), no edema over the sacrum or lower extremities, an apical impulse that is within the midclavicular line, a liver that is at the costal margin; and lung bases free of moist rales, his physician can firmly conclude that there is no congestive failure. Furthermore, if this patient has had no edema or appreciable dyspnea from exertion, orthopnea, or paroxysmal nocturnal dyspnea, all easily quantified in terms such as the number of steps climbed before shortness of breath is noted, the number of pillows the patient requires to sleep on, and so forth, the physician with only general experience can conclude with assurance that the functional capacity of his patient's heart as a pump is satisfactory. This conclusion can be firmly maintained despite the presence of murmurs or of some type of arrhythmia, determination of which may demand special experience and techniques. Generally, by such simple clinical means as those just noted, any physician should be able to estimate the gross functional capacity of a heart.

The clinical detection of venous engorgement in the neck is highly important in a number of circumstances, including congestive failure, constrictive pericarditis, pericardial effusion, and mediastinal tumors; hence, this observation should be made with great care. Occasionally the venous pressure may be markedly elevated even though the neck veins look flat; when the veins are palpated they are found to be distended. I have seen several cases of constrictive pericarditis overlooked because of failure to carefully check the venous pressure. I recall one patient who was studied for months for so-called "protein-losing enteropathy," and was found to have constrictive pericarditis when someone at last noted increased venous pressure! Hence, one should always palpate the veins in the neck, bilaterally.

In some individuals, the only indication of congestive heart failure is, for a considerable period of time, hepatic congestion, there being marked distention of the liver in the absence of peripheral edema or moisture in the lungs. Such evidence of so-called "right-sided heart failure" may be found in individuals with disorders which might ordinarily be expected to be associated only with "left-sided failure," such as systemic hypertension or myocarditis, and hence such a finding is of no differential diagnostic value.

Sometimes the only indication of such congestive hepatomegaly is a distressing sensation produced when the physician applies firm pressure in the epigastrium or along the right costal margin over the surface of the tense liver. Such a distended liver may lead to dyspeptic symptoms, often confused with primary gastrointestinal disorders, or to discomfort on bending or breathing, occasionally mistaken for pleurisy or some other cause. Distention of the liver may also produce severe anorexia and weight loss, which in the anxious and reactive elderly person may be mistaken for involutional depression, or suggest a latent new growth. A chronic, intractable cough that is worse at night, frequently misjudged to be "chronic bronchitis," is another commonly overlooked presentation of congestive failure in the elderly.

Perhaps the single most important observation in evaluating the functional capacity of the heart as a pump is the accurate estimation of its size. Therefore, the greatest care should be taken in locating the apical impulse, and in delineating the borders of the heart. If the apical impulse is not located in its usual position, one must determine if the displacement is due to some intrinsic disease of the heart or pericardium, or if it is the result of some intrathoracic abnormality, such as pneumothorax, massive atelectasis, or pleural effusion. While delineation of the heart borders is of value, it must be recognized that accurate percussion of the heart is often difficult, especially in patients with emphysema or effusion, and a chest film must be taken.

A number of factors may affect the accuracy of cardiac auscultation. These include whether the examining room is noisy or quiet; whether the chest wall is thin or there is a heavy layer of fat; the degree of emphysema; the presence of fever or some other cause of hypermetabolism with tachycardia; the existence of an arrhythmia, such as auricular fibrillation, which may cause diastolic murmurs to change their quality; of an appreciable anemia; or of congestive heart failure. One should ask oneself the question, "Under what particular circumstances am I listening to this heart?" before coming to firm conclusions about what is heard.

Experience has shown that many times an accurate evaluation of cardiac function can be made only after repeated examinations under a variety of circumstances. Furthermore, it is often impossible to correctly interpret heart sounds without an evaluation of the patient's total history and all of the other physical findings, as well as the data received from a number of special studies.

Pericardial Diseases

The presence of a pericardial effusion is easily and very often overlooked. The particular physical findings resulting from an effusion are determined largely by the major localization (anterior, posterior, or lateral) of the effusion within the pericardial sack. When an effusion is located principally anterior to the heart, the cardiac outline is wide and "water bottle" in type. The precordium is quiet, with muffled heart sounds and damping of the normal precordial movements. By contrast, with a posterior effusion the signs are those of compression of the left lower lobe of the lung, with dullness to flatness at the left base, and other alterations frequently thought to indicate a pleural effusion, pneumonia, or infarction; the precordium may be active and the heart sounds loud. Similarly, when the effusion is located in the left lateral position the precordium may be normally active and the heart sounds may be distinctly heard, the characteristic feature being extension of cardiac dullness lateral to the apical impulse. In many instances pericardial effusions distribute themselves more or less diffusely throughout the entire pericardial sac; nevertheless, an analysis of the physical alterations produced by a suspected effusion in terms of these three areas of major distribution is most helpful.

Pericardial rubs may be evanescent, changing from hour to hour. In listening for a rub, the patient should be placed in a variety of positions. One of the most helpful is to have him bent forward, in full expiration. Loud, widely dispersed pericardial rubs may be heard even in the presence of a large pericardial effusion. Clicking, metallic sounds may be heard when calcium is contained within the pericardial sac, as a result of chronic inflammation. The "crunching snow" noise mediastinal emphysema is readily differentiated once the observer has had the experience of hearing it. In brisk hyperthyroidism, a rubbing sound is sometimes heard in the second and third left interspaces: the "Mean's-Lehrman" sign.

The development of cardiac tamponade is not directly related to the size of a pericardial effusion but rather to the ability of the pericardial sac to accommodate itself to the expanding effusion. This, in turn, is related more often to the rapidity with which the fluid accumulates than to the size of the fluid collection. Signs of tamponade are restlessness, anxiety, dyspnea, tachycardia, cold, clamminess of the skin leading to shock, and progressive elevation of venous and depression of arterial blood pressures. While a pulsus paradoxus is characteristic of this condition, this particular physical sign is not too helpful in differential diagnosis, since it appears in a broad spectrum of other conditions often associated with venous in-flow blockage, such as myocarditis and mediastinal fibrosis.

Constrictive pericarditis is usually regarded as being associated with a small heart with a quiet precordium and heart sounds which are distant. Yet quite different physical findings may be present if the constriction of the pericardium is confined principally to the posterior surface of the heart at the point of entrance of the superior and inferior vena cava. In this setting there may be a marked degree of in-flow blockage due to the venous in-flow obstruction, but the precordium may continue to be active, the heart sounds distinct, and a moderate degree of cardiac enlargement may ensue. Constrictive pericarditis often presents in ways which are atypical, and it is wise to always review this condition as a possibility whenever a patient appears with manifestations which could be resulting from chronic venous in-flow blockage.

It may be thoroughly impossible on physical examination to distinguish primary myocardial disease from primary pericardial disease. There are special laboratory techniques that may be helpful, including radioisotope scanning and cardiac catheterization, but at times even these methods may fail to differentiate the two disorders.

Peripheral Arteries

One should make it a habit to feel the pulsations in the major arteries in all four extremities and in the carotids. It is equally important to record these findings in the patient's chart. If one feels for these pulsations only when there is "a definite clinical indication," the time will inevitably come when he will overlook these indications and fail to perform the one diagnostic examination that may be critical. Interpretation of the significance of an altered pulse will be much more accurate if the observer can go back and determine from the patient's record whether a particular pulse was or was not normal when previously checked. If an arterial pulse is absent, one should palpate upstream in an effort to localize the point of blockade. Contrary to popular opinion, in dissecting aortic aneurysm the peripheral pulses may be altered only intermittently; hence, repeated re-evaluation of the status of the arterial pulses is needed if this condition is suspected.

While coarctation of the aorta is usually associated with decreased or absent pulsation in the lower extremities, at times the collaterals are so extensive that the peripheral pulses are normal. Also, if the collateral circulation is sufficiently extensive, coarctation may exist in the absence of any hypertension whatsoever in the upper extremities. However, this is a very unusual occurrence. It may be hard to see the arterial pulsations or to hear the systolic bruits accompanying the increased blood flow through the intercostal arteries that are characteristic of coarctation. Having the patient roll his shoulders forward and fold his arms over his chest may facilitate observation of these important signs. A cross light is also helpful.

Peripheral Veins

As with peripheral arteries, one should always palpate carefully along the course of the veins of the lower extremities; steady, firm pressure should be applied in the femoral triangles. Discomfort so induced may be the only indication of a deep vein thrombosis. Tension should also be put on the calf muscles, as in Homan's maneuver, to see if there is tenderness.

If phlebitis is suspected, the legs should be measured repeatedly and the measurements recorded daily in the chart. The day-to-day changes in these figures may be much more significant than the original measurements.

Pulmonary Embolism

It is now recognized that pulmonary embolism occurs a great deal more frequently than hitherto had been considered, in circumstances previously unsuspected, and in clinical guises only now beginning to be recognized. Much more often than not, the classical features of embolism (pain in the chest, dyspnea, hemoptysis, varying degrees of shock) are not exhibited, and the clinical presentations are much more subtle, and even deluding.

Such presentations include the following: transient elevation of the temperature, pulse, or respiratory rates; fluctuation of blood pressure; episodes of anxiety and restlessness often regarded as "a case of nerves"; transient chest pain, cough, or dyspnea; a syncopal attack or an actual "idiopathic" seizure; a stroke (in elderly persons); an episode of acute cardiac arrhythmia; unexplained onset of heart failure or worsening of chronic failure previously under control; viral or bacterial "pneumonia"; and pleurisy with or without effusion. "Pneumonia" is confused with an embolic occurrence (and vice versa) so commonly that it is a wise clinical practice to always question the likelihood of the presence of the one before making a diagnosis of the other. Repeated pulmonary emboli may present as fever of unknown origin.

Clearly, there are no "typical" physical findings of pulmonary embolism. The clinician must always keep in mind the great commonness of this potentially fatal disorder and the myriad ways in which it may present itself. Unfortunately, a word to the wise is not always sufficient and many instances of embolism continue to be overlooked.

Abdominal Aneurysms

Abdominal aneurysms are said to be characterized by the presence of a pulsatile, expansile, abdominal mass over which a bruit is heard. In reality, however, often large abdominal aneurysms may be present with no mass being palpable, no bruit being heard, and no abnormal pulsations being felt. The peripheral pulses may be unaltered. By the same token, solid tumors or cysts lying contiguous to vigorously pulsating abdominal vessels may appear to contain an intrinsic pulsation, and bruits can be the result of arteriosclerotic plaques, misleading one into thinking that an expansile mass is vascular in origin when it is actually a solid tumor or cyst. Hence, a suspected "typical abdominal aneurysm" may be nonexistent at exploratory laparotomy. A case in point was an elderly nurse whose "aneurysm" at operation was discovered to be a remarkably ptotic liver overlying a sclerotic aorta. As already indicated in the discussion of mediastinal tumors, the most helpful physical change indicating a true aneurysm is a change in the peripheral pulses, and evidence of such a change should be carefully sought, although it is not by any means universally present.

I have noted on several occasions a significant degree of weight loss occurring in persons with abdominal aneurysms. This at times has been so progressive that it has led me to wonder whether there may be some form of hidden intra-abdominal malignancy.

Murmurs (Other Than Over the Heart)

Systolic and, less often, systolic–diastolic murmurs may be heard in a variety of locations other than over the heart. Such bruits over aneurysms of the aorta and its branches and over the skull have already been mentioned. In Paget's disease of bone, a bruit can occasionally be heard. Mycotic aneurysms may be associated with a systolic bruit, and arteriovenous aneurysms from any cause may produce a systolic or systolic–diastolic murmur.

Highly vascular solid tumors, such as chorionepithelioma or sarcoma of various sorts, or hypernephroma, may become evident through the observation of systolic murmurs in the liver, abdominal cavity, lungs, or bones. For this reason, it is always important to listen with the stethoscope over any painful or seemingly inflamed area to which the patient directs your attention. One young female, thought to have a ruptured intervertebral disk because of extremely severe pain in the lumbosacral spine, was examined, and a systolic bruit was heard in this area. She was subsequently proved to have a highly vascularized chorionepithelioma.

Arteriovenous fistulae in the lungs may produce bruits, but they are sometimes exceedingly difficult to hear, even though there are obvious changes in the x-rays.

In recent times there has been renewed interest in unilateral renal hypertension induced by vascular abnormalities. Sometimes these are associated with systolic bruits in the region of the affected kidney. To detect these, it is important to listen carefully in the kidney area not only anteriorly but also laterally, and, particularly, posteriorly as well. Occasionally, following an abdominal or pelvic operation, a patient may develop fever, tachycardia, signs of a blood stream infection, and ultimately, congestive heart failure, all the result of the accidental production by the surgeon of an arteriovenous aneurysm with secondary bacterial endocarditis. Auscultation over the operative site in some such instances has revealed a telltale bruit. An appreciable number of patients with carcinoma of the body and tail of the pancreas may have a systolic murmur heard best in the left upper abdominal quadrant. One mustn't forget, however, that a kinked, sclerotic splenic artery may also produce a systolic bruit in this area.

The Abdomen

The surface of the abdomen should be carefully inspected. For example, detecting the eruption of herpes zoster may provide a simple explanation for the pain of the patient suspected of having an acute gallbladder. Localized discoloration of the skin may be highly significant, to wit, the bluish discoloration around the umbilicus in ruptured ectopic pregnancy. The implications of a venous pattern are well known. In order to delineate the outline of any intra-abdominal mass or of peristaltic overactivity, it may be well worth the trouble to use a cross light over the patient's abdomen. Bulging in the flanks may be the only indication of intra-abdominal fluid or a cystic mass.

It is important to watch the movements of the abdomen as the patient is asked to breathe deeply and to cough. The patient with peritoneal irritation may be loath to do so, and spasm of the abdominal muscles over the affected area may be a clue to the nature of his illness.

In palpating the abdomen, the physician should take the time to get himself into a comfortable position, and of course the patient must also be comfortable so that maximal relaxation of the abdominal muscles can be assured. Palpation of the abdomen when the patient is submerged in a bathtub full of lukewarm water may achieve better relaxation, and masses not palpable otherwise may become evident. This is an old-fashioned technique, but still pays off on occasion. In an effort to relax the patient, the initial palpation should be very gentle. If probing palpation is begun too soon, the discomfort may cause the patient to protectively tense his abdomen, rendering further examination fruitless. Sometimes it is helpful to ask the patient to first palpate his own abdomen and to locate the areas that seem to cause his greatest distress. The patient may then gain enough confidence to let the physician proceed. Palpation should first be done in an area remote from the region of maximal distress; then, gradually, the most severely affected area can be approached. It is always wise to warn the patient beforehand if a particular maneuver is likely to be distressful. This is especially true when checking for rebound tenderness or point tenderness. Surprising the patient with pain will surely alienate him.

Much has been written about the "doughy-feeling" abdomen of the patient with tuberculous peritonitis. In my experience, the value of this finding is overestimated, or at least its frequency of occurrence is. More often, the patient with tuberculous peritonitis is moderately toxic and torpid, with varying degrees of fever which may be persistent or intermittent. On physical examination, the striking finding is varying degrees of abdominal distension; this characteristically waxes and wanes from period to period, the abdomen sometimes seeming to be partially obstructed, and at other times relatively flat and soft. These comings and goings of what appears to be partial obstruction are presumably due to the sticking together of inflamed loops of small gut.

Repeated physical examination is of unusual pertinence in dealing with suspected acute abdominal conditions. Questions totally unanswerable at 10 o'clock in the morning may be obvious at 3 P.M. When first examined, the patient may be too apprehensive to supply meaningful information and his over-reacting may make a shambles of the physical signs. Upon re-examination, his composure may be regained and the real clues begin to appear: physical changes, originally diffuse, become more specific and accurately interpretable. Also, the passage of time and a bowel movement may cause a "mass" to disappear.

In palpating the lower border of the liver, always remember that the liver's position has real significance only in relationship to the location of its upper border, which may be depressed downward from its normal position by emphysema or simple visceroptosis. Therefore, locate the upper border before trying to locate the true lower border.

There are other ways of estimating liver enlargement when the enlarged liver cannot be actually palpated. Such enlargement may be associated with an unpleasant sensation of fullness and tenderness felt when firm, steady pressure is applied over the epigastric notch with the flat of the hand. When the liver is enlarged because of congestion, tumor, or inflammation, the patient will frequently wince, and say, "Don't do that. It makes me nauseated." Inability to feel the normal aortic pulsation in the epigastrium in a thin person may be evidence that there is a mass in the epigastrium, perhaps an enlarged liver. It may be worthwhile, particularly with an obese patient, to place the left hand posteriorly along the costal margin while palpating with the right hand below the costal margin anteriorly. If the liver is significantly enlarged, one can sometimes compress or perform a ballottement on the mass between the two hands held in these positions. One should always begin to feel for the liver edge by starting palpation low in the abdomen, above the iliac crest, slowly moving upward toward the costal margin. In this way one can avoid missing a grossly enlarged, deep-lying liver that can be overlooked if one starts at the costal margin and palpates downward, for in so doing, one may always be on top of the organ and miss the edge.

In attempting to palpate the spleen, one must keep in mind that masses felt underneath the left costal margin are by no means always the spleen. A mass in or about the kidney or adrenal gland, a pancreatic cyst, a mesenteric cyst, a large hematoma, a tumor of the stomach, an ascending or transverse colon, and a number of other lesions may exactly mimic an enlarged spleen. As the spleen enlarges, one can usually feel just under the soft tissues a rounded, tongue-like projection extending below the left costal margin just medial to the flank. As the spleen grows, it tends to progress downward and medially, moving toward the umbilicus as its size increases. One can be fully confident that such a mass is truly the spleen only if one feels the splenic notch. Renal masses generally extend downward into the flank and gutter.

One clinical complex seen infrequently, but often enough to be important, is enlargement of the spleen in association with pancreatic carcinoma, produced by involvement of the splenic veins. Such splenomegaly may be associated with an effusion at the left base secondary to metastases to the left diaphragm, and recognized by a systolic bruit resulting from implication of the splenic arteries.

If rupture of the spleen occurs from any cause, there may develop an effusion at the left lung base, which is often hemorrhagic in nature. This may be associated with tenderness or soreness in the right shoulder.

Another clinical complex to be aware of in carcinoma of the pancreas is a peculiar anxious, depressive state which may dominate the whole presentation. For reasons he can't explain, the patient becomes "not himself." He feels restless, "down," anxious, overactive, in a turmoil. His behavior may become peculiar. These changes are often accompanied by weight loss and anorexia. In older persons, such manifestations are easily mistaken for those of serious functional disease. I recall walking into my office to find an elderly dowager sprawled in a chair with her feet on my desk. She apologized, saying, "I'm so anxious, I can't seem to control myself. I do odd things to try to overcome my depression. I upset the family at night by getting up in the early morning to stare at the moon in the garden. I'm an emotional mess, and I've lost twenty pounds." An exploratory laparotomy revealed pancreatic carcinoma.

It is surprising how many physicians carefully palpate the abdomen but rarely *listen* to it. Auscultation of the abdomen can be extremely helpful for many reasons, some of which have already been discussed. A friction rub over the liver may indicate an abscess or a tumor mass at its surface, or an area of infarction. A bruit may accompany a vascular tumor. Rubs and bruits may be heard over the spleen, and have similar connotations. Noting the quality and quantity of peristaltic activity is obviously most important.

A small collection of fluid within the abdomen is best delineated by having the patient in the knee-chest position so that the fluid will accumulate in the most dependent portion of the abdomen, about the navel. Percussion of the abdomen will then show dullness over this area with resonance above the fluid in the flanks. It is sometimes very difficult to distinguish massive ascites from a large cystic tumor. When the patient is lying on his back, ascites is generally indicated by dullness in the flanks with resonance about the umbilicus. When there is a large abdominal cyst present, the findings are generally reversed. Sometimes with large abdominal cysts one can feel a deceptive fluid wave which may suggest ascites. In the presence of massive ascites, there is often a secondary collection of fluid in the right thoracic cavity, rather than in the left, because lymph flow through the right diaphragm is more profuse.

Sometimes when one would expect distinctive evidences of peritoneal irritation to be present, there is disarmingly little indication of an acute intra-abdominal inflammatory process. However, one must not readily exclude the possibility of an intra-abdominal emergency simply because the classic signs are absent. An elderly individual may develop a ruptured appendix with few or none of the usual abdominal signs. Patients on adrenal steroids may rupture a peptic ulcer with widespread soiling of the peritoneal surfaces and yet maintain a soft abdomen. Infarction of a portion of the gut due to occlusion of a mesenteric vessel may occur with surprisingly few signs of an acute abdomen shortly after the onset of the occlusion. Patients with acute pancreatitis may have few clinical signs of a localized inflammatory process, the early changes being those of altered intestinal motility with ileus and partial obstruction. It is essential to always evaluate the abdominal findings in relation to any medication the patient may have recently received. The personality and sensitivity of the patient should also be taken into account, as already stressed. Some patients over-react to painful stimuli, and others react very little.

In contrast to the situations just described, there is a well-known group of diseases in which the physician may mistakenly conclude that the patient has an acute abdomen, because not only do the patient's symptoms indicate it but the accompanying physical alterations do as well, although the latter are more often than not equivocal. Included in this group are tabes dorsalis, porphyria, lead poisoning, abdominal migraine, acute diabetic acidosis, herpes zoster, acute glomerulonephritis, Schönlein-Henoch purpura, congenital compliment deficiency state with angioneurotic edema, black widow spider bite, and Coxsackie virus infections.

This list alone should be enough to establish the verity of the philosophical point we have stressed from the outset of this discussion of the physical examination: *To be meaningful, the findings in one organ system must be integrated with the findings derived from examination of all the other organ systems.* This is particularly true of examination of the abdomen, where the changes may be especially hard to pinpoint through purely clinical means: hence the infinite value of examining the abdomen only *after* all of the other organ systems have been meticulously checked. Clearly such an approach is essential in the differential diagnosis of the conditions just listed, as is the performance of certain definitive laboratory studies.

A special note is due about the diagnosis of acute abdominal pain caused by the Coxsackie virus, since this virus may occur epidemically in communities, especially in younger persons, exactly imitating such acute emergent conditions as appendicitis, gallbladder disease, and pancreatitis. The onset of abdominal pain is often sudden, and severe. Fever, low-grade or up to 102 degrees, may be present or entirely absent. There may be diffuse or focal abdominal tenderness, with or without spasm. Usually peritoneal signs are equivocal, and the patient's pain and distress is often out of proportion to the degree of objective findings. (While this may suggest the correct etiology of the patient's distress, it is not fully trustworthy, and should not be relied upon.) The best approach to the correct diagnosis is to discern other features of Coxsackie virus infection either in the patient or in some contact he has had. In the recent past, has the patient, or a contact, had a flu-like syndrome or a wry neck, an episode of acute muscular pain in the shoulders or around the insertion of the diaphragm, or acute pleural or pericardial pain? On physical examination, can one demonstrate focal tenderness of any of these muscle groups, particularly about the neck and upper border of the trapezia? The latter is the real payoff.

It is well to be aware of the limitations of physical diagnostic methods in dealing with some very important intra-abdominal disorders, discussed in the following paragraphs.

Few diagnoses are more difficult to establish clinically than is an intra-hepatic abscess. In fact, at any stage in the development of such an abscess, but particularly in the early stages, all of the expected physical changes may be absent, and the correct diagnosis must be discovered through some other technique—liver scan or exploratory laparotomy. The diagnosis of hepatic abscess is made doubly difficult because, contrary to older opinions, bacterial (as opposed to amebic) abscesses are more often than not primary, and not secondary to some telltale suppurative process elsewhere within the abdomen, such as a ruptured appendix. A fever of unknown origin is therefore a very frequent presentation. The fever may be high and spiking, or low-grade. There may or may not be leukocytosis. Although some degree of hepatomegaly is ultimately to be anticipated, the liver may be normal in size, particularly early in the infection. Liver tenderness—the usual hallmark of a liver abscess—though carefully and repeatedly searched for, may be consistently absent. If the abscess is close to the surface of the liver, one may hear a friction rub, but this does not occur often. If the inflammatory process in the liver involves the diaphragm, the latter may become elevated and fail to descend, and there may be pleural reaction with a small collection of fluid at the right lung base, associated with tenderness of the upper border of the right trapezius muscle. However, none of these changes can be expected if the abscess is deep within the liver.

Another diagnostic enigma is a subdiaphragmatic abscess. Again, there is sometimes no apparent reason why the patient should have acquired such a lesion in the first place. I recall a Negro female who was ultimately found to have a chronic abscess under her left diaphragm. Weeks before, she recalled having vague epigastric "hungry feelings." She proved to have leaked from an otherwise silent duodenal ulcer. For obvious reasons, the physical changes accompanying a subdiaphragmatic abscess are similar to those associated with a superficial hepatic abscess, already described. Again, the important clues are tenderness about the rim of the affected diaphragm, decreased mobility of the diaphragm, and tenderness of the associated trapezius muscles. Unfortunately, however, the appearance of such signs may be delayed, or equivocal, and one has to turn to other diagnostic methods, often surgical.

Carcinoma of the pancreas is perhaps the greatest diagnostic enigma and, for that matter, so are all retroperitoneal new growths, including sarcomas and lymphomas. One may suspect such a process by virtue of progressive anorexia, weight loss, anxiety and depression, altered bowel function, the appearance of malabsorption, hard-to-interpret abdominal pain, unexplained phlebitis, myopathy and neuropathy, and nonspecific skin changes, but its delineation by physical diagnostic means is impossible, unless the process has advanced to the stage where a mass is palpable.

In thus stressing the hardships of the clinical diagnosis of carcinoma of the pancreas I do not mean to overlook the classic presentation of carcinoma of the head of the pancreas in association with obstructive jaundice and an enlarged palpable gallbladder; of tumor of the tail of the pancreas with ascites and perhaps palpable intra-abdominal metastatic masses; or of the syndrome already described of splenomegaly and fluid at the left lung base. More often than not, however, early carcinoma of the pancreas presents more unobtrusively than by these classic signs.

Another condition which may be clinically totally occult is a perinephric abscess, the expected tenderness on both light and deep palpation and percussion about the affected kidney being absent, or of a degree difficult to accurately interpret. There is a clinical adage that if a patient who is toxic and febrile complains of pain in or about the kidney area or deep in the flanks, and one can obtain a history of an antecedent suppurative infection of the skin, such as a boil, then the patient can be anticipated to have a renal, perirenal, or retroperitoneal abscess, probably owing to the staphylococcus.

Likewise, an acutely inflamed or ruptured appendix located retrocecally may show none of the classic abdominal presentations, whatever degree of tenderness there may be being confined deep in the right flank, and suggesting renal, gallbladder, or right colonic disease.

Inflammatory disease in the pelvis, while generally readily accessible to clinical examination, can be overlooked, even by a highly competent—and confident!—examiner. I recall several instances in which I have been lulled into missing the real nature of a patient's illness by absolute assurances that "the pelvis is entirely clear." The only protection against such errors is repeated examination. In particular, suppurative or nonsuppurative pelvic phlebitis has been a diagnostic enigma.

I have seen several patients enter the hospital with chills, fever, and marked toxicity, but with no specific changes to account for these serious alterations. Ultimately (and sometimes not until a large number of expensive studies had been completed), the answer was found in a perirectal abscess. Many of these patients had leukemia or some other disorder affecting immune mechanisms. The correct diagnosis was overlooked originally either because the condition wasn't suspected and specifically searched for, or because the rectal examination was inadequately performed or was not later repeated as the process began to ripen locally.

So often these same reasons apply to other diagnostic errors. In general, a particular physical diagnostic maneuver won't pay off unless (a) the observer has a specific reason for performing it, (b) he performs it meticulously, and (c) he performs it repeatedly, if the anticipated information is not obtained the first time.

The Genitalia

The cause of a complicated systemic disorder may be overlooked as the result of a poorly accomplished, or postponed, genital examination. In polyarteritis nodosa, involvement of the testicles or epididymis or both is not uncommon, and biopsy is easily accomplished. A recent patient with a fever of unknown origin complained of tenderness in his right testicle and a biopsy revealed the diagnosis of miliary tuberculosis. Tuberculous peritonitis may originate in the female pelvic organs. In the young female, a lung abscess and especially multiple abscesses, should always raise the question of a pelvic infection with phlebitis and pulmonary emboli, frequently following a septic abortion. Hypercalcemia may be the result of bone metastases from a tumor primary in the genital tract. In young males, mediastinal masses easily mistaken for lymphoma may be the product of a malignant testicular tumor.

Skeleton

If a patient complains of pain in his back, it is not enough that his back be examined in the customary fashion while he is recumbent. He should be stripped completely and made to stand up while a number of observations are made, including study of his body conformation and his posture. It may be helpful to see him walk about. In addition, his spine should be flexed in various modalities, and his responses observed. Is he limited in any of these movements? Does any movement cause pain? Does any action result in spasm of associated muscles? The patient should be watched carefully as he gets on and off the examining table or a chair. The way he puts on his shoes and socks may tell a great deal more. The patient who complains bitterly of disabling pain in his back but subsequently hops off the table and puts on his shoes and socks and trousers without significant difficulty probably does not have any serious organic disease.

Occasionally an acute "arthritic" condition is confused with involvement of the periarticular tissues and not of the joint itself, and hence it is worthwhile to analyze the complaint of a "painful joint" with circumspection. For example, an acute cellulitis, a phlebitis, a synovitis, a bursitis, and even a peripheral neuritis can all be mistaken for an acute arthritis, as can a bone fracture and osteomyelitis. We have already discussed the need to differentiate a periostitis as observed in pulmonary osteoarthropathy.

Estimating the Severity of Illness

In addition to determining the specific cause of a patient's illness, the physician must also form a judgment about its degree of severity. *How* sick the patient is is an exceedingly important factor, often determining what must be done for the patient, and how rapidly. Sometimes it tells the physician that immediate therapeutic measures must temporarily take precedence over the quest for the specific cause of the patient's illness, as for example the realization that a patient is having sudden, severe respiratory distress due to airway obstruction.

In specific instances, accurate determination of the degree of severity of an illness depends upon several factors, including knowledge of the patient's history, the physician's clinical experience (and intuition!), and what laboratory, x-ray or other technical information may be at hand; in addition to these, evidence derived from the physical examination may be most helpful.

General Evidence

The patient's state of responsiveness is a most significant matter. Alteration of responsiveness may cover a broad spectrum, ranging from hyperirritability and anxiety to confusion, disorientation, dullness, and coma. The essential point is this: Regardless of the particular form it may assume, any appreciable deviation from the patient's usual mental state is a danger sign of serious organic or functional illness. Upon meeting a patient, the experienced clinician engages him in brief social conversation, not just to be pleasant, but also to determine his quality of response. Is he alert, bright, and sociable, or dull, confused, not quite himself?

The character and degree of the patient's spontaneous activities may be very informative. Is he extremely agitated and restless, or markedly lethargic and slowed down? He may be unable or unwilling to assume certain positions: to lie flat, for example, or to stand firmly erect. He may indicate a preference for certain positions, such as sitting up and leaning forward, or sitting with his legs drawn tightly to his abdomen. He may compulsively pace the floor, or he may insist upon lying motionless, untouched.

The patient's general appearance contains clues to his state of health. Is his coloration ashen, cyanotic, pallid, sallow, flushed, or jaundiced? Does he appear to have lost much weight recently? The severity of a patient's illness may be portrayed in his facial expression, as in the Hippocratic facies of peritonitis.

The great importance of even minor alterations in the vital signs has been stressed previously. Serious illness may be associated solely with elevation or depression of the pulse, changes in temperature and respiratory rates, and the blood pressure. These may be the only indications of the degree of severity of the illness. The most important thing is to be aware that a significant change in these factors has occurred. Next in importance is the degree of the change, and the character of the alteration. While it is significant when a patient with pneumonia has an increased respiratory rate, it is even more meaningful if he breathes stertorously, with distended nostrils and with the aid of the accessory muscles of respiration. A thready, intermittent pulse tells more than simple tachycardia.

A great deal may be learned from easily made, specific observations, such as detection of odor of the breath, indicating the presence of suppuration in the lungs, acidosis, uremia, fetor hepaticus, and so forth. One other such observation is of the turgor of the skin, affording readily available information about the patient's state of hydration.

Specific Evidence

In addition to these general signs of a severe illness, the following are specific indications of an urgent problem:

1. Excessively high fever
2. Shaking chills
3. Drenching night sweats
4. Impending or actual shock
5. Severe hypertension
6. Rapid tachycardia, or bradycardia with cerebral anoxia

7. Coma
8. Signs of increased intracranial pressure
9. Cyanosis
10. Airway obstruction
11. Pulmonary edema
12. Cardiac tamponade, or decreased pulse pressure
13. Signs of an acute abdomen
14. Nuchal rigidity

In addition to these and other clinical points indicating that a patient's problem requires immediate, specific management, it is wise to keep in mind that certain disorders are, by their very nature, always potentially hazardous to the patient's life. Hence they demand immediate and optimal handling, even though the patient when first seen may appear disarmingly well. Included among these are meningitis, subarachnoid hemorrhage, stroke, myocardial infarction, pneumonia, pulmonary embolism, hyperthyroidism, intestinal bleeding, sepsis, anuria, and an acute abdomen, to name but a few. Failure to appreciate the life-threatening potentialities of disorders such as these, and the postponement of specific therapy or the institution of less than adequate treatment, may mean that a mild episode of a potentially serious illness will be allowed to progress to a catastrophic one. One must get on top of such problems immediately.

THE PHYSICAL EXAMINATION

Determining the Blood Pressure

Bordley, J., and Eichna, L. W.: Normal blood pressure. Internat. Clin. *1* (series 48):175, 1938.
King, G. E.: Errors in clinical measurement of blood pressure in obesity. Clin. Sci. *32*:223, 1967.
Ragan, C., and Bordley, J.: The accuracy of clinical measurement of arterial blood pressure. Bull. Johns Hopkins Hosp. *69*:504, 1941.

The Integument

Anscombe, A. R., et al.: Acanthosis nigricans. G. P. *34*:93, 1966.
Aikawa, J. K.: Nature of myxedema. Ann. Intern. Med. *44*:30, 1956.
Barth, W. F., Glenner, G. G., Waldmann, T. A., and Zelis, R. F.: Primary amyloidosis. Ann. Intern. Med. *69*:787, 1968.
Bean, W. B.: Enteric bleeding in rare conditions with diagnostic lesions of the skin and mucous membranes. Proc. World Cong. Gastroenterology *2*:807, 1958.
Bean, W. B.: Vascular Spiders and Related Lesions of the Skin. Springfield, Ill., Charles C Thomas, 1958, p. 54.
Beerman, H., and Mitchell, G. H.: Nodular vasculitis. Amer. J. Med. Sci. *228*:469, 1954.
Beerman, H.: Some aspects of dermatology in neurology. Amer. J. Med. Sci. *230*:441, 1955.
Blommer, A. J., et al.: Myxedema. Arch. Intern. Med. *104*:234, 1959.
Blum, A., and Sohar, E.: The diagnosis of amyloidosis. Ancillary procedures. Lancet *1*:721, 1962
Bluefarb, S. M.: Nonspecific manifestations of the leukemia-lymphoma group and internal cancer. Post Grad. Med. *16*:6, 1954.
Bodinan, S. F., and Condemi, J. J.: Mediastinal widening in iatrogenic Cushing's syndrome. Ann. Intern. Med. *67*:399, 1967.
Braverman, I. M.: Skin Signs of Systemic Disease. Philadelphia, W. B. Saunders Company, 1970.
Burgoon, C. F., Jr.: Mast cell disease. Arch. Derm. *98*:590, 1968.
Caplan, R., and Curtis, A.: Xanthoma of the skin. JAMA *176*:859, 1961.

Capra, J. D., Winchester, R. J., and Kunkel, H. G.: Hypergammaglobulinemic purpura: studies on the unusual antiglobulins characteristic of the sera of these patients. Medicine 50:125, 1971.
Christian, C. L., et al.: Eighteenth rheumatism review. Review of American and English literature for the years 1965 and 1966. Arthritis Rheum. 11:Suppl. 11:523, 1968.
Church, R.: Disorders of hair and scalp. Brit. Med. J. 1:95, 1967.
Cohen, A. S.: Medical progress. Amyloidosis. New Eng. J. Med. 277:522, 574, 628; 1967.
Cormia, F. E., and Domonkos, A.: Cutaneous reactions to internal malignancy. Med. Clin. N. Amer. 49:655, 1965.
Cornelius, C. E., et al.: Calcinosis cutis. Arch. Derm. 98:219, 1968.
Crowe, F. W., et al.: Clinical, Pathological and Genetic Study of Multiple Neurofibromatosis. Springfield, Ill., Charles C Thomas, 1956.
Cummings, M. M., and Hammarsten, J. F.: Sarcoidosis. Ann. Rev. Med. 13:19, 1962.
Eckert, J., et al.: Hair loss in women. Brit J. Derm. 79:543, 1967.
Engleman, E. P., and Shearn, M. A.: Recent advances in rheumatic diseases. Ann. Intern. Med. 66:199, 1967.
Fitzpatrick, T. B., Sieji, M., and McGugan, A. D.: Melanin pigmentation. New Eng. J. Med. 265:328, 374, 430; 1961.
Gheksman, J. M., et al.: Gonoccocal skin lesions. Arch. Derm. 96:74, 1967.
Gimlette, T. M. D.: Pretibial myxedema. Brit. Med. J. 2:348, 1960.
Goldzieher, M. A.: Endocrinologic aspects of dermatology. New York J. Med. 67:2328, 1967.
Gordon, H.: Erythema nodosum. Review of 115 cases. Brit. J. Derm. 73:394, 1961.
Greenberg, E., Divertie, M. B., and Woolner, L. B.: Review of unusual systemic manifestations associated with carcinoma. Amer. J. Med. 36:106, 1964.
Greenberg, L. M., et al.: Scleredema adultorum. Review of world literature. Pediatrics 32:1044, 1963.
Hahn, B. H., Yardley, J. H., and Stevens, M. B.: "Rheumatoid" nodules in systemic lupus erythematosus. Ann. Intern. Med. 72:49, 1970.
Hamilton, C. R., Jr., Shelly, W. M., and Tumulty, P. A.: Giant cell arteritis. Medicine 50:1, 1971.
Hodgson, C. H. et al.: Hereditary hemorrhagic telangiectasia and pulmonary arteriovenous fistula. New Eng. J. Med. 261:625, 1959.
Kinsella, R. A., Jr.: Thyroid acropathy. Med. Clin. N. Amer. 52:393, 1968.
Kyle, R. A.: Benign hypergammaglobulinemic purpura of Waldenstrom. Medicine 50:113, 1971.
Laymon, C. W.: Cutaneous manifestations of some internal disease. Lancet 83:394, 1965.
Lerner, A. B.: Melanin pigmentation. Amer. J. Med. 19:902, 1955.
Lichtenstein, B. W.: Neurofibromatosis (von Recklinghausen's disease). Arch. Neurol. Psychiat. 62:822, 1949.
Longcope, W. T., and Freiman, D. G.: Study of sarcoidosis based on combined investigation of 160 cases including 30 autopsies from Johns Hopkins Hospital and Massachusetts General Hospital. Medicine 31:1, 1952.
Longcope, W. T., and Pearson, J. W.: Boeck's sarcoid (sarcoidosis). Bull. Johns Hopkins Hosp. 60:223, 1937.
Lorency, A. L., et al.: Cutaneous manifestations of incipient systemic disease. Med. Clin. N. Amer. 44:249, 1960.
Lucena, G. E., et al.: "Dewlap"—Corticosteroid induced episternal fatty tumor. New Eng. J. Med. 275:84, 1966.
Mayock. R. L., Bertrand, P., Morrison, C. E., and Scott, J. H.: Manifestations of sarcoidosis. Analysis of 145 patients with a review of nine series selected from the literature. Amer. J. Med. 35:67, 1963.
McAllister, A. M., Hicken, W. F., Latimer, R. G., and Condon, V. R.: Seventeen patients with Peutz-Jeghers syndrome in four generations. Amer. J. Surg. 114:839, 1967.
McCarty, J. T.: Cutaneous vasculitis. Med. Clin. N. Amer. 49:761, 1965.
McFarlin, D. E., et al.: Ataxia telangiectasia. Medicine 51:281, 1972.
McKusick, V. A.: Heritable Disorders of Connective Tissue. 4th ed. St. Louis, C. V. Mosby Co., 1972.
Muller, S. A., and Winkelmann, R. K.: Alopecia areata. Arch. Derm. 88:290, 1963.
Murray, I.: Lipodystrophy. Brit. Med. J. 2:1236, 1952.
Osler, W.: On a family form of recurring epistaxis, associated with multiple telangiectases of the skin and mucous membrane. Bull. Johns Hopkins Hosp. 12:333, 1901.

Plotz, C. M., Knowlton, A. I., and Ragan, C.: The natural history of Cushing's syndrome. A review. Amer. J. Med. *13*:597, 1952.
Preston, F. W., et al.: Cutaneous neurofibromatosis. Arch. Surg. *64*:813, 1951.
Puklin, J. E., et al.: Culture of an Osler's node. Arch. Intern. Med. *127*:296, 1971.
Reingold, I. M.: Cutaneous metastases from internal carcinoma. Cancer *19*:162, 1966.
Rowell, N. R.: Dermatological manifestations of the immunity deficiency syndromes. Brit. J. Derm. *80*:618, 1968.
Sharp, J. T., et al.: Observations on the clinical, chemical and serological manifestations of rheumatoid arthritis: 154 cases. Medicine *43*:41, 1964.
Sherwood, W. C.: Palmer varices and gastrointestinal bleeding. Arch. Intern. Med. *128*:598, 1971.
Shuman, C. P.: Relapsing pannicultis (Weber Christian Disease). Literature review. Arch. Intern. Med. *87*:669, 1951.
Shuster, S.: Systemic effect of skin diseases. Lancet *1*:907, 1967.
Smith, F. H., and Murphy, R.: Cutaneous melanosis associated with gastrointestinal disease. Med. Clin. N. Amer. *50*:349, 1966.
Steiger, W. A., et al.: Adiposis dolorosa (Dercums disease). New Eng. J. Med. *247*:393, 1952.
Stoker, J. H., et al.: Weber Christian syndrome. Amer. J. Med. Sci. *225*:446, 1953.
Szabo, G.: Melanin pigmentation. Dis. Nerv. Syst. *29*:58, 1968.
Telner, P., and Adam, J. E.: Cutaneous lesions and internal malignancy. Canad. Med. Ass. J. *93*:358, 1965.
Thomas, E. W. P.: Disorders of pigmentation. Practitioner *184*:582, 1960.
Trell, E. et al.: Osler's disease—familial pulmonary hypertension and multiple abnormalities of larger arteries. Amer. J. Med. *53*:50, 1972.
Tuffanelli, D. L., and Winklemann, R. K.: Systemic scleroderma. A clinical study of 727 cases. Arch. Derm. *84*:359, 1961.
Vallee, B. L.: Scleredema, a systemic disease. New Eng. J. Med. *235*:207, 1946.
Walker, A.: Chronic scurvy. Brit. J. Derm. *80*:625, 1968.
Walzer, R. A.: Autoimmunity and cutaneous disease. Med. Clin. N. Amer. *49*:769, 1965.
Warin, R. D.: Fungal infections of the skin. Brit. Med. J. *2*:1307, 1966.
Williams, R. C.: Dermatomyositis and malignancy, A review of the literature. Ann. Intern. Med. *50*:1174, 1959.
Winkelman, R. K., et al.: Acanthosis nigricans and endocrine disease. JAMA *174*:1145, 1966.
Watanakuna Korn, C., et al.: Myxedema. Arch. Intern. Med. *116*:183, 1964.
Yerner, A. B.: On the etiology of vitiligo and gray hair. Amer. J. Med. *51*:141, 1971.

Musculoskeletal

Banker, B. Q., and Victor, M.: Dermatomyositis of childhood. Medicine *45*:261, 1966.
Berry, T. J.: The Hand as a Mirror of Systemic Disease. Philadelphia, F. A. Davis, 1963.
Brom, B., et al.: Periostitis, aseptic necrosis and arthritis in Crohn's disease. Gastroenterology *60*:1106, 1971.
Dubois, E. L. (Ed.): Lupus Erythematosus. A review of the current status of discoid and systemic lupus erythematosus and their variants. New York, McGraw-Hill Book Co., 1966.
Farman, J., et al.: Crohn's disease and periosteal new bone formation. Gastroenterology *61*:513, 1971.
Fisher, D. S., et al.: Clubbing, a review with emphasis on hereditary acropathy. Medicine *43*:459, 1964.
Hammarsten, J. F., and O'Leary, J.: The features and significance of hypertrophic osteoarthropathy. Arch. Intern. Med. *99*:431, 1957.
Holling, H. E., and Brody, R. S.: Pulmonary hypertrophic osteoarthropathy. JAMA *178*:977, 1961.
Hueston, J. T.: Dupuytrens contracture. Baltimore, Williams & Wilkins, 1963.
Mackenzie, A. H., and Schenbel, A. L.: Connective tissue syndromes associated with carcinoma. Geriatrics *18*:745, 1963.
Newman, M. K., and Gugmo, R. J.: Neuropathies, myopathies, and occult malignancies. JAMA *190*:575, 1964.
Pattison, J. D., Jr., et al.: Hypertrophic osteoarthropathy in carcinoma of the lung. JAMA *146*:783, 1951.
Pojer, J., et al.: Dupuytrens disease associated with abnormal liver function in alcoholism and epilepsy. Arch. Intern. Med. *129*:561, 1972.
Pyke, D. A.: Finger clubbing; validity as a physical sign. Lancet *2*:352, 1954.
Ramsey, I. D.: Muscle dysfunction in hyperthyroidism. Lancet *2*:931, 1966.

Rimoin, D. L.: Pachydermoperiostosis. New Eng. J. Med. 272:923, 1965.
Ropes, M. W.: Observations on natural course of disseminated lupus erythematosus. Medicine 43:387, 1964.
Silverstein, A., and Siltzback, L. E.: Muscle involvement in sarcoidosis. Arch. Neurol. 21:235, 1969.
Williams, R. C., Jr.: Dermatomyositis and malignancy: A review of the literature. Ann. Intern. Med. 50:1174, 1959.
Wilson, J., and Walton, J. Some muscular manifestations of hypothyroidism. J. Neurol. Neurosurg. Psychiat. 22:320, 1959.

Peripherovascular

DeTakats, G., and Fowler, E. F.: Raynaud's phenomenon. JAMA 179:1, 1962.
Gifford, R. W., Jr.: Arteriospastic disorders of the extremities. Circulation 27:970, 1963.
Farmer, R. G., et al.: Raynaud's disease with sclerodactylia. Follow-up of 71 patients. Circulation 23:13, 1961.

The Eye

Pearlman, M. D.: A Catalogue of Eye Signs in Systemic Disorders. Springfield, Ill., Charles C Thomas, 1965.

Coxsackie Infections

Ager, E. A. et al.: An epidemic due to Coxsackie virus Group B, type 2. JAMA 187:251, 1964.
Artenstein, M. S., and Cadigan, F. I., Jr.: Epidemic Coxsackie virus infection with mixed clinical manifestations. Ann. Intern. Med. 60:196, 1964.
Butsch, S. J., and Harberson, J. C.: Acute virus infection with nerve root involvement simulating appendicitis. JAMA 123:405, 1945.
Cramblett, H. G., et al.: Coxsackie virus infections. J. Pediat. 64:40, 1964.
Harvey, A. M., and Tumulty, P. A.: Epidemic myalgia. Southern Med. J. 41:732, 1948.
Locke, E. A., and Farnsworth, D. L. The clinical characteristics of epidemic pleurodynia. Tr. A. Am. Physicians 51:399, 1936.
Massell, B. F., and Solomon, P.: Epidemic benign myalgia of the neck. New Eng. J. Med. 213:399, 1935.
Smith, W. G.: Adult heart disease due to Coxsackie virus Group B. Brit. Heart J. 28:204, 1966.
Sylvest, E.: Epidemic Myalgia, Bornholm Disease. London, Oxford University Press, 1934.

Pneumothorax

Davies, P. D. B.: Spontaneous pneumothorax. Practitioner 203:767, 1968.
Mills, M., and Baisch, B. F.: Spontaneous pneumothorax—400 cases. Ann. Thoracic Surg. 1:286, 1965.

Mediastinal Mass

(See references for "A Patient with a Mediastinal Mass.")

Superior Vena Cava Syndrome

Failor, H. J., et al.: Etiologic factors in obstructions of superior vena cava—a pathologic study. Proc. Staff Mayo Clin. 33:671, 1958.
Lowenbery, E. L., et al.: The superior vena cava syndrome. Dis. Chest 47:323, 1965.
McIntire, F. T., and Sykes, E. M., Jr.: Obstruction of the superior vena cava. Review of the literature. Ann. Intern. Med. 30:925, 1949.
Schechter, M. M.: The superior vena cava syndrome. Ann. J. Med. Sci. 227:46, 1954.

Pericardial Disease

Golinko, R. J., et al.: Mechanisms of pulsu paradoxus during acute pericardial tamponade. J. Clin. Invest. 42:249, 1963.
Holmes, J. C., and Fowler, N. O.: Diagnosis of pericarditis. Post Grad. Med. 44:92, 1968.
Iturrino, J. L., and Holland, R. H.: Emergency surgical management of acute pericarditis. J. Thoracic Cardiovasc. Surg. 45:324, 1963.
Madras, J. S., Jr.: Constrictive pericarditis: Diagnosis and operative management. Dis. Chest 52:746, 1967.

Morgan, B. C., et al.: Effect of blood volume on venous pressure in cardiac tamponade. J. Thoracic Cardiovasc. Surg. 51:577, 1966.
Robertson, R., and Arnold, C. R.: Constrictive pericarditis with particular reference to etiology. Circulation 26:525, 1967.
Schnabel, T. G., Jr.: Constrictive (restrictive) pericarditis. Med. Clin. N. Amer. 50:1231, 1966.
Symposium on pericarditis. Amer. J. Cardiol. 71:1961.
Wolff, L., and Wolff, R.: Diseases of the pericardium. Ann. Rev. Med. 16:21, 1965.

Myocarditis

Abelman, W. H.: Myocarditis. New Eng. J. Med. 275:832, 944; 1966.
DeGroot, L. J.: Thyroid and the heart. Mayo Clin. Proc. 47:864, 1972.
Hamby, R. I.: Primary myocardial disease, a study of 100 patients. Medicine 49:56, 1970.
Harvey, W. P., and Segal, J. P.: Primary myocardial disease. Post Grad. Med. 42:144, 1967.
Levin, S. H., and Harvey, W. P.: Clinical Auscultations of the Heart. Philadelphia, W. B. Saunders Company, 1959.

Dissecting Aortic Aneurysm

Baer, S., and Goldbrogh, H. L.: Varied clinical syndromes produced by dissecting aneurysms. Amer. Heart J. 35:198, 1948.
Cohen, S., and Littman, D.: Painless dissecting aneurysm of the aorta. New Eng. J. Med. 271:143, 1964.
Dillon, M. L., et al.: Aneurysms of the descending thoracic aorta. Ann. Thoracic Surg. 3:430, 1967.
Fomon, J. J.: Aneurysms of the aorta: Review of 249 instances. Ann. Surg. 165:557, 1967.
Hirst, A. E., Jr., et al.: Dissecting aneurysm of the aorta: A review of 505 cases. Medicine 37:217, 1958.
Julius, S., and Stewart, B. H.: Diagnostic significance of abdominal murmurs. New Eng. J. Med. 276:1175, 1967.
Lindsay, J., Jr., and Hurst, J. W.: Clinical features and prognosis in dissecting aneurysm of the aorta. Circulation 35:880, 1967.
Moersch, F. P., and Sayre, G. P.: Neurologic manifestations of dissecting aorta aneurysm. JAMA 144:1141, 1950.

Coarctation of Aorta

Hamilton, W. F., and Abbott, M. E.: Coarctation of the aorta of the adult type. Amer. Heart J. 381:574, 1928.
Reifenstein, G. H., Levine, S., and Gross, R.: Coarctation of the aorta. Amer. Heart J. 33:146, 1947.

Pulmonary Embolism

Gorham, L. W.: A study of pulmonary embolism. 100 cases. Arch. Intern. Med. 108:81. 1961.
Miller, G. A. H., and Sutton, G. C.: Acute massive pulmonary embolism. Clinical and hemodynamic findings in 23 patients studied by cardiac catheterization and pulmonary arteriography. Brit. Heart J. 32:518, 1970.
Petersdorf, R. G., and Beeson, P. B.: Fever of unexplained origin; report of 100 cases. Medicine 40:1, 1961.
Sokoff, L. A., and Rodman, T.: Acute pulmonary embolism. Amer. Heart J. 74:710, 829, 1967.

Tuberculous Peritonitis

Burock, W. R., and Hollister, R. M.: Tuberculous peritonitis. A study of 47 proved cases encountered by a general medical unit in 25 years. Amer. J. Med. 28:510, 1960.
Gonnella, J. S., et al.: Clinical patterns of tuberculous peritonitis. Arch. Intern. Med. 117:164, 1966.
Sinsh, M. M., et al.: Tuberculous peritonitis. New Eng. J. Med. 281:1091, 1969.
Sochocky, S.: Tuberculous peritonitis—a review of 100 cases. Amer. Rev. Resp. Dis. 95:398, 1967.

Carcinoma of Pancreas

Arlen, M., and Brockonier, A., Jr.: Clinical manifestations of carcinoma of the tail of the pancreas. Cancer 20:1920, 1967.

Cliffton, E. E.: Carcinoma of the pancreas. Amer. J. Med. 21:760, 1956.
Fras, I., Litin, E. M., and Bartholomew, L. G.: Mental symptoms as an aid in the early diagnosis of carcinoma of the pancreas. Gastroenterology 55:191, 1968.
Gullick, H. D.: Carcinoma of the pancreas. Review and critical study of 100 cases. Medicine 38:47, 1959.
Ingelfinger, F. J.: The diagnosis of cancer of the pancreas. New Eng. J. Med. 235:653, 1946.
Julius, S., and Stewart, B. H.: Diagnostic significance of abdominal murmurs. New Eng. J. Med. 276:1175, 1967.
Serebro, A. A.: A diagnostic sign of carcinoma of the body of the pancreas. Lancet 1:85, 1965.

Liver Abscess

Berke, J., and Pecora, C.: Diagnostic problems of pyogenic hepatic abscess. Amer. J. Surg. 111:678, 1966.
Cain, J. D., et al.: A ten year review of amebic abscess of the liver, 1956–1966. Amer. J. Digest. Dis. 13:709, 1968.
Clain, D., Wartnaby, K., and Sherlock, S.: Abdominal arterial murmurs in liver disease. Lancet 2:516, 1966.
Cronin, K.: Pyogenic abscess of the liver. Gut 2:53, 1961.
Ochsner, A., DeBakey, M., and Murray, S.: Pyogenic abscess of the liver. II. An analysis of 47 cases with review of the literature. Amer. J. Surg. 40:292, 1938.
Sherman, J. D., and Robbins, S. L.: Changing trends in casuistics of hepatic abscess. Amer. J. Med. 28:943, 1960.

Subphrenic Abscess

Davis, E. E., Jr., et al.: Subphrenic space infection—reassessment. Ann. Surg. 168:1004, 1968.
Editorial. Subphrenic abscess—a changing pattern. Lancet 2:301, 1970.
Ochsner, A., and DeBakey, M.: Subphrenic abscess: Collective review and analysis of 3608 collected and personal cases. Internatl. Abstr. Surg. 66:426, 1938.
Sherman, N. J., et al.: Subphrenic abscess: a continuing hazard. 100 patients. Amer. J. Surg. 117:117, 1969.

Appendicitis

Burgos, W. F., and Johnston, D. G.: Appendicitis: A computer study. Post Grad. Med. 44:110, 1968.
Cope, Z.: The Early Diagnosis of the Acute Abdomen. 12th ed. London, Oxford University Press, 1963.
Smith, P. H.: The diagnosis of appendicitis. Post Grad. Med. 41:1, 1965.
Thorbjarnarsm, B., and Loehr, W. J.: Acute appendicitis in patients over 60. Review of 195 patients. Surg. Gynec. Obstet. 125:1277, 1967.

The Testicles

Dahl, E. V., et al.: Testicular lesions of polyarteritis with special reference to diagnosis. Amer. J. Med. 28:222, 1960.
Martin, L. S. J., et al.: Testicular seminoma. Review of 179 patients. Arch. Surg. 90:306, 1965.

Miscellaneous

Burchell, H. B. Unusual causes of heart failure. Circulation 21:436, 1960.
Burchell, H. B.: Possible unrecognized forms of heart disease. Circulation 28:1153, 1963. Diagnostic problems in cardiology discussed as (1) rarities, (2) simulators, (3) complicators, and (4) emotionally obscured.
Capps, J. A.: An Experimental and Clinical Study of Pain in the Pleura, Pericardium and Peritoneum. New York, The Macmillan Company, 1932.
Conn, H. O., et al.: Pulmonary emphysema simulating brain tumor. Amer. J. Med. 22:524, 1957.
Cope, V. Z.: The early diagnosis of the acute abdomen. 11th ed. London, Oxford University Press, 1957, pp. 45–74.
Donner, M. W., and Weiner, S.: Diagnostic evaluation of abdominal calcifications in acute abdominal disorders. Rad. Clin. N. Amer. 2:145, 1964.
Eichna, L. W., Farber, S. J., Berger, A. R., Rader, B., Smith, W. W., and Albert, R. E.: Non-cardiac circulatory congestion simulating congestive heart failure. Tr. A. Am. Physicians 67:72, 1954.

Guinee, V. F.: Lead poisoning. Amer. J. Med. 52:283, 1972.
Hamman, L. Mediastinal emphysema. JAMA 128:1, 1945.
Klemperer, M. R., Woodworth, H. C., Rosen, F. S., and Austen, K. F.: Hereditary deficiency of the second component of complement (C'2) in man. J. Clin. Invest. 45:880, 1966.
Mellinkoff, S. M.: The Differential Diagnosis of Abdominal Pain. New York, McGraw-Hill Book Co., 1959.
Mellinkoff, S. M.: Systemic causes of abdominal pain. Amer. J. Digest. Dis. 4:642, 1959.
Mellinkoff, S. M. (Ed.): Differential Diagnosis of Diarrhea. New York, McGraw-Hill Book Co., 1964.
Roberts, W. C.: Examining the precordium and the heart. Chest 57:567, 1970.
Schempff, S. C., et al.: Rectal abscesses in cancer patients. Lancet 2:844, 1972.
Solomon, P., and Aring, C. D.: The causes of coma in patients entering a general hospital. Amer. J. Med. Sci. 188:805, 1938.
Stein, J. A., and Tschudy, D. P.: Acute intermittent porphyria—a study of 46 patients. Medicine 49:1, 1970.
Wolf, H. G., and Wolf, S.: Pain. 2nd ed. Springfield, Ill., Charles C Thomas, 1959.
Terry, J. H., Self, M. M., and Howard, J. M.: Injuries of spleen: Report of 102 patients and review of literature. Surgery 40:615, 1956.

SECTION C

Clinical Management

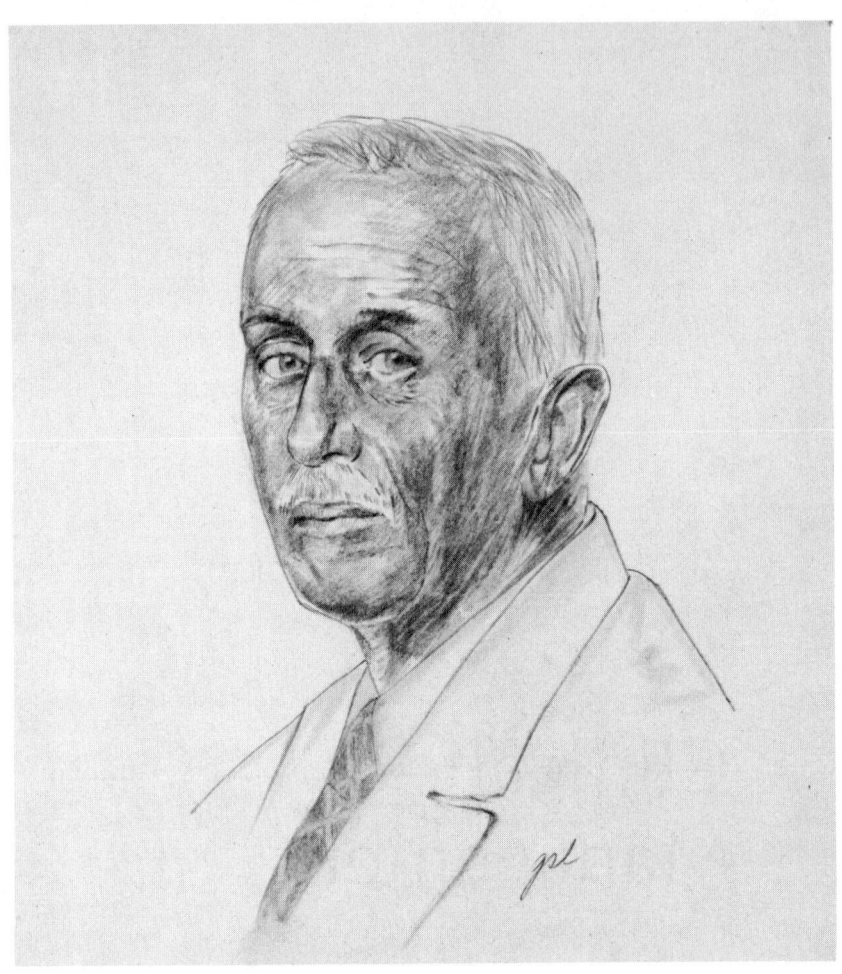

Warfield T. Longcope
PROFESSOR OF MEDICINE

Dr. Longcope is renowned for many things; his clinical observations and research in widely diversified fields remain permanent contributions. A leader of American medicine, for years his counsel in important matters was widely sought. He led many of his students and subordinates to distinguished careers as physicians, teachers, and investigators. It is no wonder, for the example he set was wholly inspiring. Genteel, dignified, charming, he was the epitome of an educated, cultured person. There was a quality about him which extracted the best from the young people who surrounded him. His own excellence was simply reflected; one dared do only one's best, although he reproved only infrequently. As a teacher, he did not attempt to indoctrinate, but preferred to stimulate original thinking through challenging discussions. His vast clinical experience and keen perception would often bring him effortlessly to the core of a complicated illness. Generally, all he required were the data obtained from the history and physical examination. His ability to recall accurately even the smallest details about the many patients seen on teaching rounds was awesome. His ward rounds were notable events, prepared meticulously in advance by the Staff, and carried out in an aura of hushed expectancy, with no little glamour. The genuine warmth and interest in the characteristic "How are you?" with which he invariably greeted each patient is one of our clearest memories. He never turned from a patient's bed without conveying his understanding and leaving behind an expression of confidence. Patients too simple to understand the caliber of a brilliant professor still recognized him as a great, good man. So did we all.

1

General Considerations in Clinical Management

As defined previously, clinical management is the progressive development of a coordinated diagnostic and therapeutic program to achieve the most effective modification of the total impact of an illness upon the patient, his family, and the community.

Clinical management of this kind is not achieved casually or precipitously or in an "off the cuff" manner. It is the product of very thoughtful analysis of the available alternatives, viewed with an in-depth knowledge of the clinical nature of the patient's problem, and a keen sensitivity for all of the different elements involved in the problem—organic, psychologic, personal, economic, and situational. There may be a variety of methods of diagnosis and treatment for the same disorder. In management, the objective is to choose those particular ones which will be the most effective for a specific patient in specific circumstances.

Effective management requires that the clinician be familiar with *all* of the elements of the patient's circumstances. It is not enough just to know that the patient has an active duodenal ulcer. What kind of a person is he? How is he emotionally constituted? What are his problems, both family and business? How effectively would he be able to adhere to an adequate medical regime? How safely could he undergo surgery? Is he the sort of person who is likely to get a good surgical result or is he the type who may continue to have persistent complaints after surgery? What kind of surgical procedure should he have if operated upon? Who could best perform the operation? What kind of anesthesia should he receive? Is he sensitive to any of the drugs he might be given? What kind of postoperative nursing care will he need? Is he a potential candidate for pulmonary embolism or heart failure or atelectasis and pneumonitis after surgery? With regard to insurance and family situation, would now be the optimum time for the patient to have an operation or would it be better to temporarily delay? How long postoperatively will the patient be unable to work, and can the family handle this? These are but some of the key questions which have to be asked and answered by the clinician in order for him to wisely manage even a relatively straightforward clinical problem.

As indicated, sound management requires familiarity with all of the various alternative ways of handling a particular problem. Since the knowledge of a single person cannot possibly encompass all clinical areas, the judicious employment of consultants who can add expertness to the the management process is essential. Hence the clinician is a coordinator of opinions, a censor of alternative viewpoints, and the selector of the best road to follow, since he, more than any of the consultants, is most familiar with the intricacies of all of the particular terrain to be travelled.

Clinical management also requires effective communication between the patient, the family, and the clinician. The best laid clinical plans cannot be consummated unilaterally. Accumulating the clinical evidence from which an optimal plan can be formulated requires communication. Likewise, "selling" the plan to the patient and family requires intercommunication. Time must be provided for explanations and questions. The patient has to understand the plan fully and to want it, and so does the family, or the plan will have failed from the very start. Therefore, before presenting any plan of management to the patient or family, a basic question is, "How acceptable will this plan be to them?" Has the stage been sufficiently set for their acceptance of it through dialogue which has made things clear and produced motivation as well?

A good sense of timing is important in presenting a plan of management to the patient and his family. What may not be acceptable today may be eagerly sought next week, or in a month or in six months. Unless a decision is urgent, the clinician should wait for the psychologically ripe time to push for a particular therapeutic goal, especially if it involves much discomfort or self-discipline or sacrifice for the patient. Time should be allowed to let problems mature, sensitivities to cool off, differing opinions to gel, and emotional walls to be torn down. There are times when it is wise to urge strongly for a particular therapeutic or diagnostic goal, but other times when gentle prodding or suggestion is the more productive course. A classic example of the need for the latter approach is colectomy in the treatment of chronic ulcerative colitis.

Unless there are no other worthwhile alternative programs, it is highly unwise to force the patient into one specific course and to insist that it be followed. There are almost always alternatives available, perhaps only differing in superficial respects. In your discussion with the patient and family, give them some latitude and choice, even as you make clear to them your reasons for preferring and advising one particular course. Then let your advice simmer for a bit. If the patient or his family members are reluctant, don't push too hard immediately; rather, take a long-term view of your relationship with the patient. By the same token, if, despite adequate dialogue, the patient or the family persistently rejects a program which you know to be the only beneficial one, and they cannot be persuaded to adopt your advice, you should then insist upon bringing in a consultant to act as referee. If the family refuses this as well, you should not continue to be responsible for management of the illness.

One of the golden rules of management is that the clinician must *himself* accumulate and examine all of the clinical evidence available on a particular problem. Before making a final diagnosis and beginning to plan management, *know all of the facts yourself.* The physician should read all of the collateral information about the patient and his problem, and what information is not at hand he must secure by telephone or correspondence. Above all, he must never accept uncritically what the patient reports about his past medical experiences: it may be grossly misleading! If the patient is in the hospital, read the entire chart, including the nurses' notes and the order sheets.

Know the facts exactly as they are! Only a very unwise physician accepts anything secondhand or takes anything for granted. One should never get into the sloppy habit of basing one's management judgments solely upon laboratory slips, x-ray reports, or consultation sheets. One must form the habit of looking at the x-rays and reviewing them with an expert, of talking to the consultants, of reviewing the biopsies with a pathologist to whom the whole problem has been explained, and of looking at the blood smears and the urinary sediment. A clinician must be an aggressive activist and a skeptic if he is to take excellent care of his patients. No approach, no effort which might induce a fuller understanding of the patient's problem can be neglected.

SELECTION OF CONSULTANTS

In selecting consultants to aid in the decision-making, there are several significant points for the clinician to review:

1. In a specific area, where do the abilities of a particular consultant lie—is his forte mainly diagnostic or technical? Which type of skill does this patient most need?

2. Is the consultant the sort of an individual you can team up with effectively?

3. Can he be relied upon to give a completely independent opinion?

4. How will the patient and the family react to his personality and approach?

Discerning selection of consultants is a must, for they may be hard to shed later. An example of what can happen if a poor choice is made is the following: Not expecting that anything serious will be found, one asks a surgical consultant to proctoscope the patient. Unhappily, a lesion requiring major bowel surgery is discovered. But the situation becomes troubled because the surgeon who did the proctoscopy is not the one you would prefer to have do major bowel surgery upon your patient. He was, indeed, a poor selection for the proctoscopy.

LISTING THE DIFFERENTIAL DIAGNOSIS

After initial analysis of all of the clinical evidence derived from the history and physical examination, as well as from any collateral sources (laboratory, x-ray, and so forth), the clinician should briefly list in order of likelihood what he considers to be the differential diagnosis. Unfortunately some clinicians are reluctant to do this for fear their preliminary judgment will later be proved incorrect. Such individuals forget, however, that in clinical diagnosis one learns progressively from one's mistakes. Hence, physicians who hedge and cover up, and refuse to commit their diagnostic judgments, never improve their analytical skills. Fear of being considered wrong stultifies learning.

By the same token, a physician should never become wedded to a particular diagnosis and cling to it despite contrary evidence. As new clinical evidence flows in, he should re-examine his judgments and be willing to revise them as reasoned analysis dictates.

NEED FOR WORKSHEET

Based upon the differential diagnosis so outlined, the clinician should next compose, in detail, a flow sheet or worksheet. This flow sheet should be a detailed, step-by-step outline of all of the studies, including consultations, judged necessary to logically scan the differential diagnosis, hopefully ultimately bringing the clinician to the most reasonable answer to the patient's problem. It is a grave error, involving waste of time, money and energy, to carry out diagnostic maneuvers in a piecemeal, helter-skelter fashion, and this inevitably results when a flow sheet is omitted. Furthermore, haphazard study of a patient's problem commonly leads to the overlooking of likely solutions to it. The clinician must have a finite, detailed plan and adhere to it. Next to each item listed on the flow sheet should be indicated the priority to be given to it—"now," "later," "perhaps," "hold," and so on.

Daily, this worksheet should be critically reviewed, and revised as new clinical evidence accumulates or as the patient's status alters.

By studying the worksheet, the clinician can always be up-to-date in planning for his patient. Perusal of it may suggest new ideas for the best moves to make next. Such a sheet is invaluable in maintaining meaningful communication between the clinician and the House Staff, and also with various consultants who may be following the patient.

SELECTING DIAGNOSTIC STUDIES

In planning each diagnostic move, the goal to keep in mind is to acquire the most telling clinical evidence with the fewest maneuvers and with the least expense, discomfort, and risk to the patient.

In trying to make these important but difficult choices, in which experience counts overwhelmingly, the following considerations are helpful:

1. In terms of the particular diagnoses considered to be the most probable, which studies are most likely to supply definitive information?

Recall that there is a great deal of difference between accumulating clinical data and acquiring definitive clinical information. Many studies will supply an abundance of the former and none of the latter. If it is thought highly likely that a patient has fever due to miliary tuberculosis, it is collecting clinical data to determine that his febrile agglutinins are negative, but it is acquiring definitive information to learn that the first strength PPD (purified protein derivative) is strongly positive. Therefore, before performing a particular study, one should ask this question: "How likely is this study to give me definitive information about this patient's disorder that will not be subject to a variety of interpretations, and will carry significant weight in allowing me to determine the probable causes of this patient's sickness? Once I have the answer from this study, will I be appreciably nearer to understanding what is wrong with this patient, or will I simply have more nonspecific data?" Granted, these are hard questions to answer. Also, it must be noted that occasionally the solution to a diagnostic dilemma springs up out of totally unexpected sources. For example, a very high serum calcium turned up in an M12 report done on a patient who was admitted in unexplained coma, leading to the diagnosis of a parathyroid crisis.

2. Is the information likely to be derived from this study actually worth the expense, discomfort and risk it will entail for the patient?

Clearly, not even a very slight risk in performing a diagnostic test can be justified unless there is sound reason to anticipate that the study will produce essential information not obtainable in some other manner involving less risk. In weighing such risks, the clinician should ask himself these questions; "Do I really *need* this piece of information to solve this patient's problem? Is it a *must*? Is there any *safer* way I could acquire similar data?"

It is a grave error to calculate the potential risk of a particular study on the optimistic assumption that all will almost surely go well during the study. Experience has shown that even the "safest" and most "uncomplicated" tests may prove to be just the opposite. What must be evaluated is the potential risk of carrying out this procedure in this particular patient should something go wrong and the unexpected happen. The potential risk of a liver punch biopsy done upon a vigorous young person is not the same as that for, the same procedure carried out on an infirm, elderly, obese patient with considerable emphysema and respiratory insufficiency. Obviously it is wrong for a clinician to order any study unless he is thoroughly familiar with the technique of the examination and is well aware of the remote as well as the immediate risks involved.

In consideration of the patient's comfort, one should never carry out even a simple study unless it is clearly required. While a gastric analysis, for example, may seem to the physician a minor item to be casually performed, to an anxious, sensitive patient this study can be a major ordeal. The golden rule should be vigorously applied in making out the worksheet!

Which Tests First?

In trying to decide which tests should be performed first, the following considerations are of value:

1. Practical issues are a most important factor, such as not confusing the radioactive iodine uptake by first doing a gallbladder series and not taking barium intestinal studies before films of the spine. Also consider how long it takes to schedule a particular test and to get the results. If a skin biopsy seems indicated the first day the patient is seen, don't waste hospital days by delaying the request for the study. If Dr. X is very busy and it will take time to get him to see the patient, call him at once. The appointment can be cancelled later if it proves unnecessary.

2. How severely ill is the patient? Obviously the studies may have to be telescoped and done less methodically if the patient is seriously ill, and starting immediate treatment is critical.

3. Always "go for where the money is"! If study A is calculated to give specific information, but test B nonspecific, study A should take precedence. Contemplation of the flow sheet and the listed diagnostic possibilities should enable one to determine which studies are central to the differential analysis and which are only peripheral. The latter should wait.

4. Often there are certain key studies, the performance of which will help to exclude an entire series of diagnostic possibilities. For example, a patient presents with the clinical complex of anasarca and an enlarged liver and ascites. The easily made determination that the venous pressure is normal will immediately eliminate all of those causes of this clinical complex which involve venous in-flow block to the right heart.

5. First priority should be given to those tests which entail the least risk, discomfort, and expense, unless it seems evident that an essential answer can be gotten only from some more complicated procedure. Sometimes valuable time is lost performing studies which provide only background data because there is unwillingness to perform a study that is more complicated but has a high degree of probability of producing definitive information. In general, however, the simple studies should be done first, and the more complicated ones later.

The Tempo of Testing

A most important consideration is the tempo at which studies should be carried out. Sometimes patients are exhausted emotionally and physically because their work-up is pushed much too hard. This can lead to serious physical consequences as well as to a loss of rapport with the patient and the family. The pace at which the diagnostic studies are performed must be suited to the patient's total circumstances. It makes no sense to conclude a clinical survey with the diagnostic possibilities magnificently studied, but with a patient who is much the worse for wear. On the other hand, one sometimes observes a patient being studied at a leisurely pace when it is all too evident that unless the correct diagnosis is quickly ascertained and specific treatment immediatly implemented, the patient's chances of recovery will be undermined.

Clearly, the proper tempo for the investigation is a matter requiring great clinical judgment. One must see the patient daily and, in terms of the basic functioning of the various organ systems, assess both the progress of the disease and the total impact upon the patient of the studies being done, attempting to wisely balance the two.

If initially a patient's story seems vague and it is not too clear exactly what is happening, and if the patient is not seriously ill, it may pay off to drag one's diagnostic legs a bit, and wait for the elements of the problem to gel. Subsequent clinical observation of the patient may make extensive studies quite unnecessary.

Know When to Stop . . .

It is important to know when to stop making studies and to return to continued clinical observation. Certainly there are diagnostic problems which cannot be solved at a particular stage of their development regardless of the intensity with which diagnostic studies are carried out. Sometimes time alone will provide the answer. In fact, time is frequently the diagnostician's strongest ally. It is essential, therefore, to know when to stop testing and to pursue instead a period of close observation. This is especially true if studies entailing a significant risk are in the offing. One must remember that the passage of time alone sometimes results in the cure of obscure illnesses; at other times, it eventually discloses what is actually wrong with the patient. An important consideration is to what degree, and how rapidly, changes are occurring in the functioning of the various organ systems, and the chances for reversibility of the disease processes.

. . . And When Not to Stop

On the other hand, there are circumstances when it is extremely unwise to discontinue a vigorous diagnostic search and to simply rely upon further observation. As is true for most critical issues in clinical medicine, there are no fixed rules in this area, and the correct decision is generated by judgment and experience. There are a few general guidelines, however.

The most important is contained in the answer to the question, "How compelling is the evidence that the patient may have some hidden disorder of a serious, progressive nature for which specific, curative therapy is available?" If the clinical evidence at hand is weighed in the affimative, then one is wise in insisting upon continued and intensified investigation. It would be the poorest clinical judgment to conclude that miliary tuberculosis, for example, is a reasonable possibility and yet not forge ahead with a panoply of studies, including a liver punch biopsy. All patients with fever of unknown origin (FUO) should be studied until the answer is found, because in most instances FUO is the result of a common disorder presenting in an uncommon fashion, and more often than not there is specific curative therapy for the underlying malady. Progessive deterioration of the function of one of the organ systems also calls for continued, progressive investigation. Among other indications of serious latent disease which should not be allowed to smoulder or slip out of sight are advancing unexplained weight loss, night sweats, changes in personality or living habits, inability of the patient to satisfactorily meet his responsibilities, persistent focal discomfort in a person previously well, altered bowel habits, and unexplained hypochromic, microcytic anemia.

PERIOD OF OBSERVATION

If continued clinical observation is decided upon, it is essential during this period not to do anything to the patient which could in any way confuse the natural course of his disorder. I have repeatedly seen the natural course of patients considered perhaps to have some collagen-vascular disease seriously confused by the giving of antibiotics or other drugs, to which the patients responded with fever, joint pains, rashes, and so on. Therefore, during this important observation period the therapeutic program should be a very simple one so that the disease can be followed in its pure and unadulterated state.

TROUBLESOME STUDIES

There are a number of diagnostic studies which should not be done until the most serious consideration has been given to their potential effects and complications.

First are studies to which the patient and the family are opposed. If their opposition is keen it may be wise to forego the study, at least for the time being, unless it is critical that it be done. For example: A patient presents with early mental deterioration thought to be caused by vascular degeneration. The family is strongly opposed to carrying out cerebral arteriography, but the examination is pushed by the physician. Afterwards, the patient "doesn't seem nearly as bright as he did before."

Such a situation can lead to serious consequences, legal and otherwise. If the clinician decides that a particular study must be done he should *not* move ahead without first explaining to the patient and family in the greatest detail the nature of the test and the potential risks involved in it. Above all, he must be accurate in his presentation. If opposition persists, he should then insist on calling in a consultant.

Second are studies involving any major risk, including an exploratory laparotomy. In the main, such maneuvers should be the *concluding* attempts to arrive at a diagnosis—not the earliest. The pros and cons of such procedures should be discussed with the patient and the family beforehand, and it is always wise to secure the concurrence of a consultant. In discussing such matters with the patient and family, although their understanding and agreement is requisite, under *no* circumstances should they be put in the position of deciding whether the study should or shouldn't be done. Such critical decisions are the clinician's responsibility, and it is unfair, unkind, and even dangerous to shift the weight of such decisions to the shoulders of the patient or family.

Third, when dealing with emotionally disturbed patients who have multiple vague complaints, one may be setting the stage for additional symptom complexes by ill-advisedly performing such maneuvers as a spinal tap or a liver punch biopsy, or by injecting peripheral nerves, and so on. Often these maneuvers become hooks on which are subsequently hung a myriad of additional complaints. It is better to forgo such studies under these circumstances unless they are deemed absolutely essential.

Fourth, an ill-timed psychiatric consultation can alienate the patient and the family from the physician, and sometimes the patient from his family. Even in this highly sophisticated world, many persons are frightened by and misinterpret a visit from a psychiatrist. They are deeply disturbed by it because they conclude that their physician thinks they are "crazy" or "imagining" or "putting on." If they are somewhat emotionally disturbed to begin with, they may now begin to panic, concluding that their strongest support, their clinician, now feels that they can no longer manage or control their own problems. A psychiatric consultation, especially if in full view of the family, can be an ego buster. Patients forced into seeing a psychiatrist may lose faith in their physicians, for they will believe that he has jumped the gun, overlooked the evidence of organic disease, or misinterpreted the data, and has chosen the easy path of concluding that their trouble is "all due to nerves."

Therefore, one must be circumspect in introducing a psychiatric consultant. The physician must have had time to develop a very solid rapport with the patient and the family; the patient's problem must be well understood and its organic aspects meticulously investigated; the physician must have had the opportunity to delicately explore significant personal factors with the patient in sufficient depth, and, in general, be familiar with his emotional sensitivities. Only then should the matter of psychiatric consultation be presented to the patient. If the physician has prepared the ground well, there will rarely be persistent opposition. There are few errors in management more serious than allowing a psychiatrist to unexpectedly pop in on a patient who hasn't been adequately prepared for his arrival.

DECISION ON HOSPITALIZATION

One of the earliest management decisions that has to be made is whether or not to hospitalize the patient. Making this decision becomes progressively more difficult as hospital costs rise—and Utilization Review Committees become more restrictive. Obviously, any patient with a serious acute or chronic illness requiring diagnostic or therapeutic care that cannot be provided on an ambulatory basis should be hospitalized.

Beyond this very broad generalization there are other groups of patients who are better managed when hospitalized, including:

1. All patients suspected of having fever of unknown origin.

2. Patients whose disease process lends itself to ambulatory study but whose general physical status is such that the stress and strain of repeated hospital visits for outpatient studies would be excessive.

3. Patients whose complaints are centered about acute, episodic, dramatic circumscribed "spells" of various sorts, during which important physiologic alterations are claimed to occur, and hence, observation and verification of an immediate sort is essential, both day and night.

4. Patients with confusing, highly complicated stories containing vague or even bizarre elements, but which nevertheless have serious implications for the patient, and it is unclear whether the process is functional or organic. In such circumstances, it is imperative that the reactions of the patient be observed very frequently at various times of the day and night, and that the clinician have ample opportunity to get to understand the patient psychologically as well as physically.

5. Patients with illnesses which, while presently mild, have the potential for suddenly becoming acutely exacerbated, sometimes quite unexpectedly. If a patient with mild hyperthyroidism acquires a severe respiratory infection, her illness can rapidly exacerbate. An alcoholic with early "mild" pneumonia is never mildly ill. There is no such thing as a "slight" heart attack or a "small" intestinal hemorrhage.

6. Patients whose illnesses require studies most effectively accomplished in the hospital, such as liver punch biopsies or cerebral arteriograms.

7. Patients who are greatly incapacitated from a functional illness and need to be removed from their present environment and into a neutral area where they will have frequent opportunities to engage in a dialogue with their physician, away from the distractions, inhibitions, and intrusions of family and daily responsibilities. Such a period of hospitalization on a medical service may very importantly serve as a kind of "halfway house" as the patient is gently introduced to psychiatric treatment.

WRITING ORDERS

If the patient is hospitalized, all orders should be funnelled through a single physician for final checking before being carried out. Dangerous confusion and conflict result when several persons leave orders on the same patient. If there is a house officer, he should be responsible for posting all orders.

In writing the general daily orders, top priority should be given to the patient's comfort. Restrictions which are not essential should not be imposed. This pertains to such items as the type of diet, bathroom privileges, and degree of bed rest. The patient should be allowed to continue to live as normally as possible. Don't leave orders which will make the patient conclude that he is sicker than he actually is!

Unless one is certain of the patient's diagnosis and highly accurate temperature recordings are not important, it is wise to insist that rectal temperatures be taken initially. We have seen very serious misinterpretations of the patient's temperature made because it was recorded only orally.

A small but important point—in writing orders, one should use as few abbreviations as possible, and then only the standard ones.

USING DRUGS

In clinical practice, it is a sound practice to use only a small number of drugs having the same pharmacological effects so that one can become thoroughly familiar with their modes of action. Instead of prescribing a wide variety of different types of digitalis or diuretic preparations, for example, a clinician should confine his choice to a few agents in each category so that he can develop a personal critique concerning their behavior. Such knowledge is difficult to acquire if one is always trying out some agent newly on the market.

It should be an unbreakable rule of clinical practice *never* to order or prescribe a drug for a patient unless the physician has a sound appreciation of both its actions and its potential toxicity. Seemingly innocuous agents sometimes turn out to be just the opposite.

I recall a salt substitute placed on the market a few years ago which was exceedingly popular for a short time. One of its main ingredients was lithium. Many who prescribed it knew little or nothing about the pharmacology of lithium, and the preparation was regarded as a harmless and useful agent. One patient who was using the material because she had hypertension and renal insufficiency abruptly developed an acute ascending paralysis. Subsequently, other similar cases were reported and the agent was removed from the market. It was revealing how many physicians, upon learning of this experience, said, "I'll bet that's what's been wrong with my patient. She's been complaining of being weak and tired. I never realized that just a salt substitute could be so poisonous." If you aren't thoroughly familiar with the pharmacologic actions of an agent, *don't* give it to a patient!

Another useful axiom is: *Don't order any drug a patient can do without!* Drugs so often produce complications. A patient's program of therapy should be kept as simple and uncomplicated as possible. The drugs a patient is receiving should be reviewed repeatedly, and any not considered essential should be eliminated. In general, drug "combinations" or "mixtures" should be avoided because the problem is compounded if the patient develops what is considered to be a drug reaction. Again, keep the program simple and pure!

One should be especially wary of running orders, and these should never be written without a definite stop order being included. Among many other instances, I recall an elderly patient with cardiorenal disease whose severe "unexplained" acidosis disappeared when her orders were checked and a running order for ammonium chloride, given as a diuretic, was cancelled.

Make certain no drugs are being given, or have recently been given, which might affect any pertinent laboratory tests that have been done or are projected for the near future.

Never give a more complicated drug that may have even occasional untoward side effects when a simpler and safer measure is available. I am repeatedly appalled by the abandon with which patients who complain of nausea of even a mild degree are given Compazine when peppermint and soda and perhaps a little tincture of belladonna would give equal relief. It is equally distressing to see a patient who is restless at night be placed at once on tranquilizers. Chloral hydrate and a glass of warm milk might be just as soothing.

The following shouldn't need to be said, but it does—Don't give *any* drug which may have direct or side effects upon the patient that would further confuse the clinical problem under study. Two classic examples (and there are so many!) of breaking this rule are the young female with mild jaundice who is given Compazine because she is nauseated, and the youngster with a suspected strep throat who is given penicillin before a throat culture is obtained. Are the fever, polyarthritis, and erythematous rash which subsequently appear due to the onset of acute rheumatic fever, or are they manifestations of a reaction to penicillin? Such a question would not have come up if the rule just discussed had been followed.

Cost of Drugs

A physician should be aware of the relative costs of the drugs he prescribes, and he should not order an expensive agent if there is a comparable drug which is cheaper. In writing prescriptions, he should take care to do so in the most economic way, not ordering larger quantities than the patient will actually require. Also, he should direct the patient to pharmacies where he can get the best buys. If the patient must take an expensive drug, such as prednisone, for a prolonged period, the physician should advise the patient to explain to the pharmacist that he must take the drug for a long time, and hence, to work out some equitable cost adjustment, if possible.

Instructing the Patient

When a patient is advised to take any drug, the reason for it and its actions should be explained in simple terms. In particular, any important side or toxic effects should be called to the patient's attention. In doing this, it is important not to so sensitize the patient to these side effects that he promptly has them: if a patient is told that iron compounds often cause nausea, he may well become nauseated. On the other hand, failure to explain common side effects in a wise, diplomatic way can cause patients a great deal of unnecessary discomfort and concern, even though such effects may not be of a serious nature. I have known patients given iron who were deeply concerned by the black color of their stools. Some patients on Maalox may develop severe diarrhea. The clinician should tell patients all they need to know to employ a drug most effectively and with the least anxiety.

By the same token, tell patients what a particular drug won't do! For example, in the public mind are all sorts of misapprehensions about the use of various steroid compounds—that they cause cancer or blood clots, change sex reactions, cause diabetes, increase body hair, make the bones get soft and shrink, and so on. While patients are oftentimes embarrassed to bring these concerns out into the open, they may be profoundly affected by them. We remember a young male who became acutely psychotic when he was given a female sex hormone because he was convinced it was "changing him," but he was ashamed to reveal his fears to his physician. In the South Pacific during the war, many soldiers hid their atabrine tablets instead of taking them because of the rampant rumor that they "destroyed your manhood." The clinician must not wait for the patient to bring such misapprehensions to the surface. He should anticipate them and meet them head on with reassurance.

Proper Administration of Drugs

The manner in which even a simple drug is administered should be double checked and not taken for granted, even when one is dealing with a well-run ward and an intelligent patient. One may find antacids being given with meals or patients being awakened to take their sleeping pills. By contrast, as simple a maneuver as leaving milk and antacids on the bedside table at night may make a major difference to the comfort and healing of a duodenal ulcer.

While some patients handle their instructions sloppily, others are overly obsessive. I can recall a number of patients who adhered to exceedingly taxing programs because they weren't instructed adequately, doing such things as awakening at 2 A.M. to "be sure I took the pill exactly four times a day, just like you told me!"

It's wise not to credit patients with much sense when it comes to following medical orders. One must be explicit in telling them what to do and what not to do. Often patients leave the doctor's office with several prescriptions clutched in their hands and a great deal of confusion in their minds. When they get home they worry and fret for fear they have not accurately recalled the oral instructions given them. They want to do just what they were told, but they aren't certain *what* they were told. Therefore, simply handing prescriptions to patients with quickly given oral advice is not enough for good management. The physician must write out in adequate detail a flow sheet for the patient to follow, with dosage and time and mode of administration clearly indicated. This can be done very quickly with practice.

If a patient has been using some simple, safe remedy for a long time and has faith that it is beneficial, don't discourage that faith. Let him continue it. On the other hand, if a patient is taking some agent the nature of which is not familiar to you, find out what it is—immediately! It could prove to be a key piece of clinical evidence. If a patient has been using a drug with reasonable success and is satisfied with it, don't change it just for the sake of change. Lastly, if a particular drug can be taken effectively orally, it makes no sense whatsoever to administer it in any other fashion.

Drug Dependence

Clinicians must be constantly on the alert to avoid starting or supporting drug dependencies in their patients. Analgesics, sedatives, and narcotics must be ordered with great care, particularly if the patient has a chronic disorder, functional illness, or if he is an unstable, immature, or hysterical type of person. Many times I have seen a patient's need for a pharmacologic crutch aided and abetted by the thoughtless prescribing of an agent such as codeine or Demerol for some vague abdominal pain or "neuritis" or "migraine." When a patient must be given narcotics, he should never be told the nature of the drug he is receiving. Running orders for such drugs should never be written.

If a patient has been chronically relying on such drugs, it is an error to precipitously halt them all. Rather, wait until rapport has been well established with the patient and his basic problems are fully understood, and some satisfying plan of management has been developed. If you "get tough" before you have established a beachhead with him and his problem, you will create resentments you won't be able to overcome. Timing is of the essence in such sensitive matters.

It is a good practice, each time a patient is seen in a progress visit, to ask oneself these questions; Must this patient take these prescribed medications? Are there any he could well do without? Are they being administered in an optimum manner and dosage?

Reactions to Drugs

If a patient is suspected of having some type of drug reaction, it is generally wise to temporarily discontinue *all* medications and not to try to guess which of the several agents might be the culprit, since any one of them might be responsible, although some statistically more so than others. If it is essential that the patient continue a particular kind of pharmacologic agent, a suitable substitute should be given for the one presently being taken.

When a patient is suspected of having a drug reaction, it is not sufficient to simply ask the patient "What drugs have you been taking?" To many patients, the words "drugs" and "medicine" have a very limited connotation. To many they imply the taking of something prescribed by a physician, or something expensive, or something given by an injection. Therefore, very specific questions should be asked: "Do you take anything for headaches? . . . for your nerves? . . . for your bowels? . . . to help you go to sleep? . . . for your menses?" We recall a physician's wife who had been miserably ill for months with recurrent erythema nodosa of unknown etiology. When asked "Have you had any drugs?" her answer was negative. But on direct, specific questioning, she recalled taking Exlax for her bowels. The erythema nodosa vanished when this "unimportant" agent was stopped.

It is a mistake to accept unchallenged the patient's claim that he is "sensitive to" or "had a reaction to" a particular agent. Many such "drug reactions" turn out not to be bona fide ones when the details of the setting in which the "reaction" occurred are carefully analyzed.

Drug Failures

By the same token, the patient's claim that a particular agent failed to help his condition should be challenged because it may become apparent on investigation that the drug was given either in an inadequate dosage or in an ineffective manner. This can be important in differential diagnosis, as in the case of "failure" of fever, rash, and arthritis to respond to adequate dosages of prednisone in a young female suspected of having systemic lupus erythematosus.

Mood Drugs

Great caution should be exercised in the dispensation of tranquilizers. They may cause peculiar and confusing sensations in some patients which can increase their depression and anxiety, and sometimes lead to panic. It should be recalled that the effects of such agents are cumulative and may be heightened or altered by the taking of other agents, such as alcohol.

I recall a charming young mother who was feeling the stress of four young and active youngsters. Given phenobarbital in daily running dosages by her physician to relax her tensions, she became progressively unsteady on her feet and thick in her speech in the evening after pre-dinner cocktails with her husband, much to the alarm of her husband and children. All of this cleared when she was given a placebo in place of the phenobarbital.

IMPORTANCE OF "LITTLE THINGS"

It is easy to become so concerned by the major complexities of a patient's illness that the "little things" are overlooked. However, sometimes these "little things" mean a great deal to the patient. Many patients are distracted by disordered bowel habits, new sleeping patterns, and worries about diet, and detailed attention to such secondary matters distinguishes the concerned and involved physician.

In taking care of a patient's major problem it is a mistake to overlook or ignore his minor complaints, for sometimes the latter actually plague a patient to a much greater degree than the former, as in the case of a patient with coronary insufficiency who is made miserable by hemorrhoids or a chronic eczematoid dermatitis. Such secondary problems should be dealt with effectively, and not passed over.

In some patients, such seemingly minor matters may assume major proportions unless they are adequately managed. A patient may receive excellent threatment for a chronic bronchial infection while a very dirty fungus infection of his feet is ignored; a patient recovering from bacterial endocarditis may have several rotten molars requiring treatment. It is distressing to observe how little attention such secondary, yet vital, issues may be given because of lopsided preoccupation with the primary problem.

DIET

Before ordering a specific diet, be sure that the patient needs it, and don't impose unnecessary restrictions. If adherence to a diet is essential or at all complicated, it is most helpful to have the patient instructed and followed by a trained dietician. Merely handing the patient a written outline is often ineffective. The dietary program must be explained in terms of the patient's particular habits and circumstances. It is senseless to demand too much of a patient with regard to his diet. If a patient must reduce, explain that you do not expect a crash program, but that you much prefer that he embark upon a twelve-month project, during which you will expect him to lose so much weight each month. Such a long term program is far more palatable and likely to be followed.

BRIEFING THE PATIENT

One of the most important obligations of a clinician is to explain to his patient in detail what it is that he plans to do to him, as well as for him. There is a gross error in management if a patient is surprised by what is done to him. If, without prior announcement, the patient is wheeled in to have a skin biopsy, or a brain scan, or a psychiatric interview, he has a

GENERAL CONSIDERATIONS IN CLINICAL MANAGEMENT

right to be resentful. The patient *must* be briefed beforehand regarding what is to be done, why, and what to anticipate. If some operative or other procedure is to be done, it should be explained in such a way as to allay the patient's fears, but at the same time in a way that will psychologically prepare him to meet whatever stresses may be involved. Fooling or "kidding" patients will backfire every time. Accurate, fair explanation of what can be anticipated breeds confidence and trust.

BIOPSIES

It is exceedingly distressing when the information that should have been obtained from a biopsy procedure goes down the drain because of lack of adequate communication between the surgeon and the internist. The surgeon should be thoroughly briefed regarding the patient's problem and, specifically, the reason for the biopsy. There should be full agreement as to exactly what tissues are to be obtained and how they are subsequently to be handled: the types of cultures to be made, stains to be done, and so forth. Nothing should be left to second guessing. Yet how many times have I seen such a relatively simple procedure botched! A patient with right-sided headache has the left temporal artery biopsied; a patient with suspected polyarteritis nodosa has a muscle biopsy, the skin and subcutaneous tissues (where the lesions often are) being carefully unmolested; a granuloma of the bowel is not cultured and the presence of tuberculosis is overlooked, and so on. As a result of the clinician's detailed conversation with the surgeon, the correct quantity of the right tissues should be obtained, and *all* of the appropriate studies carried out upon it. This may require considerable planning, and it is not to be done casually. Few things are as wasteful as an inappropriately performed biopsy.

PLANNING OPERATIONS

If a patient is to be operated upon, the matter must, of course, be discussed in detail with the prospective surgeon. It is wise not to tell the patient that a particular operative procedure is to be done until the surgeon has examined the patient and has concurred. The patient and the family may become confused and upset if there are last-minute alterations of plans.

A number of special items should be discussed with the surgeon, including what the patient has already been told about his condition, what his psychological reaction to the procedure is likely to be, and whether or not any medical problems exist that could affect the patient's course during or immediately after the operation, such as poor pulmonary toilet, heart, kidney, or liver disturbances, peripheral venous disease, history of pulmonary emboli, diabetes mellitus, or sensitivity to particular drugs (including halothane anesthesia).

If possible, the internist should be present at the operation and participate in any critical decision making. His presence will be very reassuring to both patient and family, and this can be of tremendous importance, especially if things do not go well subsequently.

Postoperatively, the patient should be followed very closely by both the physician and the surgeon, with sufficient dialogue between the two whenever questions of management arise. One quickly recognizes those surgeons in a community who are not only technically skillful but are also adept at postoperative management and, highly important, which ones are willing to work effectively as a team with the medical group. All three qualities are essential to excellent surgical care.

KNOW THE FACTS

One should never take definite action, even in an emergency, unless one has some grasp of at least the basic facts in the matter. There is always a strong impulse to do something to help a sick person, but *no* action is better than the wrong action. One can usually delay until the basic facts of the problem are known and a few key observations have been made. Plunging blindly to correct an unknown abnormality is likely to produce poor results.

In general, it is wise to be conservative in managing patients' health problems, and not to make a move unless one is reasonably certain of what the results will be. Continued observation over a sufficient period of time may clarify issues that are now obscure, and a certain percentage of patients do heal themselves. Overzealousness on the doctor's part to quickly know all, and to begin some type of specific therapy as soon as possible, may lead to unnecessary or harmful undertakings. Unless it is clear that a vital organ system is being rapidly and progressively adversely affected, and hence time is of the essence, the physician should not feel forced to take quick action. A well-planned, methodical, step-by-step approach, in which there is adequate time to digest the clinical evidence at hand, observe the patient, and plan the next most logical move, is the most profitable course of action. To be avoided is the shooting off of batteries of tests and all the implications of such expressions one so often hears as "liver profile," "running the gut," "culturing him up," and the like. Specific tests should be chosen with care to provide specific answers until the nature of the patient's malady is finally apparent. What answers are needed can only be appreciated through meticulous and constant re-evaluation of the clinical evidence derived from the history and physical examination. Repeated observation and re-analysis of the patient's present status progressively adds to the usefulness and meaningfulness of this evidence.

GENERAL CONSIDERATIONS IN CLINICAL MANAGEMENT

VALUE OF CONSERVATISM . . .

If a physician has no beneficial treatment to offer a patient at a particular stage of an illness, he should not feel obligated to offer the patient *some* therapy. Yet, many clinicians have this compulsion. If a patient has an unexplained fever, it is much harder to resist starting some kind of treatment than it is to decide to bide one's time and observe the patient for a period.

It is a peculiar fact that it is psychologically much easier to agree to give a patient some therapeutic agent (often an antibiotic) than it is to decide to withhold it and study the patient's progress. Such therapeutic activism is one of the worst features of modern medical care. And yet, to do nothing to a patient until one knows about the nature of his illness may prove to be much more therapeutic than blindly administering a "broad spectrum drug" or "covering all of the treatable possibilities."

. . . AND KNOWING WHEN TO ACT

On the other hand, there are clearly times when immediate therapeutic action is essential, and in such instances it is vital to be aware of all of the possibilities of treatment, and to design a program which will take care of those which are statistically most likely to be successful in a particular set of circumstances.

After all of the clinical evidence has been gathered, it is a good plan to reflectively sit down and ask oneself the question, "What are all of the reasonable diagnostic possibilities here, both likely and remote?" After listing these in descending order of likelihood, one then asks the question, "Which of these possibilities, unless specifically treated, can result in serious injury to any of this patient's organ systems, and at what stage in the future?" The next question to be answered is, "What specific forms of therapy are available to prevent such injury from taking place?" And finally, "What risks might be involved in using them?"

If such an analysis indicates that there is indeed reasonable diagnostic evidence that essential organ functions may soon be seriously impaired, then one is correct in employing specific forms of therapy on an empirical basis, even though some reasonable risk may be entailed. Otherwise it is much wiser to hold one's fire and continue to study the patient.

VALUE OF STABILITY

Once a particular therapeutic program has been launched, give the patient's response to it time to mature and produce clear-cut answers before it is stopped or altered. Frequently there is a tendency to alter the program every time some minor change in the patient's status is noted. The net result is that the patient is kept bouncing from one program to the next, never being granted the opportunity to reach a steady state. There are already too many variables in human disease—this is what makes clinical diagnosis so difficult. Don't add to these variables by frequent alterations in the treatment program. To do so can lead to chaos. Let the patient's condition settle down by removing as many variables as possible while his response is closely observed.

PROGRESS VISITS—HOSPITALIZED PATIENTS

It is a valuable and laudable habit for a clinician to visit his hospitalized patients daily, including Sundays. Sunday morning rounds can be very pleasant and relaxed, a time when one can catch up on details and lay plans for the coming week. In the "good old days" at Hopkins (and they were good days, when clinical excellence was given highest priority), all of the senior faculty made rounds on Sundays dressed in formal morning suits with a flower in the buttonhole. This was no mere affectation, for it helped to develop and sustain that atmosphere of dignified, thoughtful, reassuring concern that helps the clinician to have a significant influence upon his patients. While morning suits are out of style, the philosophy of patient care which led to their use should not be.

Before visiting a patient, it is of obvious importance to review the temperature chart and the clinical notes. It is also helpful to check with the head floor nurse, for she sometimes has clinical tidbits which no one else has—family attitudes, reactions and concerns of the patient, and so on. It is a mistake to ignore the "intuitions" of the nursing staff! The order book should be reviewed each day to make certain that the therapeutic program is optimal. Unfortunately, mistakes do sometimes occur, particularly in allowing running orders to continue past the time when they are no longer needed.

Before visiting the patient, one should also ask oneself what specific anxieties and concerns are likely to be in the patient's mind at this particular stage of his illness. How can these be most effectively offset by your conversation and attitude? These considerations apply to the family as well. What questions are you likely to be asked today regarding the patient's present and future status? How can you best answer these to maintain the atmosphere you believe is best for the patient and family? What do you want to tell the patient or family to bring them in a constructive and positive way through the next step of the illness? Casual, unpremeditated conversation is not likely to achieve these results satisfactorily. Frequently, off-the-cuff remarks leave the patient and family puzzled, insecure, and perhaps fearful of what is in store.

As already indicated, conversation with patients should be held with the physician seated—not standing, or propped up against the bed. Questions should be asked regarding the small, but important details of patient care:

Is the patient comfortable? How is the food? Are bowel movements satisfactory? Is sleep adequate? Are there any personal concerns? How are the children at home? . . . and so on.

Insure that the patient will not have any unpleasant or disturbing surprises by explaining what is being planned for the next day: what tests are to be done, what they will entail, what they will require of the patient, and what consultants are to be seen. In explaining the nature of tests to be done, it is a mistake to pretend "there is nothing to it" if, indeed, there *is* something to it. The patient will handle discomfort much better if he is wisely prepared for it than if he is surprised by it.

If the patient's illness presents a diagnostic problem, it is a mistake to give the patient and family information about the progress of the investigations being carried out in daily bits and snatches. Such data may not be meaningful to them, and their hopes and concerns will rise and fall depending upon their interpretations of each new piece of information. Instead of thus leaking information in brief, daily conversations, it is wiser to tell the patient and family at the very onset that your method is to sit down and hold a conference with all concerned, during which you will answer all questions, just as soon as you believe that you have some meaningful conclusions to present. Meanwhile, during your daily visits, you should reassure both patient and family that the studies are going well and that the necessary clinical data is being gathered.

Sometimes (unfortunately, not infrequently) patients, or their families, plague the physician by daily plaintively and insistently asking, "Why can't I go home tomorrow?" Insistence upon leaving the hospital too early can be destructive to good care and good relationships, for it may very well result in short cuts and hasty decisions. The very first time the patient or family starts this kind of nuisance, the physician should firmly make it clear that this is unreasonable and must not continue; that he too wants to get the patient home as soon as it is feasible; that he will give ample warning of the time of discharge so that necessary family plans can be made; but that in the meantime he will expect the patient and the family to settle down and work together with him. It should be pointed out that diagnostic studies cannot be shot off harum scarum, all at once. Diagnostic studies have to be accomplished stepwise, one clue leading to another until the answer is finally at hand. Rushing and short cuts are not the way to solve important problems or to restore the patient's health.

In any hospital setting, mistakes are bound to occur occasionally, and not everyone on the staff always responds to the needs and desires of the patients in the most desirable fashion. In addition, some patients and their families are very difficult to satisfy, and some, as already indicated, are even looking for trouble. A clinician has to learn to be the shock absorber of such unpleasantness, and he must be circumspect in handling these problems soothingly and diplomatically. To deny their existence or to "cover up," or to respond with resentment is to invite even more serious reactions. As previously indicated, any occurrence significantly affecting patient care must, for legal reasons, be recorded in the clinical record.

Daily progress visits afford the clinician an excellent opportunity to get to know the patient as a person, and to learn of his circumstances in more and more detail. In an informal, unobtrusive, comfortable way, the physician can gradually explore areas wherein the roots of functional illness may be imbedded: "What kind of a little girl were you? Did your parents bring you up strictly? What are your children like? Do you enjoy them? Can you communicate easily with your husband? Do you get a bang out of your job? Do you have much time for hobbies? What do you enjoy most in life? Have you had more than your share of problems in life?", and more questions in the same vein.

Through such visits one can learn much of value, without obviously probing. One can also sometimes learn a good deal by watching the interplay between the patient and his relatives, and his deportment with the staff on the floor.

Re-examination of the patient during progress visits is invaluable. If the patient has an organic disease, physical changes not present one day, but observed the next, may contain the essential clue to the diagnosis. Furthermore, in the management of functional illness, re-examination of the patient is essential for giving the patient reassurance, and for strengthening the position of the physician. Such re-examinations convince the patient with functional illness that the physician is not just assuming that "it is all in my mind," and that he is keeping his eyes wide open to make certain not to overlook other organic possibilities. If a patient with functional abdominal pain, for example, continues to complain of discomfort but is merely given reassurance without being re-examined, he is going to wonder, "How can my doctor be certain something isn't developing inside of me?" Five minutes spent in re-examining the patient can give much added weight to a 15-minute talk concerning relevant personal factors. Besides, sometimes the original diagnosis of functional illness is incorrect, and the patient does develop objective alterations not previously noted. In clinical medicine, it is impossible to be *too* careful.

PROGRESS NOTES

The ability to write succinct, meaningful progress notes is, unfortunately, a gift which is not widely shared. Good progress notes are a hallmark of the truly able clinician. Like all other abilities, the composition of such notes has to be learned and practiced. Too often, so-called progress notes are not that at all, but are rather a listing of studies already accomplished and of others still to be done.

Progress notes should be brief, succinct, and to the point, and yet com-

GENERAL CONSIDERATIONS IN CLINICAL MANAGEMENT

plete. They should be written daily, or at least every other day, so that every significant step in the patient's course is recorded. They must document the responsible physician's contribution to the care of the patient, for legal and insurance as well as for medical purposes. Their content should accomplish the following:

1. Describe the patient's present status.
2. Outline in adequate detail any changes which have occurred in his status since the prior note.
3. Relate the observer's interpretation of these alterations.
4. Outline the next measures to be taken (diagnostic or therapeutic) to meet the patient's problem.
5. List the major diagnostic and therapeutic maneuvers as they are accomplished, and the reasons for them.

As already discussed, since the clinical chart is both a legal and a scientific document, there is no place in the progress notes for humor or for venting one's spleen. The latter are indications of clinical immaturity. Careless, thoughtless, irresponsible notes can be a source of embarrassment, and also of litigation. One should never put *anything* into the progress notes that one would not like to have read by one's peers.

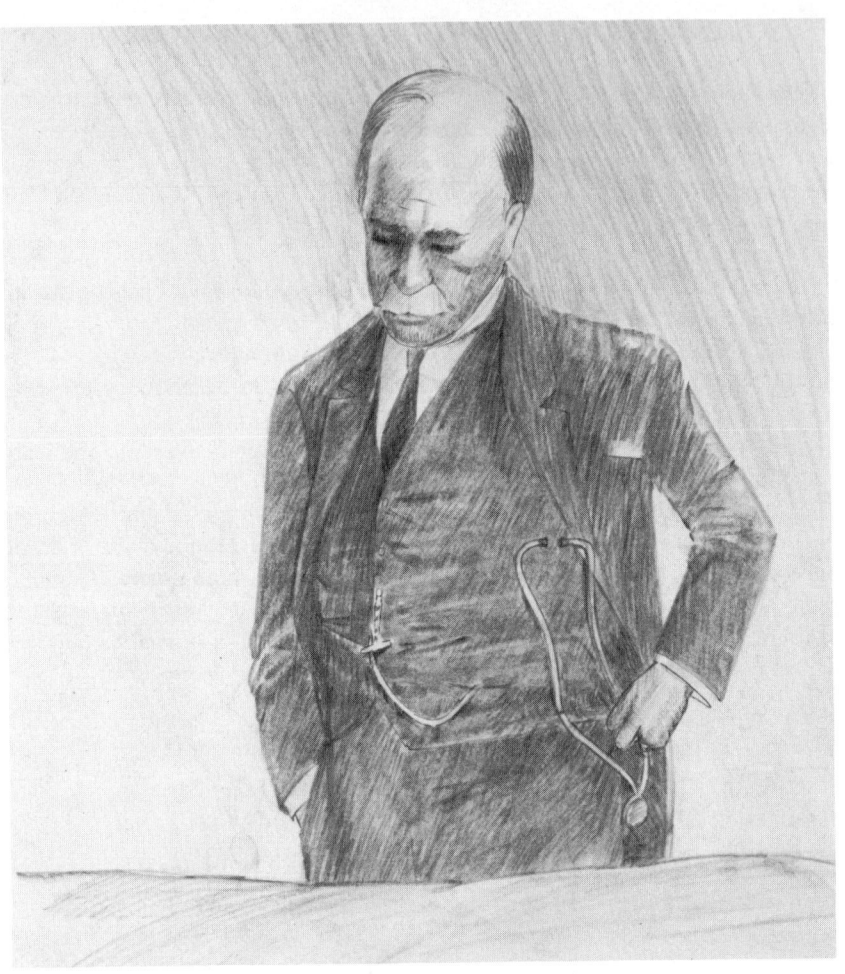

William Osler
PROFESSOR OF MEDICINE

So many words have been employed to describe Dr. Osler, both as a person and as a physician, that additional use of them for this purpose makes redundancy and repetition almost inevitable. But a single picture is "worth a thousand words," and an unposed one perhaps even many more. Surely, this sketch of an old photograph tells many things about this physician and his approach to this patient.

The atmosphere is one of thoughtful contemplation. The physician is completely involved in his patient's problem. There is an attitude of personal concern; he is not only feeling for the patient, but feeling with him as well. Most evident is the fact that the physician's chief interest seems to be an intent and scrupulous observation of the patient and his clinical chart, and one gets the impression that all which is being seen is also being analyzed, with unhurried study.

There is no evidence of precipitousness, or of haste, or of a desire for action before full thought, or of the early arrival at conclusions inadequately conceived. Observation is not being neglected for more complicated methods of gathering information. Personal concern and involvement of self in the patient's problem, meticulous and analytical observation, quiet contemplation, exclusion of haste–clearly, these are the characteristics of Dr. Osler's approach to this patient.

Men are immortalized on this earth when their good actions and qualities are imitated by those who come after. So it has been with Dr. Osler. So let it be with us.

2

The Patient with a Functional Disorder

Skill in the diagnosis and management of functional disorders is essential for anyone concerned with human disease. In a review of 500 consecutive patients seen in consultation because of problems in diagnosis, Hamman found that a third suffered solely or predominantly from functional disorders. In other studies, the minimum figure for the occurrence of purely functional illness is about 25 percent of all patients who present themselves to an internist or outpatient facility, whereas the maximum figure, which includes patients with organic problems, is as high as 80 percent. The physician who lacks interest in this kind of illness, and attempts to avoid it, cannot be effective either as a diagnostician or as a therapist. He may well become a person having only certain technical abilities.

It is my impression that many patients with such disorders are not well managed, and for a variety of reasons.

First, effective management of functional illness is exceedingly time consuming. Such patients are not disposed of quickly: repeated and prolonged visits are often required. This introduces a very practical problem, which has no solution at present; that is, that many such patients are either unable or unwilling to adequately compensate an internist for so much of his time, and neither are their medical insurance carriers, including Medicare. Clearly, the role of the internist on the health team is not adequately understood.

Second, there is a desire in all physicians to observe their patients' improvement, yet so often functional illness drags along visit after visit, getting no better, and oftentimes getting worse. The physician doesn't enjoy continuing a relationship which makes his efforts seem fruitless, and he begins to resent the patient.

Third, because so many of these patients are not helped by the kind of care they now get, they migrate from physician to physician exhibiting increasingly refractory symptoms. Their complaints grow more voluminous as each new physician becomes skeptical of his ability to change what seems to be a habit of sickness.

Fourth, there are personality factors and life settings especially productive of functional disease. Some physicians are negatively affected and "turned off" by these. I suspect some of us may see in them ourselves, and this can indeed be sensitizing.

Fifth, to benefit functional illness, a physician must extend fully his personal as well as his professional assets. Without question, the hardest cases are the functional ones. A clever diagnosis and the right medications will cure Whipple's disease, and the problem is done with. Much more is required of a clinician to favorably affect a functional illness. Included are a perceptive interest in all of the vagaries of human nature, a sophisticated familiarity with what it is that deeply moves people, an understanding of the genuine sensitivities of the human spirit, facility in communicating with patients and their families, and, just as essential, a willingness to take the time to do it, and finally, infinite patience, for it is necessary to review with the patient the same material, over and over and over again.

It is common experience that the majority of patients with purely functional disorders fail to recognize them as such, and for a variety of reasons. Many are unfamiliar with the nature of functional disorders. Others are fully convinced that they have some organic disease, and this belief has frequently been deeply imbedded by previous medical advice. Still others are inwardly afraid or ashamed to recognize such a disorder within themselves, because gross misconceptions about such illness make them think that a stigma is attached. Finally, there are patients who find it more comforting to think that their disorder is organic in nature. Therefore, in his approach to the patient with a functional disorder, the physician must realize that he is contending with more than an illness—he must also be prepared to meet ignorance, stubborn misconceptions, and a melange of fear, shame, and pride, as well as selfish motivations.

Such is the challenge of the approach to the patient with functional disease. Some of the mistakes observed most frequently in attempts to meet it are the following:

First is failure to give the patient enough time to tell her story in detail. The patient is hurried along, treated casually. She leaves the office dissatisfied, convinced she has told her story to a fixed jury. She believes that if she could only have communicated this or that piece of information, the true answer to her problem would have been unearthed. So, she starts all over again with another pair of tired ears.

Second, and one of the most serious errors, is failure of the physician to clearly explain to the patient that it is his firm conclusion that her illness is, in fact, functional in nature, even when this is indeed his final opinion. Just when the opportunity for a major therapeutic breakthrough is at hand, the physician vacillates, and draws back from "telling it like it is." Instead,

THE PATIENT WITH A FUNCTIONAL DISORDER

he merely reassures the patient about her general physical status, or worse yet, he discusses her "low blood pressure" or "hypoglycemia" or "slightly low PBI" or "ptotic kidneys" or "hiatus hernia" or "water retention." Consequently, he becomes a co-conspirator in the continuance of her crippling complaints, which time will almost surely exaggerate.

There are a number of reasons why so many physicians won't speak to their patients forthrightly about functional disease, including the following:

1. Some patients deeply resent being told that they have a functional illness, and scorn physicians making such a diagnosis. They become resentful and sometimes even hostile.

2. Again, the matter of time. A prescription can be given to the patient ever so much more quickly than insight.

3. Being insecure about his diagnosis, the physician is afraid to take a firm stand for medicolegal reasons. This is usually the by-product of hastily gathered clinical evidence.

4. The physician is convinced that the patient hasn't got the intellectual or emotional capacity to accept the truth and to build constructively upon it, and hence he feels obligated to provide a series of pseudo-organic crutches.

Whatever the reason, many patients are deprived of the opportunity to get well because the real nature of their trouble is never crystallized for them by their physician, and hence they continue to limp through life, supported by wobbly iatrogenic crutches.

Tragically, functional disease is frequently infectious and environmental, and it causes pollution so that not only is the patient made sick by it, but family members are as well. It is only the physician who can alter this destructive chain reaction.

A third common error occurs when the physician does inform the patient that he believes her sickness is functional in nature, but does so in such a manner that the impact is entirely negative. The patient forms a variety of wrong conclusions about herself, all of them anxiety-producing, such as the following:

1. The doctor thought her complaints were silly and frivolous, a waste of his time.

2. The doctor concluded she was imagining or pretending, "putting on," or even malingering.

3. The doctor regards her as inadequate or queer or different, as losing control of herself, or sick in her mind and bound to get worse. She feels trapped by her own personality and life circumstances, and sees no way out of her situation. Panic begins.

A fourth error is substituting tranquilizers for meaningful communication between patient and physician. More often than not, I have found the so-called "mood drugs" to be of disappointing value in these circumstances, and sometimes they are even harmful. They may increase the patient's depression, or produce peculiar and unfamiliar sensations of unreality and lack of control, which may lead to panic.

The role of tranquilizers in these problems should be minor; and they should be most cautiously employed, to my way of thinking.

Lastly, the diagnosis of functional disease is often followed by the advice that the patient should forthwith see a psychiatrist.

As pointed out by Dr. Louis Hamman years ago, the majority of patients with functional disorders do not need a psychiatrist, because in most instances the factors involved are quite familiar to all of us. Many we have met in our own lives. Hence, we should be capable of dealing effectively with them.

After all, the psychiatrist has no magic problem-solving wand that we do not have. In dealing with these matters, we often feel that the patient expects more of us than we can deliver, and so we draw back. We are uneasy because we can't provide ready solutions to the patient's problems. Actually, what is wanted (and a great many times, all that is needed) is sympathetic listening and understanding, and most of all, sound practical advice. These are things we should all be able to provide.

Early referral to a psychiatrist is sometimes mandatory, for it is the internist who often first sees serious personality and emotional problems.

A number of readily observed indicants of the severity of functional illness are as follows: weight loss, sleeplessness, dependence upon drugs (or alcohol), impairment of memory and concentration, inability to cope with usual responsibilities of home and job, inappropriateness of affect, peculiarities of behavior and tics, despondency accompanied by self depreciation, hysteria, and severe somatic symptoms (vomiting, diarrhea, etc.).

If the presence of any of these indicates a serious emotional or personality disorder, immediate consultation with a psychiatrist is in order.

Some of the principles of management we have found helpful are as follows:

Appropriate diagnostic studies must be carried out to exclude all pertinent organic possibilities. Unless these are eliminated to a reasonable degree by objective means, the patient will think that the physician is relying upon an "educated guess" and that he has not been given the benefit of modern diagnostic techniques that might have revealed some hidden or unusual organic disease. There is a relationship between the need for laboratory tests to satisfy the desires of the patient and the skill and carefulness with which the initial examination is carried out. The less these qualities are demonstrated at the initial interview, the greater the subsequent need for "a battery" of laboratory examinations.

It is frequently difficult and sometimes quite impossible to determine whether a particular illness is emotional or organic in origin. There are many very important organic disorders that mimic functional illness. These include the collagen vascular disorders and brain tumors and other forms of neoplasia, to name but a few. In his efforts to exclude organic illness, the physician is confronted by the difficult problem of striking a wise balance: He must avoid the two extremes of testing too little and of "shooting the works" diagnostically, and aim for the reasonable exclusion of organic disease through the performance of a small number of thoughtfully selected examinations. The ability to do this well is a hallmark of the mature clinician. Will the data obtained from this particular study significantly affect the patient's management? The answer to this question is a helpful criterion of the value of any test.

In the study of patients with functional disorders there are certain diagnostic procedures to avoid, since performance of them occasionally leads to an intensification of symptoms or the development of a new set of complaints. Only the soundest reasons should impel one to advise an exploratory operation in these circumstances, for very often it will not give a conclusive answer and instead of helping to convince the patient that he has no organic illness, it only compounds his complaints. Nor is the patient benefited by being assured that some minor or unrelated condition found at operation, such as adhesions or a cystic ovary or a retroverted uterus, is producing the presenting symptoms. Such an assurance may quiet her complaints temporarily but sooner or later she will become ill again, oftentimes worse than before, until a straightforward attack is made upon the actual basis of her emotional disorder. Operative procedures have no place in the management of suspected functional disorders unless there is no other way of excluding health-threatening organic diseases. Even then they should not be undertaken until the physician has very carefully prepared the patient emotionally to meet the stressful aftermath of the operation.

Among other procedures frequently carried out that may not be well handled by such patients are spinal puncture, myelography, and infiltration of peripheral nerves with agents such as alcohol and procaine. Although usually benign in themselves, these procedures may be followed by more severe and disabling symptomatology. This is especially true of the injection or cutting of the peripheral nerves or nerve roots. Usually, one such needling leads to another, the resulting dysesthesia aggravating the patient's emotional disorder, and a vicious circle develops. Not rarely this type of circumstance has culminated in drug addiction. I recall an exceedingly anxious, neurasthenic young woman who had persistent, localized disabling left chest pain. I was persuaded to observe the effects of an intercostal nerve block. Unfortunately, during this "simple" procedure, the patient developed a pneumothorax. Afterward the pain persisted, and in addition there was a whole new series of respiratory symptoms.

In his eagerness to come to a definite conclusion regarding the emotional or organic nature of his patient's complaints, the physician sometimes forces a diagnostic conclusion when the available facts do not yet warrant a final opinion. He would be wiser to be content to halt and observe the progress of his patient, for it is often the evolution of the patient's illness over a period of weeks or even months that finally reveals its emotional or organic character.

During this period of observation, drugs having effects that might further cloud an already confused clinical problem should be avoided. For example, a 17 year old girl with vague musculoskeletal aching and easy fatigability was recently studied in a setting of serious conflict with her parents. Although her physician strongly suspected that her illness was emotional in origin, she was given methyl-prednisone in large doses. Her subsequent course was complicated by the appearance of "moon" facies, ecchymotic patches on the legs, epigastric burning, and marked weakness in the muscles of the lower extremities. Similarly, the clinical course of a purely emotional disorder may be given a confusing and misleading organic appearance through development of a reaction to one of the antibiotic agents, sometimes administered for some minor infection.

It is distressing to hear a patient with functional pain say, "At first my doctor gave me codeine but now I have to take meperidine—although he warned me to take as few as possible." The patient with functional disease is extremely vulnerable—a sitting duck for drug addiction. A young mother seen recently with atypical facial pain that began shortly after her husband committed suicide is a case in point. Having first been treated with a number of injections into the nerve roots, she was then given codeine and now is addicted to meperidine. Her original disability has become seriously compounded.

The administration of various sorts of injections, steroids, or antibiotics and even the performance of major surgical procedures are sometimes excused on the basis of the "patient's insistence." Emotional disorders are overcome only when the patient has learned self-discipline. A physician who cannot dominate his patient's therapeutic program cannot hope to instill this essential quality in his patient.

Once the initial examination and diagnostic studies have been completed, the patient should be told the result of each test, and its significance. The normality of each result should be emphasized. It is most important not to mention results that are equivocal or dubious or of no pertinence to the present problem. A patient should not be told that her "electrocardiogram shows slight depression of the T waves" or that her cholesterol is "a little on the high side." The hastily added postscript that "these findings really do not mean anything" usually does not repair the damage done. Patients are frightened more often than not though they deny it, and inwardly they suspect the worst of themselves. Knowing little about medical affairs, they cannot dismiss "an old scar of the left apex" with the same nonchalance as their physician. A small doubt is planted, anxieties begin to grow, and new symptoms soon blossom.

The experienced clinician recognizes the fact that his words will have not only a special meaning for the patient but also a considerable effect upon him, and so he chooses them with the greatest care. Before speaking to a patient, he plans exactly what he wants that particular conversation to accomplish, and he assiduously avoids any phrase or implication that his knowledge of the patient tells him would be harmful.

The differences between organic and functional illness should then be simply and yet vividly explained to the patient. It is essential at this point to describe not only what functional disease is but also what it is not, since there are so many misconceptions about it. It should be made clear that functional illness is not "imagining you are sick," "putting on," or "wanting to be sick." It is not malingering, nor is it a manifestation of "personal weakness" or "going crazy." The *commonness* of this type of illness should be emphasized in the strongest terms. Explain that sooner or later, to a greater or lesser degree, all humans are touched by it; hence, it is best regarded as a by-product of our very human nature.

While it is something that must be brought under control, it is not to be denied, or feared, or to feel shameful about. Point out that the very human qualities which, when not well disciplined, cause functional illness, are what make human nature warm and sensitive and responsive to the needs of others. Those who never cry may also never laugh. Clarification of these points will do much to reduce the wall of shame and fear and pride that sometimes separates patient from physician.

The nature of functional illness is usually readily understood if presented to patients as a disorder of the "automatic" nervous system that controls and coordinates the function of all the organ systems of the body. It should be emphasized that although this system is independent of the human will, it is exposed to the influences of internal and external forces, including emotions and personal circumstances. The reality of this interplay of emotions and physical state can be convincingly brought home by simple illustrations of what the patient meets constantly in everyday life: When he is embarrassed, his face flushes because of the opening up of little blood vessels in the face; when he is frightened, they close, and he becomes pale; his heart beats fast when he is excited; he may vomit from fear or have diarrhea from tension; and when under stress, he passes more urine.

The patient should then be told that there is no doubt that his major disorder is functional and not organic in origin. The physician must be straightforward and not hedge if the patient voices skepticism or frank disbelief or even antagonism, as oftentimes happens. To compromise at this juncture and suggest that perhaps some physical condition such as menopause or hypothyroidism or low blood pressure may be playing a significant part frequently aids and abets a life of chronic complaints, disability and unhappiness for patient and family alike. The patient must gain a true understanding of what is really wrong; otherwise, full recovery may be impossible. If in addition to the basic emotional disorder some organic abnormalities of lesser significance are found, the patient must of course be told about them, but always in such a way that they are recognized as *minor* issues not to be substituted in any way for the major problem.

Unfortunately, some physicians are reluctant to talk to their patients in such a direct and uncompromising manner about emotional disease. They may suggest that "nerves," fatigue, tension, or worry have some role in their patient's sickness, but too often they lose a major therapeutic opportunity by lamely adding that this or that minor structural abnormality may also be a significant factor. The patient frequently retains only the part of the diagnosis that he likes, and hence, unless the physician drives home the truth uncompromisingly, there is little hope of changing the patient's sick mode of living. He must be divested of this conviction of organic disease if he is to recover; no one can do this but his doctor. Often, the physician is happily surprised by the constructive manner in which most patients ultimately accept this straightforward evaluation of their symptoms. Human beings are endowed with a faculty for recognizing the truth, even when it is distasteful, and if the true facts are thoughtfully presented to the patient, he will eventually accept them. With acceptance of the truth, progress toward recovery will have begun.

The next step is to outline for the patient what he must do to overcome his emotional illness. At this point he is often disgruntled and may state that he would much prefer something that "could be cut out" or "just treated with medicine." It is encouraging to point out to the patient that he is in reality most fortunate, since he has an illness that potentially can be completely eradicated. By contrast, many organic illnesses are either incurable or associated with varying degrees of permanent disability. Perhaps it will take a long time and large amounts of determination and self-discipline to conquer his illness, but the same things are required in coping with any chronic organic disease. His personal stake in learning to manage this illness well is exceedingly high: It means an end to his inadequate way of living (in which his entire family may share) and a return to peace, satisfaction and joy in life. The physician must emphasize that this can actually happen if the patient will only wholeheartedly take the following steps to recovery:

First, he must develop an understanding of the nature and meaning of functional illness: What it is; how its effects are produced; how it differs from organic disease; and its intimate relation to emotional and circumstantial factors in life.

Second, he must accept without reservation the assurance that his illness is in fact emotional and not some unrecognized organic process. This acceptance must be real, and not simply lip service to his physician.

Third, over a period he must acquire an understanding of the total factors both within and without himself that have led to this illness. This will not be easy, for some will be forgotten, others not recognized, and still others perhaps deeply hidden.

Many patients will still interrupt to say that although they fully understand the concept of functional disease, they could not possibly have such an illness themselves, because they "haven't a worry in the world; the children are well; my husband has a good job; we have a nice income and a fine home—what could possibly be making me sick?" To such patients, it must be pointed out that the factors generally causing functional disorders are matters dealing with interpersonal relations. These are subtle matters that affect man's deepest emotions; they are not obvious extrinsic problems such as a mortgage or an acutely ill child. They include unrequited desires, ambivalent feelings, frustrations, resentments, fears, and insecurities.

Two examples illustrate the important part played by interpersonal relations in functional illness. Through no fault of his own, a man is laid off of work because of a business recession. He may worry a great deal about this, but not become functionally ill, largely because the action that caused him to lose his job was an impersonal one, and not a direct attack upon himself or his work. Another man has been working faithfully for 15 years, with the constant goal of someday becoming foreman of his division. His friends have always told him, "Tom, you are surely slated for it." Unfortunately, a fellow worker, much his junior, is given the job "because of special technical training." In this situation, the man is likely to become functionally ill, even if given a salary raise for his "long and faithful service to the company."

Having acquired some insight into the factors that appear to have been significant in the genesis of his illness, the patient must study what may practically be done about them.

Here, many patients become profoundly disheartened because they regard themselves as trapped by factors that they cannot eliminate. It is most important, therefore, to point out that what is necessary is reasonable alteration and modification of a practical sort, and not necessarily elimination of the factors. Very few people can eliminate all the undesirable conditions of their lives. Most must alter and modify, avoid and substitute. The mark of emotional maturity and health is the willingness and ability to make such necessary personal compromises wisely and with relative facility. The attainment of this kind of emotional maturity is essential for the patient with functional illness. It is the only way he can get well. It can be acquired only through firm self-discipline.

Finally, the patient should be reminded that he need not search for a formula that will assure a blissful degree of happy living. Rather, he should set his sights considerably lower, to a level of reasonable satisfaction in living where one has to give at least as much as one gets, and sometimes more. This is the level reached by men of emotional maturity. The patient must be made to understand the difference between blissful living on the one hand and existence as a chronic emotional invalid on the other, and that the middle path, best taken, is a life containing reasonable satisfaction.

If, despite the patient's best efforts, he is unable to recognize the factors within himself or his circumstances that are causing his illness, or is unable to modify them successfully, he must seek help from someone with special training and experience in such matters. Such a person might be the patient's regular physician, a psychiatrist, or a wise minister, priest or rabbi.

In all sickness there is considerable fear, and the patient who recognizes or is told that he has a functional disorder often has very special and destructive fears—fear that he is different, or inadequate, or that he is losing control of mind and ultimately of his life. These fears can mount up to a state of panic over a given period, and hence it is essential to head them off at the earliest opportunity. I have repeatedly found that doing nothing more than removing this fear and self-depreciation almost at once results in considerable improvement. These patients, therefore, as already stressed, should be told of the great commonness of functional illness—that it is indeed a rare person who at some time in life does not endure it, to a greater or lesser degree. It is an illness shared by all beings. From a therapeutic standpoint, it is most beneficial to foster in the patient the conviction that although he may be sailing through rough waters, he has a steady hand on the helm and is in full control.

It is a singularly difficult management problem when the physician strongly suspects that the patient's illness is emotional, but is not yet in a position to altogether exclude the possibility of some obscure organic disease. In such a precarious position, the physician may be reluctant to lean in one direction or the other. His resultant neutrality may do great harm to the patient, who may seize upon this lack of decisiveness as tacit confirmation of his fears that there actually is some hidden organic disease.

In these circumstances, the physician must have the patient's full confidence. His judgment must carry great weight, and his opinion must be final. In this regard, nothing creates more confidence within a patient than allowing him adequate time to tell his whole story, followed by a meticulous physical examination. The physician who *listens patiently, questions thoughtfully,* and *examines carefully* is never without the confidence of his patients.

After the examination results have been reviewed with the patient, it is a good plan to then state that in your opinion all the evidence very strongly points to a functional disorder, although in all frankness circumstances do not immediately permit the absolute exclusion of some latent organic disease. Furthermore (and this point should be driven home emphatically), the meticulous examination just completed has failed to disclose any significant abnormality in any of the organ systems. Hence, even if the passage of time should disclose some organic condition, there is no *present* evidence whatsoever that any deterioration of the patient's general physical status has occurred.

The physician is now in a position to discuss the nature of functional disease, and how such disorders can be overcome. He should give the patient a simple, supportive, symptomatic program to follow, and advise him to return for periodic check-ups.

This approach leaves both physican and patient in a satisfying position. The patient has been given a definite opinion about his complaints, albeit not necessarily a final one. The door has been opened wide for fruitful discussion of possible emotional factors in the patient's illness. Additional time is available for latent structural disease to become evident. The value of this watchful period is not impaired by the use of therapy having confusing side effects. Having taken note of the great care with which all of the evidence was gathered and analyzed, the patient feels secure and confident of the future.

Obviously, the effective accomplishment of this approach to patients with functional disorders places very heavy demands upon the physician. He must be able to exclude with skill and certainty important organic disease from problems that are often highly complex. Even more, he must be able to induce the frequently reluctant patient to accept and pursue a therapeutic program based upon firm self-discipline. No other clinical problems require more of the physician. As Hamman (1939) has so well stated:

> It takes little time and is no tax at all upon the mind to order numerous tests and swiftly tabulate the morbid conditions they reveal; whereas it requires great patience and much serious thought to gather the particulars of a patient's constitution and environment and to assemble these data into a background for the illness. The busy practitioner seeing 20 or 30 patients a day cannot afford the necessary time, and as a rule the consultant is preoccupied with the search for recondite lesions. Every physician who interests himself, even if only a little, in these matters, is well aware of the trying and exhausting nature of the diagnosis and treatment of psychoneurotics.

Finally, I would like to re-emphasize the economic dilemma in which physicians who care for patients with functional disease find themselves. They desire to use the type of approach described here, and yet the patient often cannot afford to pay them adequately for the considerable time that this approach requires. The alternatives—to treat the patient symptomatically for some minor or supposed organic disorder and avoid the basic issues, or to refer him immediately to a local psychiatrist—are thoroughly unsatisfactory for both physician and patient.

This problem is but one of a large number that remain a challenge in the care of patients with functional illness. The importance of rehabilitating these patients is incalculable. They are legion, and because of their emotional sensitivity they are often highly gifted. Functional illness is frequently destructive to the healthful, happy, and productive living of both the patient and his family. Effective treatment of it can lead to a restoration of happiness for all concerned.

THE PATIENT WITH A FUNCTIONAL DISORDER

Allan, F. N., and Kaufman, M.: Nervous factors in general practice. JAMA 138:1135, 1948.
Hamman, L.: Relationship of psychiatry to internal medicine. Ment. Hyg. 23:177–189, 1939.
Myer, E.: Psychosomatic concept—use and abuse. J. Chronic Dis. 9:298, 1959.
Roberts, B. H., and Norton, N. M.: Prevalence of psychiatric illness in medical outpatient clinics. New Eng. J. Med. 246:82, 1962.
Tumulty, P. A.: The approach to patients with functional disorders. New Eng. J. Med. 263:123, 1960.

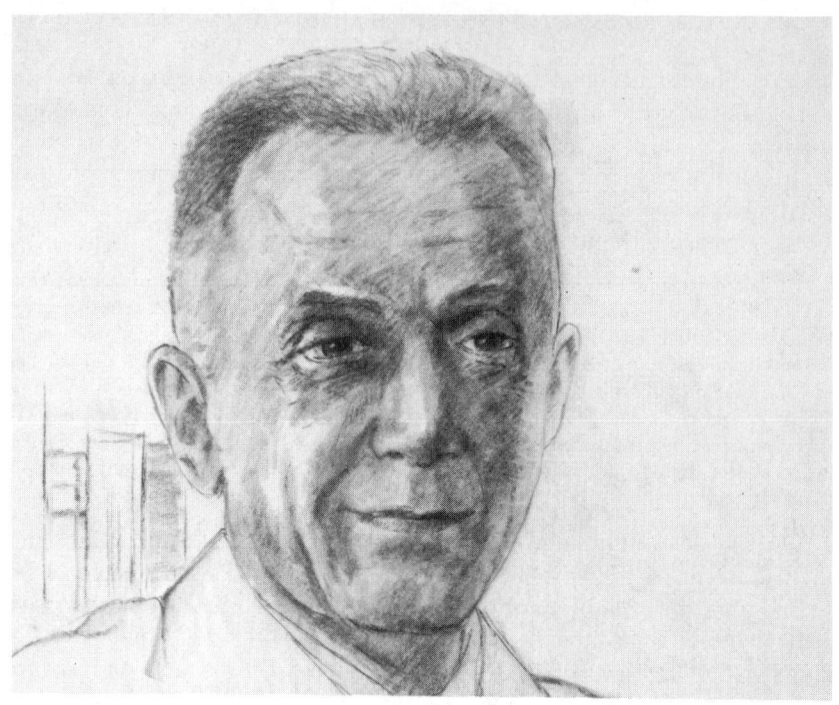

Arnold R. Rich
PROFESSOR OF PATHOLOGY

Dr. Rich was brilliant, and he brightened wherever he was; he gave vitality and enthusiasm to whatever he was doing. One so eminent might have been aloof, or too self-occupied, but no matter how cluttered his day, he would find time to push back his chair from his desk to discuss questions, ideas, and problems, often brought by those just commencing their scientific careers. He would be critical and viewpoints had to be defended, but he challenged the questions constructively and took pains not to discourage or deflate. Most of all, he infused determination to get to the truth. He was particularly tolerant of the enthusiasm of the beginner and did not awe or overwhelm him. He had high respect for new and imaginative thinking, even the most innovative.

He loved to converse and found pleasure in discussing almost any subject. Open debate and vigorous discussion were his forte; he relished having the last word, but when bested, he would give in with supreme aplomb.

Dr. Rich contributed to our fundamental knowledge in many areas, and his points of view carried great weight. He spoke with authority, yet as one still seeking the answers. Some of the brightest sessions many can recall were his Monday afternoon conferences and his Wednesday CPC's. During these, he was incomparable, imaginative, exciting, challenging, and dramatic, with the flair of the showman. He enjoyed to the full, and so did the crowded audiences, this splendid delivery of information and discussion of ideas. One easily learned a great deal from him, and what one learned was difficult to forget.

Dr. Rich left behind an example and inspiration. The example: that we teach best what we are learning ourselves, and this through associations with persons younger than we are. The inspiration: his vitality, his blithe spirit, the breadth of his concern, and above all, his devotion to the quest for truth and to the enrichment of younger people through teaching.

3

The Patient with Fever of Unknown Origin (FUO)

INTRODUCTION

Few clinical problems are as challenging and difficult as that presented by the patient who has had a febrile illness for more than 10 to 15 days, the origin of which remains obscure. No type of illness puts to a stronger test the physician's ability to approach a clinical problem effectively and to manage it proficiently, hence the inclusion of this chapter, devoted solely to a discussion of fever of unknown origin, or *FUO*.

BODY TEMPERATURE

The *normal body temperature* undergoes a diurnal (daily) variation from about 97.5° F. during the early morning hours of sleep to as high as 99.2° in late afternoon or early evening. In most patients with fever, the temperature curve—although above normal—still tends to follow the same pattern, with higher levels occurring in late evening. This is also the time when the spikes of a widely swinging or hectic fever usually occur. Rectal temperature tends to be about a degree higher and axillary temperature about a degree lower than the oral reading. In most seriously ill patients the rectal temperature should be followed, since it is more accurate.

Factors Affecting Body Temperature. Factors (other than disease) that tend to raise body temperature include exercise, hard work, and emotion. Children generally manifest greater variations in normal temperatures than adults. Dehydration may result in a significant fever in infants, but generally not in adults unless it is of a marked degree.

Certain individuals, predominantly female, normally exhibit a low-grade elevation in temperature (up to 100.5° F.) in late afternoon. Such patients with habitual hyperthermia also tend to react to emotional stimuli by slight elevations in temperature. This leads to the question of whether anxious depression alone can produce an FUO. In my experience it never has, if one defines "fever" as an alteration of body temperature greater than the evening physiological variations just described. Many depressed persons exaggerate the significance (and at times the degree) of these normal diurnal swings.

Patients with extensive skin disorders may have disturbances in the heat-dissipating mechanisms and accordingly tend to become febrile in hot weather. Patients who have undergone sympathectomy or who are taking atropine or related drugs may show a similar phenomenon, which may also be induced by some of the drugs used in the treatment of parkinsonism, and some of the ganglionic blocking agents.

Fever Pattern. Fever tends to have a particular pattern. The types of fever pattern usually observed are: (1) *sustained* or continuous fever with little or no variation throughout the day; (2) *remittent* fever with greater than one degree variation during the day but with the temperature remaining above normal; (3) *intermittent* or *quotidian* fever with daily elevations but with the temperature returning to normal each day; and (4) *relapsing* or *recurrent* fever characterized by a day or more of fever interspersed with one or more days of normal temperature.

The heat-regulating mechanisms operating through the peripheral circulation and sweat glands can generally prevent excessive elevations of body temperature that might threaten life. Thus, oral temperatures exceeding 106° F. are unusual. Marked hyperthermia is most often observed in patients with meningitis, cerebrovascular accidents, encephalitis, tumors of the hypothalamus, after brain surgery, or following trauma to the upper cervical spinal cord. Other conditions sometimes causing elevations above 106° F. are lymphomas, acute yellow atrophy of the liver, thyroid crises, and fulminant pancreatitis. Infections often associated with fevers above 105° F. are those of the urinary tract due to gram negative bacilli, typhoid, brucellosis, tularemia, tuberculosis, malaria, relapsing fever, and leptospirosis. By contrast, some infections are characterized by low-grade or even no fever. Diphtheria may not cause elevations above 102° F., and cutaneous anthrax and sporotrichosis are often associated with a mild febrile response. In general, however, the degree and type of fever pattern is of no great aid in differential diagnosis, as will be brought out later.

THE DIFFICULTIES OF DIAGNOSIS

There are a wide variety of causes of FUO, categorized as follows:

1. Infections
   a. Localized
   b. Generalized

2. New growths
3. "Collagen-vascular" or "auto-immune" disorders
4. Drug reactions
5. Granulomatous processes (sarcoid)
6. Hyperthyroidism
7. Blood dyscrasias
8. Nonspecific enterocolitis
9. Malingering (factitious)
10. Liver disease
11. Central nervous system (CNS) disease
12. Peculiar disorders of unknown etiology, such as Mediterranean fever, periodic fever, Waldenström's macroglobulinemia, Whipple's disease.

The differential diagnosis between these can be exceedingly difficult, and at times it may be impossible to establish the specific cause of such an illness by clinical means alone. This is because many of the diseases of diverse origin that commonly present with prolonged, undiagnosed fever have identical clinical manifestations. Chronic infections, new growths, collagen-vascular disorders, drug hypersensitivity states, enterocolitis, leukemias and granulomas—the most common causes of FUO—may all be associated with irritability, malaise, headaches, anorexia, weight loss, chills, sweats, various skin eruptions, arthritis, myositis, neuritis, enlargement of the spleen, liver, or lymph glands, alteration in blood elements, such as hemolytic anemia and thrombopenia, and abnormalities in the serum proteins and, in particular, hypergammaglobulinemia.

The sameness of many of these clinical manifestations is due to the fact that all of these disease states are capable of similarly affecting immune mechanisms, and the resultant clinical or laboratory alterations are often the products of these commonly shared immune effects. There may be absolutely nothing specific about these effects and the resultant clinical or laboratory changes they produce. For instance, identical mucocutaneous eruptions may be seen in all of the widely differing disease states listed above—erythema nodosum, purpura, Sjögren's syndrome, migratory polyarthritis, myositis, a marked increase in gammaglobulins, or the appearance of macroglobulins and other peculiar proteins, including antibodies against red blood cells or platelets, or amyloidosis. Repeatedly one is confronted by a number of changes each of which could be associated with a wide variety of quite different types of disease processes, all of which have the capability of presenting to the physician with chronic fever. One has to look through these nonspecific changes and try to discover the *specific* nature of the underlying process. This can be extremely difficult. The problem is made even more complex by the fact that, for varying periods of time—months, and sometimes even years—the only clinical evidence of these kinds of disorders may be fever of varying degrees and duration, perhaps associated with such general symptoms as irritability, malaise, easy fatigability, headaches, anorexia, and so forth.

An appreciation of the complete lack of specificity of most of the clinical alterations associated with disorders presenting as undiagnosed fevers is basic to their proper evaluation and sorting out.

While a number of laboratory, x-ray, and other procedures may be helpful, and the importance of laboratory tests is not to be minimized, the mainstay of the clinical approach to the problem of the patient with FUO remains the analysis of the data derived from an accurate, complete history and physical examination. The meticulous collection and analysis of such data should be the physician's primary concern.

THE PATIENT'S HISTORY

Family History

Information on the health status of family members may be helpful, as the patient may have acquired his illness through such a contact. A family history of tuberculosis, hepatitis, or typhoid fever, among other conditions, may be significant. The patient may also have acquired his illness by exposure to some common cause of illness that has affected other members of the family, as for example, faulty plumbing, a sick parakeet, or some industrial intoxication.

Some disorders previously regarded as individual occurrences may have a hereditary basis. One example is systemic lupus erythematosus, which may be a genetically determined state expressing itself in a variety of clinical syndromes in different members of the same family. The family history of a patient with systemic lupus erythematosus (SLE) may disclose members who have had rheumatic fever, rheumatoid arthritis, scleroderma, Sjögren's syndrome, hemolytic anemia or thrombopenia, goiter due to Hashimoto's disease, agammaglobulinemia, or a false positive test for syphilis. One 36 year old woman entered the hospital with a high fever of three weeks' duration, and musculoskeletal aching. The examination was unrevealing, as were all the routine studies. She had a sister with rheumatoid arthritis, an aunt who had had her spleen removed because of a "queer" anemia, and a mother who had a goiter removed which "had a funny Oriental name." Studies for LE cells were positive.

Past History

A detailed knowledge of the patient's past health is of special importance. The "collagen-vascular" or "auto-immune" disorders, of which systemic lupus

THE PATIENT WITH FEVER OF UNKNOWN ORIGIN (FUO) 141

erythematosus is an example, now rank among the more common causes of obscure prolonged or episodic fever. Their natural course is commonly drawn out over many years, with episodic appearances of active disease. Over a span of 15 to 20 years or longer, a patient may have episodic involvement of the skin, joints, muscles, serosal surfaces, kidneys, or bone marrow elements, among others, either singly or in confusing combinations.

Since unexplained fever is a common clinical presentation of these disorders, the importance of a searching historical system review is clear. A 44 year old female with chronic fever, malaise and a purpuric rash is a case in point. Some 15 years prior to admission she was thought to have rheumatoid arthritis. This subsided, and she had been well for five years when she had an episode of pneumonitis in her right mid-lung zone. This persisted for several months, and was designated a "virus pneumonia." About five years later, a period of good health was interrupted by the development of dry eyes and mouth and parotid swelling, which was diagnosed as Sjögren's syndrome. Three weeks before admission, she was given penicillin for some minor infection, following which she developed a persistent fever and a purpuric rash, considered to be a reaction to the penicillin. She was admitted for study because of a persistence of fever. By searching back into this patient's history and discovering the earlier episodes, one can readily surmise that the present fever and purpura is not an isolated illness, but rather another chapter in a long, drawn-out illness that is now expressing itself with these symptoms. The logical answer to this patient's undiagnosed fever—systemic lupus erythematosus—is indeed what she was found to have.

THE PRESENT ILLNESS

In obtaining the history of the present illness, it is imperative to pay strict attention to even the smallest details concerning the onset of the symptoms, for trivial details may hold the answer: Where was the patient when the illness began? Precisely what was he doing? Where had he been? Had he had any contact with animals or other possible carriers of disease?

Patients tend to start their stories not at the beginning (which is often not specific or dramatic) but at a later period. A patient may begin his account with a description of pleurisy in the right chest of three weeks' duration, and ignore the fact that for four months he has been cranky, unable to get his job done, and experienced sweating at night. The physician/historian must constantly press the patient to go back to the earliest and most insidious beginning of his illness. He must not merely accept uncritically what the patient thinks to be the onset.

One must also be wary of casting aside as "silly" or "inconsequential" little details that patients (or their relatives) have come to believe may be pertinent to their illness. There is a tendency among physicians to accept as valid information only that data which make sense to us. *All* of the data must be taken and weighed, and a diagnosis reached which fits *all* of the facts.

Finally, it is often profitable to repeatedly review the history with the patient. One may feel after taking the history that this part of the patient's work-up is completed, and that attention can now be turned to other diagnostic approaches. On the contrary, new information gathered from a variety of sources should make new lines of questioning pertinent. Repeated questioning of the patient is a basic approach to the study of unexplained fever.

While all of these points have been discussed previously in the chapter on history-taking, repetition of them is not superfluous, for they are vital to the disclosure of the real cause of an FUO.

The Physical Examination

Repeated, even daily physical examination of the patient is yet another basic approach to this difficult clinical problem. A physical alteration not present one day but noted the next may disclose the answer. As with items in the history, it is oftentimes the seemingly small, unimportant and unobstrusive physical changes that are the valuable clues. These are frequently transient alterations, such as petechiae, or changes requiring time for their development, such as a murmur in acute bacterial endocarditis. Unless the patient is completely examined each day until the reason for the fever has been ascertained, vital information may be overlooked. The details of physical examination are discussed in Section B, Chapter 1.

The Temperature Course

It is essential at the very outset to study the course of the patient's temperature. There are several items worth noting.

First and foremost, on specifically *what day* of the patient's illness are you examining him? This is of vital significance because during the early phase of an illness the symptoms and signs that are present may be quite different from those characteristic of a later period of the same process. During the first week of typhoid fever, for example, there is usually little or no evidence of an intestinal infection, the earliest manifestations generally being cough, fever, and malaise. Only during the second week may the intestinal alterations appear. Early in acute staphylococcal endocarditis there may be no cardiac murmur or anemia, whereas later in the course of this infection the absence of a murmur or anemia would be unusual. Hence, the question, "At what precise stage of his illness am I seeing this patient?" is always to be asked. The answer should strongly influence the observer's interpretation of the clinical phenomena at hand.

Whether the fever has been constant or episodic, what the patient's physical status has been during periods of remission, and the duration of the remissions may be very revealing. Hodgkin's disease is one of the more common causes of intermittent periods of fever occurring over a period of many months or even years, with relatively good health during the intervals. Bronchiectasis, various forms of viral or granulomatous pleurisy, pericarditis, Charcot's fever due to intermittent biliary obstruction, urinary tract infections, diverticulitis, systemic lupus erythematosus, Crohn's disease, ulcerative colitis, and drug reactions are other common causes of recurrent periods of fever intermingled with periods of relatively good health.

The height of the fever is not consistently helpful in diagnosis: sensitivity to phenobarbital may produce just as elevated a temperature as a pneumococcal septicemia.

The pattern of the daily temperature elevations may give limited information. For example, a daily high spiking temperature is generally regarded as indicative of a septic process, particularly of pus under confinement. Yet the same sort of daily spikes are seen in some patients with drug reactions, systemic lupus erythematosus, lymphoma, hypernephroma, and so forth. One elderly female had spiking fever with shaking chills every third day of her illness for many weeks. She was considered to have tertian malaria and was treated accordingly, but eventually a hypernephroma was discovered. A temperature curve that is highest in the morning is said to be most often associated with miliary tuberculosis, although Bennett finds it frequently in Salmonella bacteremia, among other disorders. A fever spiking twice each 24 hours (double quotidian) is characteristic of gonococcal endocarditis, but is also observed in miliary tuberculosis and other infections.

Knowledge of the drugs the patient has been receiving is very important in reviewing a patient's temperature course, since so many drugs may induce fever, or alter its course. From a diagnostic standpoint, it is helpful to know whether or not, and to what extent, a particular agent has been effective in lowering fever. Thus, failure of adequate salicylate therapy to affect the fever of a patient with polyarthritis would cast doubt upon the diagnosis of acute rheumatic fever.

While shaking chills occur more frequently in bacterial infections and with blood stream invasion in particular, they may also occur in other febrile disorders, including viral infections, drug reactions, new growths, "collagen" disorders, and others, and they are therefore of limited help in distinguishing the cause of a febrile illness. Whether a patient chills or not in response to fever seems a very individual matter indeed.

TUBERCULOSIS

Tuberculosis continues to be one of the major causes of FUO and heads the list of those most frequently overlooked. There is a tendency to dismiss tuberculosis as being no longer a common problem, and to recognize its presence only when it appears in one of its more classic guises. Again and again, patients suspected of having had some esoteric disorder are found at post mortem examination to have actually had some form of tuberculosis. In dealing with FUO, the wise physician persistently acts on the assumption that tuberculosis mut be excluded before another diagnosis is accepted.

Contrary to earlier experience, tuberculosis now occurs most frequently in elderly individuals, usually male. In this setting of old age, the constitutional accompaniments of tuberculosis are easily mistaken for those associated with the aging process itself, or perhaps with some hidden neoplastic process common in this age group. Fatigability, irritability, musculoskeletal aching and soreness, and low-grade anemia have such broad connotations in the elderly that their significance in terms of tuberculosis may be overlooked.

It may be particularly difficult to recognize tuberculosis in its disseminated form when there are no localized phenomena pointing to the diagnosis. Tuberculosis may masquerade in many guises, including that of monocytic leukemia. Its symptoms are usually totally nonspecific and the physical alterations produced are ones common to a very wide variety of disorders. Included among these nonspecific changes are uveitis, chorioretinitis, lymph gland enlargement, hepatomegaly, splenomegaly, muscle wasting, arthritis, erythema nodosum, hemolytic anemia, hypergammaglobulinemia, leukopenia or leukocytosis, and thrombopenia or thrombocytosis. The old clinical axiom that miliary tuberculosis is always associated with miliary changes in the lungs is thoroughly incorrect: the patient's course may conclude with persistently clear lung fields. The point is that the dissemination may be limited. Commonly, the liver is the first organ affected, and I have repeatedly found that thorough investigation of the liver provides the final answer in the clinical diagnosis of miliary tuberculosis, or for that matter, in any other form of miliary granulomatous infection.

Disseminated tuberculosis may run a much longer and milder course than is generally realized. Some patients continue their work for a year or longer with active disseminated tuberculosis. The extreme mildness of a patient's course may disarm the physician and delude him into excluding the possibility of tuberculosis because the patient "doesn't look sick enough."

Tuberculosis is one of the so-called opportunistic infections—those infections likely to develop in individuals with some defect in their immune mechanisms. Included among those susceptible to such infections are patients with neoplasms, blood dyscrasias, "collagen" disorders, liver disease, and diabetes mellitus.

In patients with these disorders, the clinical indications of tuberculous infection may be completely submerged by the changes of the parent disease, and hence the coexistence of tuberculosis may not be appreciated until revealed by post mortem examination. In some instances, a therapeutic trial with antituberculous agents is the only safe way of excluding this curable infection.

As already mentioned, tuberculosis may mimic monocytic leukemia, and it may be impossible to differentiate between the two on clinical grounds. This problem is intensified by the fact that the final stages of monocytic leukemia are frequently complicated by the development of tuberculosis, which is often the final chapter in the course of the former disease.

Patients receiving corticosteroids are candidates for disseminated tuberculosis, and the usual manifestations of this infection—including fever and malaise—may be masked by the steroid effect.

Biopsy of the liver, obtained either by needle punch or at laparotomy, has proven to be one of the most effective ways of establishing the diagnosis of disseminated tuberculosis. Biopsy may be positive even when all liver function tests are normal. Finding of a grossly normal liver at laparotomy should not deter biopsy since granuloma or other changes may be found on biopsy, even though the surgeon reports "a normal liver." For example, a 56 year old pharmacist who had had recurrent periods of fever and malaise for several years underwent laparotomy, and the surgeon reported all organs to be normal. A biopsy of the liver was taken anyway, and many tubercles were found. The patient recovered when given antituberculous therapy. His liver function studies had been repeatedly normal.

The finding of granulomata in the liver by no means necessarily indicates tuberculosis, for there are a number of other disorders that may produce hepatic granulomata. Included among these are drug reactions, sarcoidosis, brucellosis, tularemia, histoplasmosis or other fungus infections, and polyarteritis nodosa. Only when typical acid-fast bacilli are stained in the tissues, or cultured therefrom, can a definitive diagnosis of tuberculosis be made. The tubercle bacillus may also be sought in smears and cultures of the bone marrow.

Tuberculin skin tests are helpful but may occasionally be negative despite active disease. If there are sound reasons for suspecting tuberculosis, a negative tuberculin skin test, even when correctly performed, does not exclude such a possibility, although clearly the likelihood is reduced.

OTHER GRANULOMAS

Until recently, histoplasmosis was seriously considered a diagnostic likelihood only if the patient had been living in certain geographic areas. Now it is appreciated that the infection is much more widespread than had been previously envisioned, and its importance as a cause of FUO is greatly magnified.

As far as the clinical alterations of histoplasmosis are concerned, it has the same propensities as tuberculosis. In fact, all disseminated granulomatous infections—including all yeast and fungus infections—have similar clinical potentialities. Oftentimes, on clinical grounds alone, one can predict only that the patient probably has some kind of a granulomatous process, the determination of the specific nature of the granuloma being a biological rather than a clinical matter—hence the importance of properly performing the various skin, serological and other tests, and in particular, of demonstrating the agent in biopsy material, if possible, either by stain on culture as in tuberculosis, in which the liver is a useful site for biopsy.

Sarcoidosis is generally represented as a disorder characterized by little or no constitutional reaction. While this is correct in many instances, there are occasions when sarcoidosis is associated with a marked degree of wasting and prolonged, hectic fever. In my experience, this has been particularly true of individuals with hepatic sarcoidosis.

The appearance of severe constitutional signs in a setting of sarcoidosis should raise the question of whether the course of this initial disorder has become complicated by the imposition of another process, such as disseminated tuberculosis or fungus. This is not a rare eventuality. Again, liver biopsy is helpful in establishing the diagnosis, as are biopsies of muscle, lymph glands, conjunctivae, and skin lesions, and the Kveim test.

OTHER INFECTIONS

Brucellosis is frequently given a high diagnostic priority as a cause of FUO; yet this infection is highly unlikely in the absence of a history of contact with an infected source. In the United States, the disease is almost entirely confined to farmers, abattoir workers, veterinarians, dairy employees, and persons drinking raw milk.

Tularemia, on the other hand, does not depend on exposure to rabbits or other rodents since this infection can be transmitted by the bite of a variety of insects to which one may be exposed, or even by eating improperly cooked rabbit.

Salmonella infections are common and may follow a typhoidal course, with continual fever and chills for several weeks. Metastatic abscesses may be formed in a variety of tissues, and endocarditis may ensue. There is an increased incidence of salmonella infections in thalassemia, sickle cell disease, leukemia, cirrhosis of the liver, neoplastic disease, and after gastric surgery. The organism can localize in neoplasms or hematomas.

Very often septicemia due to Staphylococcus or Streptococcus begins without any locus of origin being evident. An insignificant puncture or abrasion may be the starting point. It is always wise, therefore, to question a patient with such a septicemia about boils, minor injuries, squeezing pimples, or pulling hairs in the recent past.

Infections due to Bacteroides are of special importance. They occur considerably more often than is generally realized, and their presence is often overlooked because they are strict anaerobes, and may be difficult to culture—particularly if the cultures are discarded too soon, as the organisms may grow

THE PATIENT WITH FEVER OF UNKNOWN ORIGIN (FUO) 147

very slowly. It is a good idea to test for Bacteroides when the setting of an illness strongly suggests infection but no organism can be isolated. A wide variety of focal infections may be produced by this organism, including retropharyngeal abscess, endocarditis, pneumonitis, urinary tract infections, osteomyelitis, and intra-abdominal abscesses located in the liver and other loci.

Recently there has been a resurgence of meningococcal infections. These may take a number of clinical forms with or without meningitis, and their presentations may be extremely disarming. For example, a 44 year old white male was seen who had had chills and fever precisely every third day for 10 months. In the intervals he felt well enough, but during the paroxysms of fever his bones would "feel like they were breaking," and he would develop peculiar hivelike lesions of varying size all over his body, particularly over the lower extremities. Blood cultures produced meningococci. This course of events is not unusual in meningococcemia.

Leptospiral infections tend to be overlooked unless the patient has a story and signs compatible with classic Weil's disease. While Weil's disease is an uncommon infection, largely confined to those who come into contact with rats, it should be recalled that there are other members of this family of organisms (L. pomona, L. autumnalis, L. canicola) that can produce an illness quite unlike the classic Weil's disease. Sterile meningitis, "pretibial fever," and flu-like illnesses are some of the clinical presentations that infections due to these organisms may have.

Another common disorder very often overlooked in cases of FUO is infectious mononucleosis. About 20 percent of those having this disorder present with only fever, malaise, and vague musculoskeletal aching, and the classic features are absent. While the febrile period usually lasts only seven to 14 days days, occasionally it may be prolonged for several weeks. The characteristic blood and serologic alterations may not make their appearance until later in the course of the disease, so that initially it may be very difficult to arrive at the correct diagnosis.

FOCAL INFECTIONS

In analyzing the likelihood of a focal infection, the observer should have a well-systematized approach so that no possibility is overlooked. It is helpful, to review in progression the pros and cons of there being a localized infection first in the brain, and then in the meninges, the pharynx, the mediastinum, the pericardium, the endocardium, the thoracic cavity, below the diaphragms, in the liver or spleen, in and about the kidneys, the abdominal cavity, the pelvis, the perirectal area, the prostate, the bones and joints, and finally, the soft tissues. If one does not adhere to such a systematized analysis, and if each possible focus is not ruled in or out in an orderly fashion, the origin of the patient's fever is apt to be overlooked.

Some of these localized infections deserve special note here. In Section

B on the Physical Examination, I commented on the difficulties encountered in establishing the presence of a hepatic or a subdiaphragmatic abscess by clinical means alone. I also stressed how easily a pelvic or even a perirectal abscess can be overlooked, and the confusing signs produced by a retroperitoneal abscess. The now widespread practice of routinely giving patients broad spectrum antibiotics postoperatively, even though the operation is deemed "clean," leads to the early obscuring of the usual clinical signs of such localized intra-abdominal (as well as intrathoracic) infections.

Charcot's fever, due to intermittent blockage of the biliary excretory ducts by any cause, is a common agency of periodic fever. Success in diagnosis of this condition depends upon one's ability to detect transient elevations of the bilirubin or serum alkaline phosphatase, or both. Therefore, as soon as the condition is suspected, base line determinations of the serum alkaline phosphatase, bilirubin, and serum amylase should be obtained with directions to the patient that he must notify the physician immediately if another episode of illness seems to be occurring. When this happens, prompt determinations of serum amylase, alkaline phosphatase, and bilirubin should be gotten, and repeated again after 12 and 24 hours. Often, a mild and very transient rise in one of these determinations tells the story. It is not unusual for the only alteration to be a brief and undramatic rise of alkaline phosphatase alone.

DRUG FEVER

Drug reactions are such an increasingly important cause of prolonged fever that the possibility of a drug-induced fever must always be an early consideration in dealing with puzzling febrile illnesses.

While some drugs are more likely to cause fever than others, it must be realized that *any* drug has the capacity to produce fever if it is given to a person who is hypersensitive to it.

A detailed drug history is essential. At the outset, the physician should explain to the patient that literally any drug or toxic agent is potentially capable of producing fever, and hence the patient must give him a detailed account of every drug ingested and all possible contacts with toxic materials. The patient should be prompted by direct questions such as, "What do you take for your bowels? For headaches? For menses?" It is surprising how often a patient will deny that he is taking a drug, only to have it become apparent later that he is sensitive to the phenobarbital in his "nerve tonic." When confronted by the fact, he may say, "But that's not medicine, and I've been taking it for years, anyway." Patients (and some physicians) fail to appreciate that a drug well tolerated for many years may abruptly begin to induce unfavorable reactions, including fever.

In the hospital it is a good practice to review the order sheets and nursing notes. Sometimes an order is left for a drug that ultimately turns out to be responsible for a persistent fever, and everyone has forgotten that the patient is still receiving it. I recall a patient who was given massive doses of antibiotics for several weeks on the suspicion that she had developed staphylococcal endocarditis after a mitral valve operation. Eventually it was realized that a running order for secobarbital at bedtime had been overlooked. When this order was stopped, the fever vanished.

Drug fevers may affect a patient's clinical course in several different ways. First, drug sensitivity may be responsible for fever de nouveau. Second, if a patient with some basic, underlying illness such as rheumatoid arthritis is given a drug, he may develop a fever that is actually due to drug hypersensitivity but is erroneously regarded as part of the basic disorder. This may lead to unfruitful investigations and the administration of still more drugs, to which additional reactions may develop. Third, occasionally a drug hypersensitivity that initially expressed itself only with fever may later become associated with the onset of a diffuse and progressive arteritis. This, of course, will markely affect the course of the underlying disorder, and may well be mistaken for it. Fourth, some disorders are associated with a predisposition to develop a variety of drug reactions, including fever. Patients with systemic lupus erythematosus are often reactive to a variety of agents. Hence, a history of drug fever or other types of drug reaction should suggest the possibility that perhaps the patient has SLE.

Drug hypersensitivity states may produce clinical changes that commonly occur in the so-called collagen disorders, as well as in neoplastic disorders, blood dyscrasias, and granulomatous infections, among others. Such drug reactions are often confused with these processes. Often the problem can be clarified only by withdrawing *all* medications, or by substituting new drugs of a dissimilar structure—for example, substitution of chloralhydrate for a barbiturate. To be absolutely avoided is the practice so frequently followed of adding more and more drugs as the course becomes more and more complicated. Clinical chaos results.

The giving of a drug may complicate a patient's clinical course not merely by the direct effects of the agent per se but also by the method of its administration. Frequently, patients given parenteral antibiotics for more than a short time begin to run a low-grade fever which often gets higher as the course progresses. This occurrence may be mistakenly interpreted as an indication of treatment failure, and another agent may be substituted, or the dosage may be increased. Unfortunately, it is not realized that the actual cause of the fever is at the site of administration of the drug, where localized necroses of soft tissues and muscle, an abscess, or cellulitis or phlebitis have developed. Secondary bacterial or fungal infections are sometimes produced in such areas by such resistant and invasive organisms as the Staphylococcus, Pseudomonas pyocyanea or other gram-negative bacilli, and various fungi. When these complications are recognized for what they are, and appropriate measures are taken, the perplexing "FUO" disappears.

NEOPLASMS

Tumors rank among the most common causes of obscure fever. While tumors of the kidney and liver, as well as lymphomas, are more likely to present with fever than some others, it is important to keep in mind that any malignant tumor has the capacity to induce fever. Fever associated with tumors may be produced in a variety of ways, such as through tissue necrosis, by involvement of the temperature regulating center, by hemorrhage, by secondary infection resulting from impaired resistance, by so-called autoimmune mechanisms, or by obstruction of a bronchus, ureter, or bile duct by the tumor mass.

The temperature may be high and swinging, and associated with chills, exactly mimicking a septic process, or it may be low-grade and indolent. Sweats may accompany the febrile periods. The long, drawn-out, intermittent course of fevers accompanying certain tumors, such as lymphomas, is well recognized. I have observed such episodes extending over a period as long as seven to eight years, with reasonably good health in between.

The possibility of tumor as the cause of fever may be overlooked for a variety of reasons. First, the frequency with which tumors present with fever may be underestimated. Second, there is often no historical or physical data pointing to the presence of a neoplasm, and laboratory changes are often nonspecific. Finally, the tumor is often not detectable as a mass lesion, even with the aid of special radiological techniques. Its presence may be heralded by peripheral manifestations suggesting a different type of disease. Bronchogenic carcinoma may present initially with severe joint pains (osteoarthropathy) that can be mistaken for rheumatoid arthritis. Lymphomas may be associated with a variety of skin eruptions; pancreatic carcinoma with polyphlebitis; carcinoma of the breast with peculiar neurological alterations; and ovarian cancer with a polymyositis; and so on. One must be highly familiar with these general disturbances produced by new growths.

Fever associated with neoplasms of all sorts, including the leukemias, is often not due to the new growth itself, but to some accompanying infection. Patients with neoplasms often have an impaired immune response which predisposes them to infection; once acquired, such infections may run rampant. For this reason, the finding of a new growth in a patient with fever does not necessarily mean that the true cause of the fever has been discovered.

Conversely, the discovery of certain types of infections in particular settings should suggest the possibility that there is an associated new growth. For example, herpes zoster and pneumococcal infections may be associated with myeloma. Underlying bronchogenic carcinoma should be considered in any male past the age of 40 who presents with a focal pulmonary infection. Amebic colitis may accompany carcinoma of the colon.

Certain "opportunistic" infections are particularly prone to occur in a setting of neoplastic disease. These include tuberculosis, the various fungal infections, pneumocystitis carinii, amebiasis, herpes zoster, herpes simplex, pneumococcal and staphylococcal infections, salmonellosis, and gram-negative sepsis.

Such infections may be dramatic in their appearance, masquerading as primary illnesses. The underlying neoplastic process may be overshadowed by the manifestations of the acute infectious process.

COLLAGEN-VASCULAR DISORDERS

If one compares the incidence of various types of diseases responsible for FUO today with that encountered some 30 years ago, two striking differences are the increased evidence of FUO induced by drugs, already discussed, and that due to the so-called collagen-vascular diseases. I believe that in most clinicians' experience, this latter group of disorders ranks with infections, new growths, and drug reactions as causes of FUO.

Any of this spectrum of disorders may present as a problem in fever, although some more so than others. Thus, prolonged fever is generally not a prominent feature of scleroderma, though it is characteristic of systemic lupus erythematosus. Many times fever—persistent or episodic, low- or high-grade, steady or swinging—is the one and only clinical change in patients with these conditions. A youngster with juvenile rheumatoid arthritis may show only fever for weeks, the rheumatic features of his illness not appearing until much later.

Again, it must be stressed that the early clinical accompaniments of these disorders may be thoroughly nonspecific, and common to a host of other entirely different disease mechanisms. Therefore, they mimic and are mimicked by a large number of other types of diseases. In polyarteritis, for example, the earliest changes are usually progressive weight loss, malaise, anorexia, and vague arthralgia and myalgia. The fever may be spiking, suggesting sepsis. The white blood cell count may be very high or very low. There may be a variety of nonspecific serological studies.

There are no easy answers to these diagnostic dilemmas. All that the clinician can do is to (a) appreciate the very high incidence of these disorders as causes of FUO; (b) understand how clinically identical their early presentations can be to one another, and to other types of diseases responsible for FUO (particularly infections and new growths); and (c) perform the appropriate diagnostic studies, recognizing that early in the course of all of these illnesses the expected specific diagnostic alterations may be absent, and may become apparent only after the passage of much time. These points stress the need for the clinician to be well versed with the many clinical vagaries of these disorders, which may unfold episodically over a long period of time—hence the need for repeated re-observation and re-evaluation of such patients.

Recently we have become aware of the great importance of another member of this family of diseases as a cause of FUO, particularly in patients past 50 years; namely, giant cell arteritis. Unexplained, chronic fever, persistent or episodic, high- or low-grade, sometimes indicative of sepsis, and associated with such nonspecific changes as anorexia, fatigue, weight loss, vague myalgia and arthalgia, depression and anxiety, and a normochromic, normocytic anemia, are all clinical features we have repeatedly observed in patients with giant cell arteritis. Some of these patients have other classic localized features of this disorder, such as temporal arteritis and polymyalgia rheumatica, and evidence for these should always be sought, but other patients present with FUO alone. To overlook giant cell arteritis—now recognized as not at all uncommon in incidence—is appalling, for it is readily controlled by appropriate treatment with prednisone. Even when all of the clinical indications of temporal arteritis are absent, it may still be diagnosed by a temporal artery biopsy.

PULMONARY EMBOLISM

When I originally read Beeson's account of 100 patients with FUO, I was surprised to find listed three patients whose fever was regarded as due to multiple pulmonary emboli. I wondered how this could be. However, in the past two years, I have encountered three similar instances. As already emphasized, presentation of pulmonary embolism is often atypical. FUO is just one more confusing clinical presentation of this common disorder.

CROHN'S DISEASE

I have become much impressed by the high incidence of Crohn's disease, and particularly by how often its initial clinical appearance is *not* associated with the gut changes one might anticipate. Rather, it presents with the nonspecific manifestations common to other types of inflammatory processes, including malaise, easy fatiguability, depression, iron deficiency anemia, malabsorption, arthralgia or arthritis, a variety of skin eruptions, including erythema nodosum, and unexplained fevers. Hence, Crohn's disease must be regarded as a potential cause of FUO even in the total absence of any of the usual intestinal features of this malady. Furthermore, the classic x-ray features of this condition are easily overlooked, if they are present at all, the cause of the patient's FUO being determined only by an exploratory laparotomy. Even with laparotomy, however, it can still be overlooked, or confused

THE PATIENT WITH FEVER OF UNKNOWN ORIGIN (FUO) 153

with other conditions involving the small or large intestine. One should recall that Crohn's disease may be familial, especially in Jewish patients.

A variety of conditions other than Crohn's disease may produce alterations confined to the terminal ileum and the cecum, and may present with FUO as the dominant problem. These include granulomatous tuberculosis of the intestine, lymphoma or other new growths, sarcoidosis, Whipple's disease, amyloidosis, and a chronic appendiceal abscess. Therefore, this region of the gut may be a highly productive one to investigate clinically, radiologically, and at exploratory laparotomy.

Yersinia enterocolitica

WHIPPLE'S DISEASE

Whipple's disease is one of the more unusual disorders often listed in the initial differential diagnoses of patients with FUO, but seldom established as the real cause of the patient's problem. There are a number of reasons for this, including the fact that this is not a commonly encountered disorder, but some clinicians may not be familiar with the two phases of the real life story of this interesting disease. One hears it said that, "I thought about Whipple's disease, but the patient hasn't had any gastrointestinal features such as malabsorption."

The life story of Whipple's disease is contained in two chapters. In the first, the obvious features of the disease are recurrent episodes of fever (sometimes with chills), glandular enlargement, pleurisy, pericarditis, pneumonitis, arthralgia and arthritis, a variety of nonspecific skin eruptions, hepato- and splenomegaly, myositis, weight loss, depression, alterations of the central nervous system, and anemia—in other words, all the clinical appearances generally attributed to a patient with some sort of collagen-vascular or immune disorder. The reason for these changes is that the patient has become chronically inhabited by a bacterial organism to which he recurrently responds in an immunologically reactive way. This organism, however, is one that is noninvasive and nondestructive; and hence it produces no suppurative alterations.

Not until the second chapter of Whipple's disease, which may be long delayed, does the patient develop gastrointestinal manifestation. These may be very mild and go undetected unless special studies are performed to disclose malabsorption or other alterations. Such gut changes are presumably due to implication of the lymphatics of the small intestine by the inflammatory reaction induced by the chronically infecting organisms already mentioned. The problem in Whipple's disease is that the second stage may take an exceedingly long time—often several years—to develop. Therefore, the early manifestations of Whipple's disease are entirely gutless. Perhaps if the clinical course of Whipple's disease were better understood, it would become a more commonly diagnosed cause of FUO.

FACTITIOUS FEVER

Probably no other single physical finding is so readily accepted on its face value as being incontrovertible evidence of organic disease as fever. However, malingering may be encountered when least expected—a patient may produce elevation of the thermometer reading by one means or another. It is therefore wise to give this possibility early consideration when dealing with a puzzling fever. It may be difficult and at times almost impossible to detect the manner in which the patient produces factitious fever. Such factitious fevers are most commonly seen in medical and paramedical personnel, or members of their families; this is also true in other types of factitious diseases.

Factitious illnesses are often a manifestation of some deep-seated psychological illness and may call for expert psychiatric management. Inexperienced management, especially brusque confrontation of the patient with the fact of his malingering, may lead to pronounced worsening of the emotional illness. Consultation with a qualified psychiatrist is therefore advisable.

Precautions to be taken in determining the patient's temperature when factitious fever is suspected have already been outlined in the chapter on The Physical Examination. Some other points which may call attention to the possibility of factitious fever are: (1) failure of the temperature curve to follow the normal diurnal variation, being higher in the morning than in the afternoon; (2) failure of the pulse to accelerate with sudden spikes of fever; and (3) rapid defervescence without sweating.

It is unfortunate when a patient who does not have actual fever, but is either malingering or is overly concerned about a normal daily physiological variation of the body temperature, is seen by a physician who fails to recognize the true nature of the problem. The physician may well start the patient on an unnecessary program of therapy—usually one or more antibiotics—obscuring the real problem, and perhaps even creating new problems; all of which could have been avoided by more careful study of the patient in the first place.

THERAPEUTIC TRIAL

As already indicated, it is frequently difficult and sometimes impossible to determine on clinical grounds alone the specific cause of an illness presenting with undiagnosed fever, and in such circumstances the question of the wisdom and usefulness of a therapeutic trial often arises.

There are pros and cons to the use of a therapeutic trial in FUO. Unfortunately, too often a therapeutic trial is too quickly substituted for a thorough investigation of the patient's illness, and such trials do more harm than good. Clearly, effective management of a patient's illness requires knowledge of its

THE PATIENT WITH FEVER OF UNKNOWN ORIGIN (FUO)

specific nature; mere suspicions, or hunches—even very canny ones—are not sound bases for definitive therapy. As a general rule, therefore, one should *not* resort to therapeutic trial in FUO, except in certain very well-defined circumstances.

A therapeutic trial in FUO usually entails the use of either antibiotics, various steroids, or antitumor agents, including radiation. All have potentially deleterious side effects that may greatly complicate an already confused problem, through the production of more fever, skin rashes, jaundice, alterations in the blood, and so on. In managing an FUO, a basic principle is *simplification of the problem.* Usually, a therapeutic trial only complicates it.

Not only may the patient's course be confused by the harmful side effects of such therapy, but any nonspecific beneficial effects which these agents have may mislead the physician, and may even lull him into a false sense of achievement. For example, a patient with a hidden liver abscess may seem to improve when given steroids, and hence valuable time is lost in bringing to bear truly effective therapy.

A therapeutic trial may also have a negative psychological effect upon the patient and the family as the patient's illness progresses. Naturally, they are all looking for the simplest way out of the problem, and the giving of some agent which produces transient improvement may induce false hopes, and dampen their willingness to embark upon some harder course, such as a longer period of observation, or an exploratory operation—which may actually be the only avenues to recovery. A therapeutic trial can become a delaying action when pushing ahead to definite information holds the single hope of recovery. If clinical judgment indicates that none of the organ systems (heart, kidneys, and so on) is being seriously impaired by the underlying process, there is no reason whatsoever to rush into a therapeutic trial. Fever alone is no cause for haste. Too often, fever becomes an alarm, leading to actions that would never be taken if a calm second thought were given to the problem.

On the other hand, rapidly advancing, life-threatening disease clearly demands the use of a therapeutic trial, but even in these circumstances there is always time to secure material for basic observations, such as blood cultures and the like.

Besides life-threatening disease, there is one other situation that may call for a therapeutic trial. There may be cases where the patient has a continuing and progressive illness, the cause of which remains obscure despite the performance of all reasonably indicated tests, and the diagnostic possibilities have been narrowed down to one or two that contain some hope of responding to specific therapy. Because of the patient's general status, a tissue diagnosis by exploratory operation or other means is not considered feasible. A specific example is that of an elderly patient with severe cardiopulmonary disease who as a result of studies completed is believed to have either disseminated tuberculosis or metastatic carcinoma. Exploratory laparotomy is considered too risky, and liver and other biopsies have not been helpful. As all other possibilities have been exhausted, giving antituberculosis therapy would seem a reasonable course of action at this juncture.

If the decision is reached to attempt a therapeutic trial, several important considerations enter into the selection of an agent. First, it should be one to which the patient is not likely to be sensitive. Second, its administration should entail the smallest possible risk for the patient. Third, to give the therapeutic trial differential diagnostic significance, the agent should be one of *limited* and, if possible, *specific* therapeutic effectiveness. Clearly, if an agent having a broad therapeutic valency is used, the patient's response to it will be of little diagnostic value. An obvious exception to this dictum is the critically ill patient for whom adequacy of treatment must be assured from the very start. In such instances, the desire to establish a specific diagnosis must take second place, and the need to rescue the patient from his critical state becomes paramount. Therefore, treatment of broad therapeutic valency must be devised so that no treatable possibilities are overlooked, since there may not be time for second attempts.

In addition to selecting the most effective agent for the particular problem at hand, one must be sure to give it in a dosage that will be effective, and hence give a clear-cut, definitive result. If a patient is suspected of having systemic lupus erythematosus, it is an error to start a therapeutic trial at a dosage level of only 20 mg., since in some instances this level of dosage is inadequate to control the disorder. Give enough of a drug to be certain of its efficacy, or lack of it. Clearly, it is also essential to continue the drug for a sufficient period of time and not halt it prematurely.

Furthermore, it is essential that the observer fully understand the various ways in which the therapeutic trial employed may affect the course of the suspected disease for which it is being given. Some patients with tuberculosis who are treated with PAS may have a sustained temperature course converted into a swinging, septic type of curve shortly after the drug has been started. This is then followed by gradual defervescence. Unless one is aware of this effect, one may reach the mistaken conclusion that the patient is becoming even sicker, and that the wrong diagnosis is being pursued.

EXPLORATORY LAPAROTOMY

The value of exploratory laparotomy in determining the cause of an FUO in some instances has been well confirmed, and it is important to consider whether such a procedure might be helpful. If the clinical evidence clearly points to a localized intra-abdominal disorder, a laparotomy is obviously in order. Often, however, there is little or no evidence pointing to intra-abdominal disease, and yet at operation the answer to the prolonged fever is discovered.

THE PATIENT WITH FEVER OF UNKNOWN ORIGIN (FUO)

A wide variety of intra-abdominal conditions may have undiagnosed fever as their single or predominant clinical feature. These include all types of intra-abdominal abscesses, various kinds of new growths, granulomatous processes such as those due to tuberculosis, fungus infections and sarcoidosis, lymphomata, granulomatous processes of unknown etiology, including regional enteritis, and immune disorders such as polyarteritis. Each of these processes and many others are capable of inducing persistent or intermittent fever, sometimes over a period of many years, and they may lie dormant within the abdominal cavity all the while. Even the most searching series of studies, repeated over a span of months and even years, may fail to disclose the presence of such processes. For example, a 16 year old boy had recurrent fever and musculoskeletal aching for 18 months. In addition to weight loss and debility, his only other complaint was of occasional loose bowel movements. Physical examination was unrevealing, as were two radiologic studies of the gut. Yet at operation he was found to have Crohn's disease.

A California real estate agent had recurrent chills and fever for seven years, although physical examination and extensive studies gave no reason for this. At operation, retroperitoneal lymph glands were found to be involved by Hodgkin's disease. It is in such circumstances, where there is little or no evidence of intra-abdominal disease, that wise judgement is needed to determine at what point the patient has been studied and observed enough and the time for laparotomy has arrived. As in all matters involving clinical judgment, only general principles can be outlined and not specific rules.

There is no such thing as a "simple" exploratory operation. Every operation has its hazards and advising a patient to undergo an operative procedure is always a serious matter. In considering the advisability of an operation, it is wise to consider not only the risks entailed if all goes well, but also what may happen if one or more complications should eventuate. The "simple operation" can easily become a complicated one.

I recall a patient whose renal studies suggested a tumor at the lower pole of the left kidney. Exploration of this was advised and a benign cyst was found. Postoperatively, the patient developed a staphylococcal wound infection after which his wound dehisced and he partially eviscerated with resultant shock. He later developed a prolonged hypersensitivity reaction to penicillin. Thus, the effects of this "simple" operation multiplied, entailing many additional weeks of hospitalization with great discomfort and at much cost to the patient.

The risks entailed in an exploratory operation are determined not only by the patient's general physical status but by what may be required surgically should a particular abnormality be discovered. It is most important that the internist and surgeon come to a clear-cut agreement beforehand as to the manner in which the various conditions revealed at the operation will be managed. It is not enough to decide that the patient can withstand just an exploration. Of equal significance is a decision regarding the patient's ability to survive various types of handling of whatever may be discovered. For example, if the clinical evidence indicates that a patient has right-sided colitis, but his general condition prohibits surgical treatment of this, it may be meaningless to prove the diagnosis by an exploratory laparotomy, and further medical treatment may be preferable. There are potential as well as immediate dangers in an exploratory laparotomy. Both must be evaluated and balanced against the benefits likely to be derived.

Thus, exploratory laparotomy should not be pursued until *all* indirect methods affording a reasonable chance of establishing a specific etiology of the FUO have been tried and have failed. Included among these methods are not only the history and physical examination, laboratory, x-ray and other special procedures but also, and most importantly, a period of searching clinical observation, during which the patient is thoughtfully re-questioned and re-examined. It is important that such a period not become a time when the patient is allowed to drift, or used as a time to add confusing forms of therapy.

The decision of when to terminate such an observation period and advise an exploratory laparotomy is a very difficult one. The physician should not jump the gun, nor should he delay too long. One must estimate the degree to which the FUO has already significantly affected the patient, or is likely to do so in the near future. Such an evaluation must encompass not only the physical effects of the illness but also the personal ones. Not being able to do one's job, recurrently "dropping out" of normal living, the psychological effects of being ill, and the financial drain of chronic or recurrent illness are all factors that should be weighed. From the physical standpoint, what is the evidence that any of the organ systems are being affected deleteriously? Clearly, significant progressive alterations in any of these systems would call for an immediate decision.

Another thing to consider is the likelihood that prolonged waiting may cause a condition that is now curable—or at least that can be held in check for a significant period—to pass to an uncontrollable stage. A decision on this point of course depends upon the diagnostic possibilities being considered.

Sometimes, despite impelling reasons for advising exploratory operation as the next step, the physician elects to "wait a little longer." Unfortunately, this wait sometimes drags on indefinitely, and it is not always employed usefully as a time of continuous clinical observation. The final chapter in this unhappy story often begins when the patient reappears, now having changes which demand immediate intervention, and which at this stage of the illness may be irreversible.

A number of factors lead to this unfortunate sequence. The patient or his family may be reluctant to embark upon an operation, the potential beneficial results of which must necessarily be presented as somewhat tenuous by the physician. However, if the physician has been meticulous in his study of the patient, has taken the time to explain each step of the way to him and the family in terms they can understand, and has by his attitude created

THE PATIENT WITH FEVER OF UNKNOWN ORIGIN (FUO)

an atmosphere of interest and competence, he should have no trouble in this regard.

More often, unwillingness to proceed with an exploratory operation stems from the physician's failure to recognize the fact that specific diagnostic information is frequently obtained from laparotomy, even in instances in which there are no clinical or other indications of intra-abdominal abnormalities. He is skeptical, and afraid to take odds which he inwardly feels are stacked against him, and so he elects to postpone an unpleasant decision. Or he chooses a therapeutic trial, with the false self-assurance that "at least we won't be making the patient any worse." When dealing with the problem of prolonged unexplained fever, the overall dangers to the patient of postponing exploratory operation, once the acceptable time for it has come, are generally much greater than the surgical risks entailed in operating upon an individual considered a reasonable surgical risk, measured by the usual criteria.

Having decided upon an exploratory operation, how should this be accomplished so that the needed information can be forthcoming? It is always most unfortunate when, after persuading a patient to undergo such a procedure, the operation is done in such a way that invaluable information is overlooked or discarded.

The internist should discuss the patient's illness in detail with the surgeon, so that there is full agreement between the two regarding the clinical possibilities to be searched for and the management of any eventualities. If possible, the physician should be present at the operation, so that he can confer with the surgeon as the operation proceeds. Having the surgical pathologist at hand for advice may also be most helpful.

Baker, based upon experiences at Johns Hopkins, has advised the following technical approach to the performance of exploratory laparotomy in FUO:

"We have routinely employed a midline incision in cases of fever of unknown etiology. This incision can be opened and closed rapidly and extended longitudinally to obtain access to any part of the peritoneal cavity. Once entering the peritoneal cavity, the liver is examined first. If any abnormality is noted, a biopsy and frozen section of the lesion is performed. In the absence of any gross abnormalities, a generous liver biopsy is obtained and sent to pathology for frozen section. A methodical examination of the abdomen is then undertaken. The gastrointestinal tract is examined first, beginning at the esophagus and examining the stomach and duodenum. The entire small bowel and its mesentery are thoroughly examined by removing these structures from the peritoneal cavity; the retroperitoneal area including lymph nodes along the iliac vessels, inferior vena cava and aorta are visualized and palpated. The cecum is exposed and palpated as is the appendix. The entire large bowel is visualized and carefully palpated for evidence of either tumor or inflammatory lesions. The spleen is exposed and examined. The lesser peritoneal sac is opened and the pancreas is visualized and carefully palpated. The gallbladder and common duct are carefully palpated for stones and other abnormalities. If the common duct is at all dilated or there is previous suspicion of partial biliary obstruction, an operative cholangiogram is performed. Both kidneys are carefully palpated and the ureters and bladder also examined. If any abnormalities are found, the involved tissue is either biopsied or removed and another frozen section obtained. These histologic sections are examined to document a histologic diagnosis which might lead to further examination of other organs. In addition, we would also like to have assurance from the pathologist that an adequate specimen is available for permanent study. In addition to the specimens for histologic examination, a second specimen is also obtained and divided into three parts for bacteriologic study. Smears and cultures of these specimens are obtained for bacteria, fungi, and acid fast organisms, regardless of the appearance of the gross lesion. Special media for anaerobic culture and media for unusual organisms, such as protoplast, should also be available. Thus, if the pathologist is unable to make a specific histologic diagnosis from a liver biopsy, a specific diagnosis might be established from the culture of the specimen in appropriate media."

Inflammatory disease is sometimes extremely difficult and even impossible to distinguish from new growth. Biopsy confirmation must be obtained. For example, carcinoma of the pancreas may be mistaken for pancreatitis, and vice versa. Terminal ileitis may not be Crohn's disease at all, but granulomatous tuberculosis. Hard lymph glands can be the product of a number of processes. New growths of all sorts may become associated with a very proliferative, nonspecific inflammatory reaction, and the hidden malignancy may not be included in the biopsy specimen. The erroneous diagnosis of nonspecific inflammatory process may be reached.

A not uncommon error is failure to adequately study the material obtained at surgery. For example, because a mass lesion is thought to represent a tumor, it is not cultured, or is cultured in only a routine way. Biopsy of the liver may be done, but the specimen may be dropped in formalin by the nurse before a piece of it can be sent for culture. A granulomatous mass due to Bacteroides, or tuberculosis or one of the fungi may be called "nonspecific" only because it has never been cultured on appropriate media. Once the abdomen is open, it is imperative that all material which should be studied is obtained, and in a form in which it can be most effectively examined. The biopsy specimen must be large enough to process in a variety of ways; the cultures must not be dried out, and must be placed on the proper media; material requiring special handling must not be regarded as "routine." The material must be put directly into the proper hands for study. Nor does the responsibility of those in charge of the patient end with such delivery. They must consult with those studying the material (pathologist, bacteriologist, etc.) to make certain that they understand fully the patient's clinical course and all of the diagnostic possibilities, so that all the necessary lines of investigation can be pursued. There is no place for the "routine" handling of specimens obtained at exploratory laparotomy.

In some instances the only abnormality found at exploratory laparotomy is an enlarged or abnormal appearing spleen. We have seen several such patients in whom the decision was made to close the abdomen without removal of the spleen, only to discover at post mortem examination later that the answer to the problem was indeed contained in the spleen. For this reason, if an enlarged or abnormal appearing spleen is the only unusual finding at operation, serious thought should be given to the advisability of removing it. In these circumstances, the special complications which may accompany removal of the spleen must obviously be weighed in the balance.

A biopsy of the skin, subcutaneous tissue and muscle, can easily be accomplished while doing an exploratory laparotomy. It is most unfortunate if the patient has to undergo a muscle biopsy at a later date to establish the diagnosis of polyarteritis.

The principles discussed for exploratory laparotomy also apply in general to exploration of the chest, mediastinum or pericardium. However, there are two matters deserving special note.

The first of these matters is exemplified by a patient who presents with a fever and a mass lesion in his right middle lobe. All studies fail to give a specific diagnosis. The suggestion is made to take a look at the lesion in his chest. The implication is that the lesion will be examined by the surgeon, palpated, a biopsy performed and the specimen cultured and then the chest will be closed. It sounds readily accomplished, but not infrequently when the chest is opened it is discovered that the only way the lesion can be adequately examined is by removal in toto. This may require a segmental resection, or even a lobectomy. Hence, if the plan is to open the chest, be certain that the patient is physically able to withstand much more than "a look," for the chances are it will be much more. Also, be certain that the patient and family fully understand how extensive the exploration may ultimately be.

The second matter refers to a diagnostic dilemma, namely, the fact that there are occasions when a specific diagnosis can't be made even though the surgeon secures a very adequate piece of representative tissue which is then studied thoroughly, histologically and biologically. This is especially true of granulomatous lesions of the lung, pleura, pericardium and mediastinum. The reason for this dilemma is that a wide variety of infectious agents, including tuberculosis, syphilis, various fungi, parasites, and certain malignant tumors, in addition to some chemical agents, may call forth an exceedingly flamboyant granulomatous inflammatory response, which is totally nonspecific and which may become so widespread as to completely outdistance the parent process. The original etiologic agent becomes a needle in a haystack of granulomatous reaction. Unless the surgeon is fortunate enough to extract this needle in the material he removes, and the pathologist is lucky enough to locate it in his searchings, the diagnosis remains obscure. This is the reason why so many punch biopsies of the pleura and small biopsies of the pericardium are valueless as far as specific diagnosis is concerned. The entire pericardium may be removed in instances of chronic pericarditis, and yet a definite etiology may not be established.

In summary, there are many different causes of fever of undetermined origin. Ultimately, in most instances, the cause is discovered to be some very common disorder, but one which is presenting in an unusual or unfamiliar manner, and only infrequently is a rare disease process responsible.

Thus, in a series of 100 consecutive patients with obscure fever studied at Yale by Beeson and Petersdorf, the following diagnoses were ultimately established:

THE CAUSE OF FUO IN 100 PATIENTS

Infections—36
Tuberculosis—11
Liver and biliary tract—7
Endocarditis—5
Abdominal abscess—4
Pyelonephritis—3
Psittacosis—2
Brucellosis—1
Gonococcal arthritis—1
Malaria—1
Cirrhosis with bacteremia—1

Hypersensitivity States—4
Granulomatous hepatitis—2
Erythema multiforme—1
Drug fever—1

Miscellaneous Disease—16
Pulmonary embolization—3
Benign nonspecific pericarditis—2
Sarcoidosis—2
Periodic disease—5
Weber-Christian disease—1
Thyroiditis—1
Myelofibrosis—1
Ruptured spleen—1

New Growths—19
Carcinomatosis—7
Localized tumor—2
Lymphoma leukemia—8
Unclassified—2

Collagen Disease—15
Rheumatic fever—6
Systemic lupus erythematosus—5
Cranial arteritis—2
Unclassified—2

Factitious Fever—3

Undiagnosed—7

Not infrequently, in managing a patient with obscure fever, there comes a time when, despite one's best diagnostic efforts, the cause of the patient's fever remains hidden. Then the difficult question has to be faced—should I treat the patient blindly, or should I take the final diagnostic step, an exploratory laparotomy?

The Mayo Clinic reported its experiences with 70 patients who were laparotomized because of FUO. We stress the fact that 30 of these 70 patients had no subjective or objective indication of intra-abdominal disease. In summary, laparotomy produced positive information in 80 percent of the 70 patients, and a definite diagnosis was established in 60 percent. In only 20 percent was nothing found. At the Cleveland Clinic 60 patients with obscure

THE PATIENT WITH FEVER OF UNKNOWN ORIGIN (FUO)   163

fever were studied. Exploratory laparotomy established the diagnosis in 51 percent. At Johns Hopkins exploratory laparotomy resulted in determination of the cause of the fever in 57 percent of 28 patients operated upon. In all but one instance, the cause of the fever could be treated, and the fever subsided on appropriate therapy.

In these three series, the morbidity and mortality due primarily to the operative procedure were said to be negligible.

Of the 100 consecutive patients with FUO studied by Beeson and Petersdorf, 32 percent died. Of those who did ultimately recover, 38 percent were considered to have done so only because the exact cause of their disease was discovered, which led to the administration of specific therapy. This experience underlines the need to exhaust every reasonable means to establish the specific diagnosis in patients with obscure fever. Otherwise, treatment is likely to be more miss than hit. The grave potentials of such therapeutic misses is further emphasized by what was discovered at autopsy in nine of the patients in Beeson's series:

> Monocytic leukemia—2
> Miliary tuberculosis—1
> Liver abscess—1
> Subphrenic abscess—1
> Ascending cholangitis—1
> Bacterial endocarditis—1
> Multiple pulmonary emboli—2

Clearly, an exploratory laparotomy is sometimes of great value in disclosing the specific cause of a fever of obscure origin. Wise judgment, however, is needed to determine the appropriate time and circumstances to turn to this procedure. If the clinical evidence at hand, whether obtained from the history, physical examination, laboratory tests or x-ray, clearly points to some type of intra-abdominal disorder, the decision for a laparotomy is a relatively easy one.

We must urge a word of caution, however, in the interpretation of symptoms and signs which seem to point to intra-abdominal disease in patients with obscure fevers, for many such disorders, although originating outside of the abdominal cavity, may be accompanied by disturbances of bowel function, nausea, distention, vague abdominal pain, soreness or tenderness, and other deceptive alterations, and, of course, mild enlargement of the liver and spleen are common to a host of extra-abdominal disorders. Therefore, unless the clinical evidence pointing to intra-abdominal disease is solid, exploratory laparotomy should not be performed until all pertinent, diagnostic studies have been completed.

The diagnostic approach must include not only various laboratory, x-ray and other special procedures but also, and above all else, a period of searching clinical observation during which the patient is thoughtfully requestioned and re-examined. Such a period must not become a time when the patient is allowed to drift, or when confusing forms of therapy are added. The art of the clinical management of patients with FUO is knowning when to terminate such an observation period, being neither hasty nor delaying too long. Against hastiness is the fact that some 20 percent of patients with FUO in Beeson's series eventually recovered spontaneously without any specific therapy. Also, we are all much too familiar with the sad fact that the decision to take "just a little peek inside" sometimes brings unforeseen hardships, and even death, upon the patient.

In general, the less objective clinical evidence there is of some type of intra-abdominal abnormality, the longer should be this period of undisturbed clinical observation. As one observes the patient, the question should be recurrently asked: To what degree is this FUO significantly affecting this patient, not only in terms of physical effects but in terms of personal effects as well? From the physical standpoint, the key question is whether any of the organ systems are being importantly affected in a deleterious manner. Clearly, *progressive* alterations call for an immediate decision. In our opinion, therapeutic trials in FUO are to be deprecated except in very well delineated circumstances, already outlined.

As previously stated, it should be re-emphasized that, when dealing with the problem of prolonged unexplained fever, the over-all dangers to the patient of postponing exploratory operation, once the acceptable time for it appears at hand, are generally much greater than the surgical risks entailed in operating upon an individual considered a reasonable surgical risk, as measured by the usual criteria.

THE PATIENT WITH FEVER OF UNKNOWN ORIGIN (FUO)

General

Petersdorf, R. B., and Beeson, P.: Fever of unexplained origin: Report of 100 cases, Medicine *40*:1, 1961.

Tumulty, P. A.: The patient with fever of undetermined origin: A diagnostic challenge. Johns Hopkins Med. J. *120*:95, 1967.

Systemic Lupus Erythematosus

Brunjes, S., Zike, K., and Julian, R.: Familial systemic lupus. Review of literature. Amer. J. Med. *30*:529, 1961.

Dubois, E. L.: Lupus Erythematosus: A Review of Current Status. New York, Blakiston Div. of McGraw-Hill Book Co., 1966.

Harvey, A. M., Shulman, L., Tumulty, P. A., Conley, C. L., and Schoenrich, E. H.: Natural course of systemic lupus. Medicine *33*:291, 1954.

Ropes, M. W.: Observations on the natural course of SLE. Medicine *43*:387, 1964.

Tuberculosis

Glasser, R., et al.: The significance of hematalogic abnormalities in patients with tuberculosis. Arch. Intern. Med. *135*:691, 1970.

Holden, M., et al.: Negative intermediate strength tuberculin sensitivity in active tuberculosis. New Eng. J. Med. 205:1506, 1971.
Munt, P. W.: Miliary tuberculosis in the chemotherapy era. Medicine 51:139, 1972.
Smith, D. T.: Diagnostic and prognostic significance of the quantitative tuberculin tests. Ann. Intern. Med. 67:919, 1967.
Stead, W. W.: The pathogenesis of tuberculosis among older persons. Ann. Rev. Resp. Dis. 91:811, 1965.
Stead, W. W.: The clinical spectrum of primary tuberculosis in adults. Ann. Intern. Med. 68:731, 1968.

Fungus and Other "Opportunistic" Infections

Baum, G. L., and Schwartz, J.: Chronic pulmonary histoplasmosis. Amer. J. Med. 33:873, 1962.
Baum, J. L., and Schwartz, J.: Coccidiodomycosis: A review. Amer. J. Med. Sci. 230:82, 1955.
Bennett, D. E.: Histoplasmosis of the oral cavity and larynx: A clinicopathologic study. Arch. Intern. Med. 120:417, 1967.
Bindschadler, D. D., and Bennett, J. E.: Serology of human cryptococcosis. Ann. Intern. Med. 69:45, 1968.
Blizzard, R. M., and Gibbs, J. H.: Candidiasis: association with endocrinopathies and pernicious anemia. Pediatrics 42:231, 1968.
Bodey, G. P.: Fungal infections complicating acute leukemia. J. Chronic Dis. 19:667, 1966.
Campbell, G. D.: Primary pulmonary cryptococcosis. Amer. Rev. Resp. Dis. 94:236, 1966.
Candill, R. G., Smith, C. E., and Reinary, J. A.: Corcidiodal meningitis. Amer. J. Med. 49:360, 1970.
Esterly, J. A., and Warner, N. E.: Pneumocystis carinii pneumonia. Twelve cases in patients with neoplastic lymphoreticular disease. Arch. Path. 80:433, 1965.
Fair, J. R.: Congenital toxoplasmosis—diagnostic importance of chronic retinitis. JAMA 168:250, 1958.
Goodell, B., Jacobs, J. B., and Powell, R. D.: Pneumocystic carinii: the spectrum of diffuse interstitial pneumonia in patients with neoplastic diseases. Ann. Intern. Med. 72:337, 1970.
Green, W. R., and Bennett, J. E.: Coccidioidomycosis. Retinal lesions in dissemination. Arch. Opth. 77:337, 1967.
Harvey, J. C., et al.: Actinomycosis: Its recognition and treatment. Ann. Intern. Med. 46:868, 1957.
Hathaway, B. M., and Mason, K. N.: Nocardiosis—study of 14 cases. Amer. J. Med. 32:903, 1962.
Heffernan, A. G. A., and Asper, S. P., Jr.: Insidious fungal disease. A clinicopathological study of secondary aspergillosis. Bull. Johns Hopkins Hosp. 118:10, 1966.
Hyde, L.: Coccidiodal pulmonary cavitation. Dis. Chest 54:273, 1968.
Khoo, T. K., et al.: Disseminated aspergillosis. Review of world literature. Amer. J. Clin. Path. 45:697, 1966.
Krogstad, D. J., et al.: Toxoplasmosis. Ann. Intern. Med. 77:773, 1972.
Lewis, J. L., and Rabinovich, S. The wide spectrum of cryptococcal infections. Amer. J. Med. 53:315, 1972.
Littman, M. C., and Walter, J. E. Cryptococcosis—current status. Amer. J. Med. 45:922, 1968.
Long, E. L., and Weiss, D. L.: Cerebral mucormyosis. Amer. J. Med. 26:625, 1959.
Louria, D. B., Stitt, D. P., and Bennett, B.: Disseminated moniliasis in the adult. Medicine 41:307, 1962.
Remington, J. S., Jacobs, L., and Kaufman, H. E.: Toxoplasmosis in the adult. New Eng. J. Med. 262:180, 1960.
Rickert, J. H., and Campbell, C. C.: Significance of skin and serologic tests in the diagnosis of pulmonary residuals of histoplasmosis. Ann. Rev. Resp. Dis. 88:381, 1962.
Rifkind, D., Faris, T. D., and Hill, R. B., Jr.: Pneumocystis carinii pneumonia. Studies on the diagnosis and treatment. Ann. Intern. Med. 65:943, 1966.
Rifkind, D., et al.: Infectious diseases associated with renal homotransplantation. I. Incidence, types and predisposing factors. JAMA 189:397, 1967. II. Differential diagnosis and management. JAMA 189:402, 1967.
Rifkind, D., et al.: Systemic fungal infection complicating renal transplantation and immunosuppressive therapy. Amer. J. Med. 43:28, 1967.

Rogers, D. E.; The spectrum of histoplasmosis in man. Med. Times 94:664, 1966.
Rubin, H., Furcolow, M. L., Yates, J. L., and Brusher, C. A.: Seminar on myocotic infections: The course and prognosis of histoplasmosis. Amer. J. Med. 27:278, 1959.
Salvin, T. B.: Current concepts of diagnostic serology and skin hypersensitivity in the mycoses. Amer. J. Med. 27:97, 1959.
Sarosi, G. A., et al.: Disseminated histoplasmosis: Results of long term follow-up. Ann. Intern. Med. 75:511, 1971.
Schwartz, J., and Baum, G. L.: Histoplasmosis, 1962. Arch. Intern. Med. 111:710, 1963.
Seelig, M. S.: The role of antibiotics in the pathogenesis of Candida infection. Amer. J. Med. 40:887, 1966.
Sutliff, W. D., et al.: Active chronic pulmonary histoplasmosis. Arch. Intern. Med. 92:571, 1953.
Utz, J. P.: The spectrum of opportunistic fungus infections. Lab. Invest. 2:1018, 1962.
Vanek, J., and Schwartz, J.: The gamut of histoplasmosis. Amer. J. Med. 50:89, 1971.
Wilson, D. E., et al.: Clinical features of extracutaneous sporotrichosis. Medicine 46:265, 1967.
Witorsch, P., and Utz, J. P.: North American blastomyocosis: A study of 40 patients. Medicine 47:169, 1968.
Young, R. R., et al.: Aspergillosis—the disease in 98 patients. Medicine 49:147, 1970.

Sarcoidosis

Camp, W. A., and Frierson, J. G.: Sarcoidosis of central nervous system. Arch. Neurol. 7:432, 1962.
Coburn, J. W.: Granulomatous sarcoid nephritis. Amer. J. Med. 42:273, 1967.
Emergil, C., Sobol, B. J., and Williams, M. H., Jr.: Long term study of pulmonary sarcoidosis. Effect of steroid treatment. J. Chronic Dis. 72:69, 1969.
Ghosh, P.: Myocardial sarcoidosis. Brit. Heart J. 34:769, 1972.
Gozo, E. G., Jr., et al.: The heart in sarcoidosis. Chest 60:379, 1971.
Hirsch, J. G., et al.: Evaluation of the Kveim reaction in sarcoidosis. New Eng. J. Med. 265:827, 1961.
Israel, H. L., and Sones, M.: Selections of biopsy procedures for sarcoidosis diagnosis. Arch. Intern. Med. 113:255, 1964.
Jefferson, M.: Sarcoidosis of nervous system. Brain 80:540, 1957.
Maddrey, W. C., Johns, C. J., Boitnott, J. K., and Iber, F. L.: Sarcoidosis and chronic hepatic disease: A clinical and pathologic study of twenty patients. Medicine 49:375, 1970.
Nolan, J. P., and Klatskin, G.: Fever of sarcoidosis. Ann. Intern. Med. 61:455, 1964.
Siltzbach, L. E.: Current thoughts on epidemiology and etiology of sarcoidosis. Amer. J. Med. 39:361, 1965.
Silverstein, A., and Siltzback, L. E.: Muscle involvement in sarcoidosis. Arch. Neurol. 21:235, 1969.
Sones, M., and Israel, H. L.: Course and prognosis of sarcoidosis. Observations on 211 patients for average of 5.8 years. Amer. J. Med. 29:84, 1960.
Spilberg, I., Siltzbach, L. E., and McEwen, C.: The arthritis of sarcoidosis. Arthritis Rheum. 12:126, 1969.

Salmonella Infections

Black, P. H., Kunz, L. J., and Swartz, M. N.: Salmonellosis—a review of some unusual aspects. New Eng. J. Med. 262:811, 1960.
Harvey, A. M.: Salmonella suis pestifer infections in human beings. Arch. Intern. Med. 59:118, 1937.
Stuart, B. M., and Pullen, R. L.: Typhoid—clinical analysis of 360 cases. Arch. Intern. Med. 78:629, 1946.
Waisbren, B. A.: Bacteremia due to gram-negative bacilli other than salmonella: Clinical and therapeutic study. Arch. Intern. Med. 88:467, 1951.

Bacteroides Infections

Bodner, S. J., Koenig, M. G., and Goodman, J. S.: Bacteremic bacteroides infections. Ann. Intern. Med. 73:537, 1970.
Felner, J. M., and Dowell, V. R., Jr.: Bacteroides bacteremia. Amer. J. Med. 50:787, 1971.

Meningococcal Infections

Carpenter, R. R., and Petersdorf, R. G.: The clinical spectrum of bacterial meningitis. Amer. J. Med. 33:262, 1962.
Hardman, J. M.: Fatal meningococcal infections. Changing picture in the 60's. Milit. Med. 133:951, 1968.
Hardman, J. M., and Earle, K. M.: Myocarditis in 200 fatal cases of meningococcal infections. Arch. Path. 87:318, 1969.
Wolf, R. E., and Birbara, C. A.: Meningococcal infections at an Army training center. Amer. J. Med. 44:243, 1968.

Leptospiral Infections

Allen, G. L., et al.: Clinical picture of leptospirosis in American soldiers in Vietnam. Milit. Med. 133:275, 1968.
Beeson, P. B., and Hankey, D. D.: Leptospiral meningitis. Arch. Intern. Med. 89:575, 1952.
Diesch, S. E., et al.: Human leptospirosis acquired from squirrels. New Eng. J. Med. 276:838, 1967.
Edwards, G. A.: Clinical characteristics of leptospirosis. Amer. J. Med. 27:4, 1959.
Heath, C. W., Jr., Alexander, A. D., and Galton, M. M.: Leptospirosis in the United States. Analysis of 483 cases, 1949–61. New Eng. J. Med. 273:857, 915; 1965.
Heath, C. W., et al.: Leptospirosis in the United States. Analysis of 483 cases. New Eng. J. Med. 273:857, 1965.
Lawson, J. H., and Michna, S. W.: Canicola fever in man and animals. Brit. Med. J. 2:336, 1966.

Infectious Mononucleosis

Clark, B. F., and Davies, S. H.: Severe thrombocytopenia in infectious mononucleosis. Amer. J. Med. Sci. 248:703, 1964.
Hoagland, R. J.: Mononucleosis and heart disease. Amer. J. Med. Sci. 248:1, 1964.
Hoagland, R. J.: Infectious Mononucleosis. New York, Grune & Stratton, 1967.
Leading Article. The cause of glandular fever. Lancet 1:576, 1968.
Penman, H. G.: Extreme neutropenia in glandular fever. J. Clin. Path. 21:48, 1968.
Penman, H. G.: Seronegative glandular fever. J. Clin. Path. 21:50, 1968.
Webster, S. G. P.: Jaundice in infectious mononucleosis. Brit. Med. J. 3:411, 1968.

Brucella

Spink, W. W. What is chronic brucellosis? Ann. Intern. Med. 35:358, 1951.

Liver and Biliary Tract

Aust, J. B., et al.: Biliary structure. Surgery 62:601, 1967.
Glenn, F.: Diagnosis in obstruction of the common duct. JAMA 191:470, 1965.
Guckian, J. C., and Perry, J. E.: Granulomatous hepatitis. Ann. Intern. Med. 65:1081, 1966.
Hanpert, A. P., et al.: Acute suppurative cholangitis. Arch. Surg. 94:460, 1967.
Howard, F. M., et al.: Common duct stone producing Charcot's hepatic fever without jaundice. Arch. Intern. Med. 103:565, 1959.
Manesis, J. G., and Sullivan, J. F.: Primary sclerosing cholangitis. Arch. Intern. Med. 115:139, 1965.
McSherry, C. K., et al.; The significance of air in the biliary system and liver. Surg. Gynec. Obstet. 128:49, 1969.
Mellinkoff, S. M., Tumulty, P. A., and Harvey, A. M.: Differentiation of parenchymal liver disease and mechanical biliary obstructions. New Eng. J. Med. 246:729, 1952.
Sherlock, S.: Diseases of the Liver and Biliary System. Oxford, Blackwell Scientific Publications, 1958.
Sherlock, S.: Primary biliary cirrhosis. Gastroenterology 37:574, 1959.
Sherlock, S.: Jaundice. Brit. Med. J. 1:1359, 1963.
Snell, A. M., and Comfort, M. W.: Unusual clinical syndromes associated with stone in the common bile duct. Amer. J. Digest. Dis. 1:312, 1934.

Tisdale, W. A., and Klatskin, G.: Fever of Laennec's cirrhosis. Yale J. Biol. Med. 33:94, 1960.
Van Heerden, J. A., et al.: Carcinoma of the extrahepatic bile ducts. Amer. J. Surg. 113:49, 1967.
Waddell, G. F.: Acute obstructive cholangitis. Scot. Med. J. 11:137, 1966.
Warren, K. W., et al.: Primary neoplasia of the gallbladder. Surg. Gynec. Obstet. 126:1036, 1968.
Watson, C. J.: Regurgitation jaundice: clinical differentiation of common forms. JAMA 114:2427, 1940.
Wenckert, A., and Robertson, B.: The natural course of gallstone disease. 781 nonoperated cases. Gastroenterology 50:376, 1966.
Zollinger, R. M., et al.: Diagnosis and management of biliary tract disease. New Eng. J. Med. 252:203, 1955.

Drug Fever

Cluff, L. E., and Johnson, J. E.: Drug fever. Progr. Allerg. 8:149, 1964.

Arteritis

Hamilton, C. R., Shelley, W. M., and Tumulty, P. A.: Giant cell arteritis: including temporal arteritis and polymyalgia rheumatica. Medicine 50:1, 1971.

Crohn's Disease

Daffner, J. E., and Brown, C. H.: Regional enteritis: clinical aspects and diagnosis in 100 patients. Ann. Intern. Med. 49:580, 1958.
Howell, J. S., and Kwapton, P. J. Ileocaecal tuberculosis. Gut 5:524, 1964.
Law, D. H.: Regional enteritis. Gastroenterology 56:1086, 1969.
Lockhart-Mommery, H. E., and Morson, B. C.: Crohn's disease of the large intestine. Gut 5:493, 1964.

Whipple's Disease

Charache, P., et al.: A typical bacteria in Whipple's Disease. Trans. Ass. Amer. Physicians 79:399, 1966.
Chears, W. C., et al.: Whipple's disease. Amer. J. Med. 30:226, 1961.
Farnan, P.: Whipple's disease—the clinical aspects. Quart. J. Med. 28:163, 1959.
Maizd, H., et al.: Whipple's disease: A review of 19 patients and the literature. Medicine 49:175, 1970.
Ruffin, J. M. Whipple's disease—evolution of current concepts. Amer. J. Digest. Dis. 11:580, 1960.
Trier, J. S., Phelps, P. C. Eidelman, S., and Rubin, C. E.: Whipple's disease; light and electron microscopic correlations. Gastroenterology 48:684, 1965.
Whipple, G. H. A hitherto undescribed disease characterized anatomically by deposits of fat and fatty acids in the intestinal and mesenteric tissues. Bull. Johns Hopkins Hosp. 18:382, 1907.
Yardley, J. H., and Hendrix, T. R.: Combined electron and light microscopy in Whipple's disease. Bull. Johns Hopkins Hosp. 109:80, 1961.

New Growths

Boggs, D. R., and Frei, E.: Clinical studies of fever and infection in cancer. Cancer 13:1240, 1960.
Browder, A. A., Huff, J. W., and Petersdorf, R. G.: Significance of fever in neoplastic disease. Ann. Intern. Med. 55:932, 1961.

Factitious Fever

Bunin, J. J.: Factitious disease: Clinical staff conference at the National Institute of Health. Ann. Intern. Med. 48:1328, 1958.

Exploratory Laparotomy

Baker, R. R., Tumulty, P. A., and Shelley, W. M.: The value of exploratory laparotomy in fever of undetermined etiology. Johns Hopkins Med. J. *125*:159, 1969.

Geraci, J. E., Weed, L. A., and Nickols, D. R.: Fever of obscure origin—the value of abdominal exploration in diagnosis, JAMA *169*:1305, 1959.

Scott, P. J., et al.: Benefits and hazards of laparotomy for medical patients. Lancet 2:941, 1970.

Sheon, R. P., and Ommen, R. A.: Fever of obscure origin. Amer. J. Med. *34*:486, 1963.

Miscellaneous

Markowitz, M., and Gordis, L.: Rheumatic Fever. 2nd ed. Philadelphia, W. B. Saunders Company, 1972.

Reiman, H. A.: Habitual hyperthermia. A clinical study of 4 cases with long continued low grade fever. Arch. Intern. Med. *55*:792, 1935.

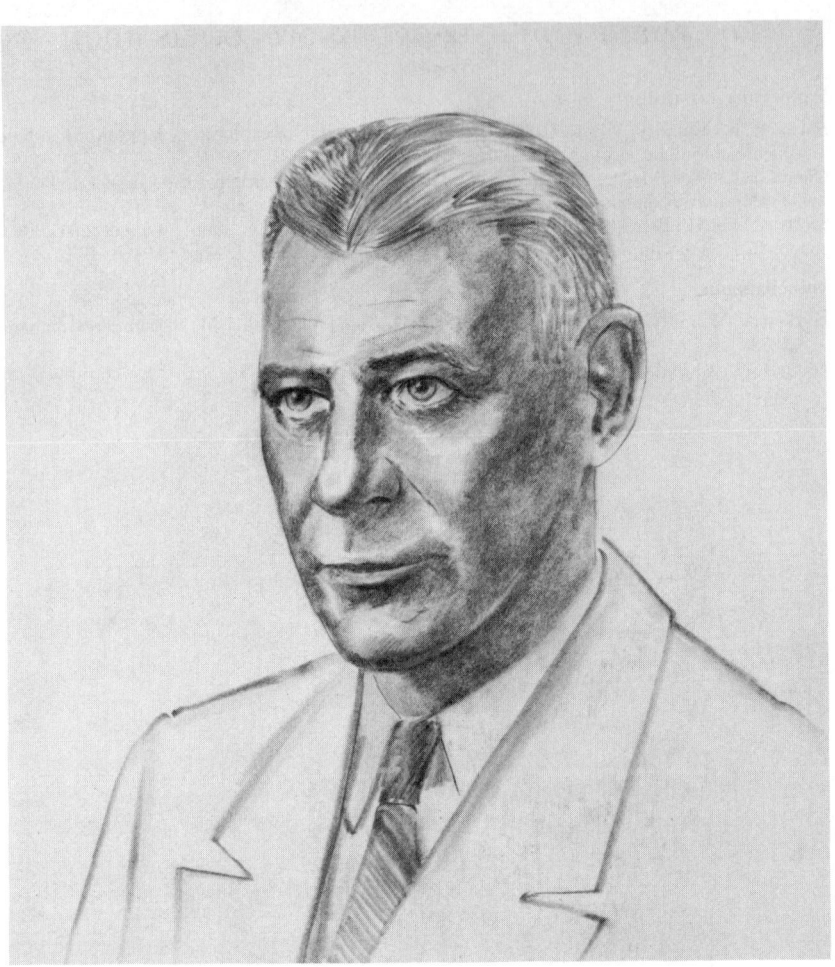

Alexander Schaffer
PROFESSOR OF PEDIATRICS

Although a pediatrician by bent (and such a superb one!), it was no effort for this brilliant man to become, of necessity, Chief of Medicine of the 18th General Hospital, the Johns Hopkins unit serving in the Southwest Pacific and the China-Burma-India theaters in World War II. Dynamic and forceful, he began creative work the moment the unit landed, helping to bring scientific order and sense out of a chaotic state of malaria control. Dr. Schaffer was ebullient, precise, direct, far-reaching in his interests and knowledge, and in some very dismal weather and times, he sustained the group's clinical sharpness, and kindled its desire to continue to learn. He challenged us by his own superb performance. Later, he returned to Baltimore to practice and to teach pediatrics. Fortunate were the mothers and youngsters who received his care—and he gave it to them wisely and gently, from a background of the most sophisticated clinical experience. To anxious, frightened parents he brought assurance, for he so patently knew precisely how to go about treating even the most difficult illnesses. To the flustered new mothers, he gave comfort and confidence, for he took the time to explain in detail the nature of even the simplest malady, and satisfied their simplest questions. His book, Diseases of the Newborn, virtually established the new speciality of neonatology, and continues to be its classic reference.

4

The Patient with Incurable, Progressive or Fatal Illness

INTRODUCTION

The clinical problem of incurable, progressive or fatal illness is one in which the science of medicine oftentimes must play a role secondary to the art of practice. To conduct a patient "successfully" through such an illness, the practice of medicine must be more than either a science or an art—it must be a *vocation*, for to treat such a patient places heavy demands upon the physician in terms of psychological stress and expenditure of time. Clearly it is hard to keep plugging along, consistently putting out one's best efforts, when confronted by a completely hopeless situation. Unfortunately, once the diagnosis of incurable, progressive or fatal illness has been established, there is sometimes a tendency for the physician to "let down"—to allow his interest and efforts to diminish. He may find himself inadvertently and subconsciously attempting to see the patient less and less frequently and to make the visits as short as possible. He may begin to feel that he is meeting his responsibilities fully with just a quick visit during which he gives the patient a pat of encouragement.

What is actually meant by conducting a patient through this kind of illness "successfully"? The expression includes two fundamental items: First, the total *physical effects* of the illness must be modified and kept under control as effectively as possible, to the very end. Secondly, the patient's equanimity must be sustained throughout the illness. This means the instillation of *hope*.

Hope is one of the essential ingredients of human existence, without which life is dark and cold and frustrating. It maintains strength and gives substance to courage. In the presence of hope, suffering of all sorts still has some positive qualities. In its absence, suffering is a completely negative experience. With even a modicum of hope, one can tolerate hardships, and still dream, and still imagine, and still plan, and still reach out for life. Without hope, none of these things makes sense. If I can hope, I can live. If not, I'd be better dead.

REQUIREMENTS OF SUCCESSFUL MANAGEMENT

What does the successful management of this kind of illness impose upon the clinician?

1. The investment of a great deal of his time.

2. Selfless devotion to a problem with which he doesn't get "results" in the usual sense of the word. The result to be sought is the maximal degree of betterment of the patient's condition. One may have to settle for very little, sometimes, but to a patient with chronic discomfort and disability, a 10 percent improvement or relief may have a 100 percent psychological impact.

3. Great ingenuity, for the physical and psychological effects of this sort of illness may be most difficult to modify, and the physician who is not imaginative and relies upon the obvious, or is readily discouraged, or who does not aggressively seek out new therapeutic approaches, will have little success. He must strive for any degree of relief of his patient's condition with the same inquiring zeal as he would for full recovery in other circumstances. In dealing with fatal illness, there is no room for complacent, sad shaking of the head. Thoughtful, inventive, aggressive attempts to better the patient's state to any degree possible is what is required.

4. A perceptive understanding of human nature, for the clinician will have to out-guess and pre-guess the patient's questions and reactions.

5. Bottomless patience, for individuals with fatal or progressive disease often become very demanding and fretful and querulous. They and their families may lose faith in their physicians, and at times even become antagonistic.

6. The clinician will have to support not only the patient but the family as well, and not infrequently the family will require far more support than the patient.

7. The physician must learn to employ the technique of "gradualism." By this is meant that he must have a comprehensive understanding of the natural course of his patient's illness and the changes that may occur in his patient during it. He must be able to foresee how the patient will react both physically and psychologically. He must always be prepared to support the patient to a maximal degree, both physically and emotionally. He must understand that one and the same illness may follow a variety of courses in different patients, and that various patients react in different ways to one and the same physical alteration. The physician must be able to meet all changes in an illness in a step-wise fashion and to even anticipate them before they happen, so that he is in a position to prepare the patient for the changes and thus to modify their impact.

WHAT TO TELL THE PATIENT

I disagree with the philosophy that many physicians espouse of spelling out "the whole truth" to the patient with incurable, progressive, fatal illness.

In my experience, it is a very rare individual indeed who can manage "the truth" well if it does not entail at least some degree of hope. Many patients insist that they want to be told "everything." When this is done, the results may be far from salutary. Often such patients immediately begin to hear the bell toll. They become depressed and fretful, overconscious of their physical condition, frustrated, resentful, and querulous. They may feel compelled to read about their condition and to ruminate about what has happened to other patients whom they know or have heard about with the same disease. Some respond by persistently looking for the miracle cure, journeying from clinic to clinic, searching for the impossible answer, and with each fruitless visit becoming more resentful and despondent. Their fears and frustrations increase. With the sword of Damocles poised over their heads, they can't even enjoy what time they may have remaining.

It is regrettable to see a patient who could have six months or a year or even longer of reasonably happy and productive living deprived of this experience because he has "been told all." With the development of chronic depression and anxiety, and often a new set of symptoms, such patients frequently find it quite impossible to carry on normal family relationships. How can they possibly be natural, gay, and nonchalant in their relationships with their spouses and families when always in the background is the awareness that "I know that you know that I know. . ."? For example, it becomes impossible for a husband and wife to pretend or to dream or to imagine together. Planning ahead becomes a ridiculous, empty thing, for there, between them, constantly sits the spectre of progressive, fatal illness.

Obviously, what the patient should be informed about his illness differs greatly from circumstance to circumstance depending upon the following: (1) the nature of his illness; (2) the particular circumstances of the illness; (3) the age of the patient; (4) his intelligence and perceptiveness; (5) his emotional makeup; and (6) what the patient's expressed desires are in the matter (again, one has to be very cautious because many patients insist that their physician "tell me all" although they really don't want to be told anything that isn't good news); (7) the family setting; (8) the kind of treatment the patient will have to undergo in the future, as for example, a major operative procedure or cobalt therapy; (9) the realistic outlook for the future; and (10) the type of disabilities the patient may develop in the future, likely complications, and so forth.

The physician has to review and analyze all of these factors as he asks himself the question: "How can I present to this patient an explanation of what I know to be the facts regarding his health status in such a way as to accomplish most effectively the following?"

1. To give the patient enough insight to satisfy his intellectual curiosity and to answer his immediate questions;

2. To motivate the patient to do whatever must be done to manage his problem medically in the best possible way;

3. To set the stage to meet future exigencies as changes in the course of the patient's illness take place;

4. To establish within the patient the belief that the future still contains some reasonable degree of hope.

This approach may at times entail withholding the truth from the patient altogether, as for example when chronic lymphocytic leukemia is discovered in an elderly person who is handling his disorder very well; or it may entail varying degrees of *molding* the truth. The latter approach substitutes for instant, complete and detailed frankness, long-term, compassionate management of the psychologic and physical problems of the patient and his family.

In explaining the patient's health status to him, the following 10 points are worthwhile keeping in mind:

1. Make the explanation simple and uncomplicated.

2. Explain the illness so that it makes sense in terms of what has happened to the patient in the past, what is happening to him now, and what is likely to happen to him in the future.

3. Do not attempt to explain any more than the present circumstances demand and do not answer questions the patient hasn't yet brought up. Here we again emphasize the value of "gradualism." As the patient's illness advances and changes, new questions will come up and new answers will have to be given. But wait for the questions to arise and then give the answers. Don't try to foretell everything here and now. Stick with "Chapter 1" of the patient's disease, and explain the others as the pages turn.

4. Don't use the name of the disease or technical expressions unless absolutely forced to do so. Such expressions as systemic lupus erythematosus, myeloma, multiple sclerosis, and so forth are all phrases which may engender fear. Thus, multiple sclerosis is better described to the patient as "a chemical or metabolic change in some of the nerve cells that prevents them from conducting nervous impulses normally." In this explanation the word *some* and not *all* (of the nerve cells) should be stressed, as well as the fact that at times this defect is overcome and the nerves begin to conduct normally again. Again, myeloma, rather than being described as a malignant tumor, may be portrayed as a disorder in which the scavenger cells of the bone marrow—the plasma cells—reduplicate excessively and overgrow some of the other cells in the marrow. It should be emphasized that treatment is available to make such cells behave, and that, as a matter of fact, such cells often spontaneously control themselves: stress that long good health is not incompatible with the condition. In other words, mold the facts to accent the positive and to generate confidence for the future.

5. Emphasize the *good* features of the patient's present health status. For instance, a patient with a tumor in his colon may be reassured by being told that his blood picture is normal, that his blood chemistry shows no abnormalities, that his heart and lungs are clear, and that his liver is functioning normally, and so forth, even though these normalities may have little or no bearing on the basic problem.

INCURABLE, PROGRESSIVE OR FATAL ILLNESS

6. Stress the *commonness* of the patient's condition so that he doesn't conclude that he has some unique disorder that may be unfamiliar and baffling to the medical profession. It is comforting to know that one has something that many other individuals have had, for this implies that a great deal must be known about it and that it can't be so thoroughly horrible after all. Inform the patient that a very great deal is known about his condition even though knowledge of its specific cause may not be at hand. It must be terrifying to realize that one has a progressive disease that is rare and obscure, with little known about it or its management.

7. Explain carefully to the patient that all diseases have a *spectrum of severity*. Thus, on the one hand, an important disease may be very mild and affect a person's health minimally, whereas on the other hand the same disease may be widespread and advance rapidly and progressively. The example of a well-known disease such as tuberculosis is helpful in this regard, it being explained that one patient may have only a little spot of tuberculosis in his lung, which doesn't affect his health appreciably, and in another patient the tuberculous infection may be disseminated and progressively destructive. The patient is then reassured that in assaying the severity of his particular illness all indications are that his disorder is not on that part of the spectrum where rapid advancement has occurred or is anticipated. Meanwhile, measures will be taken to prevent advancement of the disease in the future. Assure the patient that many individuals who have his kind of disorder handle it very well indeed, and lead happy and productive lives, and that there is sound reason to anticipate that he will have the same good fortune.

8. Mention that a great deal of research is being carried on in an effort to learn more about the patient's particular disorder and its effective treatment, and that you are familiar with these developments and will make certain that the very latest information is brought to bear in handling his illness.

9. Reaffirm that although it is true that it is not possible to cure the patient's illness in the sense of eradicating it completely, nevertheless, a great deal can be done to keep it within bounds and to relieve the symptoms that it produces.

10. Finally, emphasize to the patient that you will make sure that an optimum program of management is worked out for him, and that you will see to it that he gets all that modern medicine can provide.

Some of the common arguments in the philosophy of "telling the facts just as they are" include (1) the patient may need to see a priest or a minister or a rabbi, or to get his business in order; (2) he may have some things that he desperately wants to do before he becomes incapacitated; (3) he may lose confidence in you, his physician, when he begins to suspect that you are stringing him along, and not being frank.

In my experience, most sensible patients guess what is going on, and quietly, in their own way and in their own time, get themselves ready to meet death. The thoughtful patient guesses the truth and prepares himself for the eventualities without having them brought out into the garish light of inevitability. He plays games with himself, with his physician, and with his family. The advantage of this technique of *not* being totally frank is that the patient *can* play games: his own games with his own rules. When the physician confronts the patient with the blunt truth, there can be no games, no imagining, no pretending. Inevitability makes all of these impossible.

It is one thing to be told hard, immutable facts by one's physician, who is after all the expert and therefore knows what he is saying, and quite another to just *suspect* the truth. How many of us would be able to carry with equanimity all of the burdens that life ultimately piles on top of our backs if we knew from the beginning that they were coming, and had them clearly predicted and described and pointed out to us beforehand. To some extent, we are able to bear them because they have been hidden from us and have come out of the unknown, unheralded and unpredicted. It is a fact of living that we are all each day dying, one step nearer to the inevitable. "We know not the day nor the hour," but the fact that the exact time and nature of our end is shrouded in clouds of indefiniteness enables us to maintain a certain unspoken conviction of invincibility. Deep inside, we all feel that somehow "I'll escape, I'll get by, it's not going to happen to me." A physician who always frankly speaks the whole truth strips away this indefiniteness from death and ends this dream of invincibility.

What is the difference between being informed that you have a cancer that will run a fatal course in a predictably short time and being told by a judge that you must "hang by your neck until dead on such and such a date"? No doubt, there is an occasional patient who will resent anything less than the blunt, factual approach. However, at the very start of one's career in clinical medicine one must adopt philosophical commitments about recurrent matters of great significance, and follow them consistently. It is my conviction that over the great span of one's clinical work, the type of approach outlined here will bring more peace to more patients with progressive, incurable, fatal disorders than will the approach of confronting them with the implacable truth.

Note carefully that the family and any other physicians who may be involved in the care of the patient must be briefed regarding precisely what the patient is going to be told and what the philosophy of his management is to be. There must be complete mutual agreement about this. Confusion can be ruinous to the patient's morale. One has to be particularly careful in informing surgeons, other consultants, and members of the clergy.

GENERAL PRINCIPLES OF MANAGEMENT

A number of general principles that may be of considerable helpfulness in managing progressive, incurable, or fatal illness have evolved from my experiences.

The patient should be examined carefully each time he has a new specific complaint even though it may be minor in nature. Not to do so, and to simply reassure the patient by saying, "I'm certain that doesn't mean anything," suggests to him that either his physician is no longer interested or, even worse, that he believes that the patient is in such a hopeless state that it is no longer worth bothering to investigate his complaints and to effectuate appropriate treatment.

Depending upon his status, the patient should be seen at frequent intervals—but not *too* frequent, lest the patient gain the impression that he is really not deriving very much improvement from his visits to the physician and that he is "getting the run-around." It must not appear that the physician is ineffective and really doing little more than stalling for time. Thus, there may be real psychological value in saying to the patient "You are now doing so well that I won't need to see you for six to eight weeks," or "I want to see you every four weeks or so in the future and then, as you improve, we can spread the visits out at longer intervals." Such remarks give the patient the impression that things must be going fairly well after all and that there is no frightening urgency to his illness.

In talking to the patient, it is imperative that the physician seem casual and confident regarding the patient's future. He may say, for example, "Why of course you can take a trip—why in the world shouldn't you?" Such a remark, casually delivered, will help to give the patient self-confidence and will support the conviction that he is not in any immediate likelihood of getting into serious trouble after all. It will give him an important feeling of independence.

The treatment program, whatever it is, should be changed from time to time, even if in only a very simple and unimportant way. If the program is never altered, the patient may quickly come to the conclusion that he is "sunk" because he isn't getting symptomatically better, or perhaps he is getting even worse, and yet his physician is continuing the same old program. The patient is led to conclude that all therapeutic possibilities have been exhausted and that it is just a matter of time before his illness will become terminal. On the other hand, changing the program, even in unimportant ways, will give the patient the impression that his illness is still subject to change, and that there are still things that can be done to affect it with some hope of betterment yet in the offing.

The physician should be psychologically prepared to adequately meet the changes that he knows are going to occur in the patient as the illness progresses and he should properly prepare the patient for them. For example, the physician should say to the patient, "For a while you may find that you have some distention of your abdomen and looseness of your bowels" or "The pain may get worse in your arm because of the inflammation produced by the treatment." It is essential that the patient not be shocked or surprised by events when they do happen. The physician must try to outguess the patient's questions and have at hand simple, reasonable answers for him so that he won't panic.

When some unfortunate new development does appear, the clinician must not act overly concerned but rather handle things in a confident and even casual fashion. He might say, for example, "This sort of development is not at all infrequent in your kind of illness and is one that we are well familiar with; we can take care of it in time," or "We anticipated that this might happen, so don't be dismayed—we can handle it."

The patient should be given plenty of time and opportunity to vocalize all of his questions and fears. The answers should not be complicated, long-winded, or involved, but rather simple and direct statements that make plausible sense to the patient. Technical expressions should always be avoided.

It is important not to over-restrict the patient or to over-treat him. If he will be happier and have less discomfort with Plan A but perhaps not live as long as if placed on Plan B, by all means follow Plan A.

The patient should be kept in his own environment doing ordinary, everyday things for as long as is practically possible. The clinician should attempt to get the patient to develop new interests and hobbies to supplant any that are no longer possible.

Only essential drugs should be given to such patients. The so-called "mood" drugs are sometimes helpful, but they may do more harm than good by inducing peculiar sensations that can increase the patient's depression, lead to panic, and create the conviction that he is losing control of himself. The use of narcotics must be paced very carefully so that they will not be least effective at the time the patient needs them most. Under no circumstances should the patient ever be told the actual nature of the drugs he is getting for the relief of discomfort. Sometimes the use of alcohol in moderate quantities may be beneficial in relaxing the patient and in giving him a sense of well-being. At times, prednisone has general beneficial effects. When the end is drawing near, drugs that give a sense of euphoria should be used. Don't give sedatives when what the patient needs is some agent to relieve pain, and vice versa. Whatever drug is being used, give a dose large enough to be effective. To assist the patient during his final decline, the use of drugs that relieve discomfort and create a sensation of well-being is much better than any form of treatment associated with significant discomfort.

When seeing his patient in a progress visit, the physician should stress and dwell upon any little betterment of his condition, even though it may not really be very important. For example, it can be comforting to say to a patient, "Your heart certainly sounds fine today and your circulation is first-rate" or "Your lungs are much clearer than they were" or "This rash seems to be disappearing" or "Your blood chemistry is better than it was."

It should be recalled that all illnesses, no matter what their nature, have natural ups and downs. Even fatal disorders wax and wane. It is the physician's job to minimize the downs and to maximize the ups. Thus it may be helpful at the outset to explain to the patient: "This type of condition may persist for a long time. We can't look ahead and tell you just how long. During its course, you will have some ups and downs. There will be times when you will feel much better and others when you will feel less well. When you feel under par, remember days will follow when you will begin to feel better. It will take time and much patience on your part, but eventually there will be more good days and fewer bad ones. Meanwhile, we will work together."

In dealing with progressive, fatal illness, so-called "heroic" forms of treatment should be assiduously avoided unless there is some reasonable chance of significantly bettering the patient's outlook. The psychological and physical comfort of the patient should be the main guidelines of management—not how long his physician can keep him alive through use of the latest scientific maneuvers. In some situations the continuance of life is not nearly so important as the conclusion of an existence free from the miseries of physical and psychological discomfort. By the same token, the physician must realize that to some patients even a few months of additional life may be exceedingly precious for a whole host of reasons, and if the patient can be given this additional time to live in reasonable comfort, he obviously *must* be given it. I recall a lovely young wife with four youngsters whose husband began to drink and philander. The wife and children were made miserable. When told that his wife had cancer, the husband stopped drinking and once again became a devoted husband and father. The family had 12 months of happy togetherness before death finally came.

It is exceedingly unfair for the clinician to ever put the family in the position of making final decisions regarding the longevity of the patient. They may express their feelings and the physician should gently and carefully sound them out, but in the end it is a decision *for the physician alone* to make. Bringing the family into such a decision is asking them to make a judgment they are not qualified to make, since they cannot possibly understand the patient's medical problem with the insight available only to his physician. One thing that must not happen is that the family be left with any sort of guilt feelings when the patient finally makes his departure.

The clinician should recall that "fatal" or progressive illnesses occasionally take a surprising and even amazing turn for the better, and the patient may fare better than anyone thought possible. Therefore the physician should never assume for himself the role of God in making critical decisions or pronunciamientos as if he were omniscient.

This brings us to a consideration of what a physician's attitude should be regarding *letting the patient die.*

Here again, and most importantly, we are dealing with a matter of career-long philosophical commitment. The physician's basic responsibility is to support life whenever possible and to relieve suffering, both mental and physical, at *all* times. It is wrong for a physician to regard himself as a judge or an arbiter in these matters. He cannot say to himself, "This patient I save; this patient I let die." It is easy to let oneself become less cautious about such matters and to make more and more judgments of a critical sort with less and less reason and balance. Surely we have all seen so-called "hopelessly ill" patients live whom we were certain would die. The clinician is not a sociologist or a priest or a judge. He is combating death and trying to support life not in the abstract but in the case of John Smith, who for this or that reason may not have much community or other value. In making his judgment, the clinician must not consider any issue other than his basic responsibility to this particular patient.

It is clear-cut that a clinician must never cause death directly by a positive act. On the other hand, there are times when the use of extraordinary means to support life is cruel, and all religions permit physicians to let the natural course of events proceed in such circumstances. Thus, a physician is not required at all times to do everything possible to continue life through the employment of every available means.

When does this principle apply?—when death is inevitably at hand because of processes which cannot be significantly altered, and the patient is undergoing mental or physical suffering which cannot be controlled with ordinary means. To fit this definition, the following conditions must be fulfilled:

1. The physician must be positive that the patient has an immutable process which cannot be effectively altered. This judgment must not be just a casual estimate. It is one of the most serious decisions that a physician can possibly make, and therefore, he *must* seek consultation in arriving at it.

2. Death must be immediately at hand—not remote or just probable.

3. Ordinary means to secure comfort and support for the patient must have been exhausted; again, consultation should affirm that this is a fact.

4. There must be a note in the clinical chart by the responsible physician, and also by the consultant, stating the reasons for their decision.

THE FAMILY IN INCURABLE, PROGRESSIVE OR FATAL ILLNESS

General Considerations

The essential goal as far as the family is concerned is that the patient be enabled to maintain reasonably normal relationships with them for whatever time he has left. Again, it seems very unlikely that he will be able to do this if the family is given a completely hopeless view of his future by the physician. Members of the family need at least some hope in meeting his critical situation just as does the patient. Despair can become infectious and epidemic—and so can hope and optimism. Hence, the physician should communicate whatever must be told the family with as much hope as he can possibly dredge up out of the situation, even if it is very meager. Stark realism is often more than the family can withstand. Thus it may be necessary to "mold" the truth somewhat. Here again, "gradualism" may be helpful: The total truth is revealed in small doses as the illness unfolds, affording the family the opportunity to get its feet under itself before another blow falls. Dumping the total truth upon the entire family early in the game and depicting in stark

INCURABLE, PROGRESSIVE OR FATAL ILLNESS

realism what lies ahead can be devastating. The patient and the family need to be eased into the truth—not slugged with it.

Specific Suggestions

Here are some specific suggestions that have been found to be beneficial:

The physician should speak in general terms and be judiciously vague in some of the things that he tells the family. He might say, for instance, "Some patients with this type of disease at times surprise us and do very well indeed for a long period of time," and make other statements in the same vein.

Technical terms should always be avoided, as well as involved, detailed descriptions. The physician should say enough to establish understanding and insight, but he should not deliver a medical synopsis.

The physician should never let himself be put in the position of predicting when this or that event is going to befall the patient. One of the first questions that families always ask is "How long will he live?" and this is one question the physician should generally avoid answering. Experience shows that such predictions are often incorrect, many patients living for a much longer or shorter time than the physician has calculated, and the setting of such dates only increases the despair and panic of the family. On the other hand, if the patient has an illness associated with a great deal of disability and discomfort, and prolongation of life may mean only continued misery, it is important for the physician to make it clear that this will not have to be endured indefinitely.

There are some issues on which the physician should be very specific and positive and certain in speaking with the family. These include the following:

1. He should make it clear that he does, indeed, know the nature of the patient's illness, that the diagnosis has been soundly established, and that he has embarked upon the best form of treatment for the patient. There is nothing sadder than witnessing a patient and his family shopping around the country searching for "the magic cure." It is imperative that the family be convinced that the diagnosis is known and that the form of treatment being carried out is optimal. Just knowing these two items may be a great comfort and support to a family.

2. It should be emphatically explained to the family that henceforth the two all-important considerations in caring for the patient will be maintaining his physical comfort and supporting his morale, since any thought of curing his illness is now impossible.

3. It should be made clear that the whole family must support the patient and cooperate fully in this undertaking.

4. The physician should assure the family that he will back them up, and guide and direct the patient's care to the very last. This is important, for often at this juncture families are frightened that they will be left alone

to deal with a problem with which they have had no previous experience and which has them overwhelmed.

If the news about the patient's condition is unalterably black, often a member of the family will ask, "How can I possibly accept what you say? How can I look at him in the future? How can I talk with him? How can I smile at him? How can I live with him? I am afraid that I will break down every time that I see him. I am afraid that I can't take it."

When this occurs, the physician should gently but firmly point out that the information he has just delivered is a fact, and hence must be accepted, although with understandable sorrow and reluctance. Secondly, he should point out to the family that they should realize that the last, and yet the greatest, gift that they could give to the patient would be to accompany him through this most difficult period in such a fashion that his morale is maintained. Therefore, in a very real sense, sorrow and depression, if evident to the patient, would be selfish. Clearly, in this sort of situation, it is the patient's feelings that must be given first priority and not one's own: "Therefore, when you feel you are about to show your emotions, say to yourself, 'If I do, what will the effect be on *him*?'" It should be emphasized to the family that if they can handle this illness in such a way that they are always supporting the patient, then they will have given a great deal to the person they love, and they should always be grateful and proud for having done it. It should be made clear to the family that they *must* be successful, and that by making the necessary effort, they will gain the needed strength. Stress that this will be one of the most significant and important acts of their spiritual lives and that they will rarely be called upon to give so much of themselves again.

There are certain questions that family members nearly always ask at this point; these should be foreseen and answered by the physician, even if they are not vocalized directly by the family. Among the questions that may be asked are: (1) Does this sickness run in the family? (2) Is it catching? (3) Will the patient suffer a great deal? (4) What will be the manner of his death? Will it be one filled with anguished suffering? (5) How much longer will the patient live?

Sometimes it is wise to select one especially reasonable member of the family to confide the real nature of the patient's illness to, suggesting that the total information not be shared with the whole family since it is difficult for families to keep secrets and their anxieties and depression might be transmitted inadvertently to the patient. This is usually avoided by having only one or two members of the family cognizant of what the real situation is.

As the patient's illness progresses, bringing him closer and closer to death, it is vital that he be seen daily by his physician in order that adequate support be given not only to the patient but to the family as well.

It is imperative that the physician manage this kind of illness in such a way that when the patient finally dies the family is not left with any guilt feelings. The family should continue on with the conviction that they did everything they possibly could, both medically and psychologically, to help the patient. During the course of the illness, the family may have a wide variety of suggestions and ideas and reactions, some of which may be quite weird and unusual. It is cruel for the physician not to hear them out.

The physician who handles this last chapter of a patient's illness well will rarely ever have difficulty getting permission for a post mortem examination, nor will he need to be concerned about being sued for malpractice.

WHEN DEATH FINALLY COMES

When death is near at hand, the patient should be seen frequently to make certain that every means of making him comfortable and peaceful is being employed. It is a source of great consolation to the family if the physician can be in attendance at or near the time of actual death.

It is the very serious responsibility of the physician to see to it that religious support is given to the patient and family at this time.

The family should be kept in close touch with all developments. In simple terms, they should be told what is happening, what is being done, and why. As already discussed, the physician should be careful not to be forced into answering the question, "When will he die?"

The physician should make special efforts to reassure the family that the patient is not consciously aware of his predicament, and in particular that he is not suffering, for this will be their major concern.

If death comes suddenly and unexpectedly, the physician may find himself in a very sensitive position with regard to the family. For this reason, it is essential that early in the course of any major, serious illness, the physician thoughtfully and gently prepare the family for the various eventualities that might be likely to occur during the patient's illness. Thus, if the patient has had an acute myocardial infarction, such complications as a pulmonary embolus or an acute arrhythmia should be mentioned to the family so that, should they occur, the family will not be swept off its feet and have their confidence in their physician undermined. However, if the physician has managed the patient thoughtfully and has had satisfying relationships with the family, such shocks can almost always be absorbed. If resuscitative methods are used, these should be explained to the family in detail. In any event, after sudden death has occurred the patient's history and the nature of his illness should be reviewed with the family, pointing out that in these particular circumstances death sometimes does occur unexpectedly. The care with which the patient was studied should be emphasized, including the fact that he was seen by various consultants. If the patient had a disease with an unhappy outlook, emphasize that it is actually fortunate that the patient's disabling illness came to a premature conclusion.

If the final stages of death are long and drawn out, the physician should urge the family to get adequate rest, suggesting that they make only short, periodic visits to the patient's room, and, if possible, that they get out of the hospital during the intervals and rest at home. The family should be assured that the doctor will call them whenever there are significant changes in the patient's status. It should be remembered, however, that many families will deeply resent not being with the patient at the time of death, and it is imperative for the physician to make every effort to see to it that they are present at the very end, if he senses that this is what the family wants.

After the patient's death, the family should be given an adequate opportunity to quiet their emotions. It is exceedingly distressing to them to have a doctor rush in at such times with a request for an autopsy or to discuss insurance matters and the like.

The physician should go out of his way to show kindness to the family. Some members may want to view the body while it is still in the room, and they should be given this opportunity. The use of a telephone should be made available. If necessary, members of the family may be given sedatives or offered coffee or tea. The physician should offer his assistance in breaking the news to others in the family, such as children or the aged or infirm, if a family member feels unable to do so.

The physician should *sit down* with the family and discuss the following critical topics:

1. The nature of the patient's illness. The family must understand exactly what has transpired and what the course of events has been.

2. Any guilt feelings that may be present in members of the family. It should be stressed that "You did more than could have been expected; you did all that anyone could do. You gave your fullest support very generously in all areas to the patient." Such reassurances are essential in eradicating hidden feelings that may be sources of emotional illness in years ahead. Families ask themselves such questions as: "Why didn't we bring him to you sooner? Why didn't we pay more attention to his complaints? Did we do all we should have done; were we secretly hoping that this long illness would end?" A physician *must* foresee these questions and try to stamp them out before they get deeply rooted.

3. The disposition of the patient's body. Many families have never encountered death before, and they haven't the faintest idea of how to proceed. They are shaken and confused. The matter of getting the body out of the hospital and into burial may seem overwhelmingly complex. Many will not know where to turn or what to do. Panic and hysteria may develop. The physician should explain to the family that it is all relatively simple, and that he will be happy to advise and to guide them and to help them with any problems they may have. The names of several good morticians might be suggested for their selection. It is unwise to recommend one particular mortician over the others, for a family may not be satisfied with the handling of the funeral and this can lead to misunderstanding. It should be stressed that there is adequate time to make sound plans and that there is no need to rush, a delay until the following day being easily feasible if desired.

4. The physician should volunteer to help the family with any insurance or other problems arising from the patient's sickness and death.

5. Assurance should be given to the family that a priest or other religious leader visited the patient in his final hours, if this appears to be important to the family.

6. Family fears that the patient might have had some kind of infectious disease or "family weakness" should be thoroughly eradicated.

SECTION D

Clinical Problem Analysis

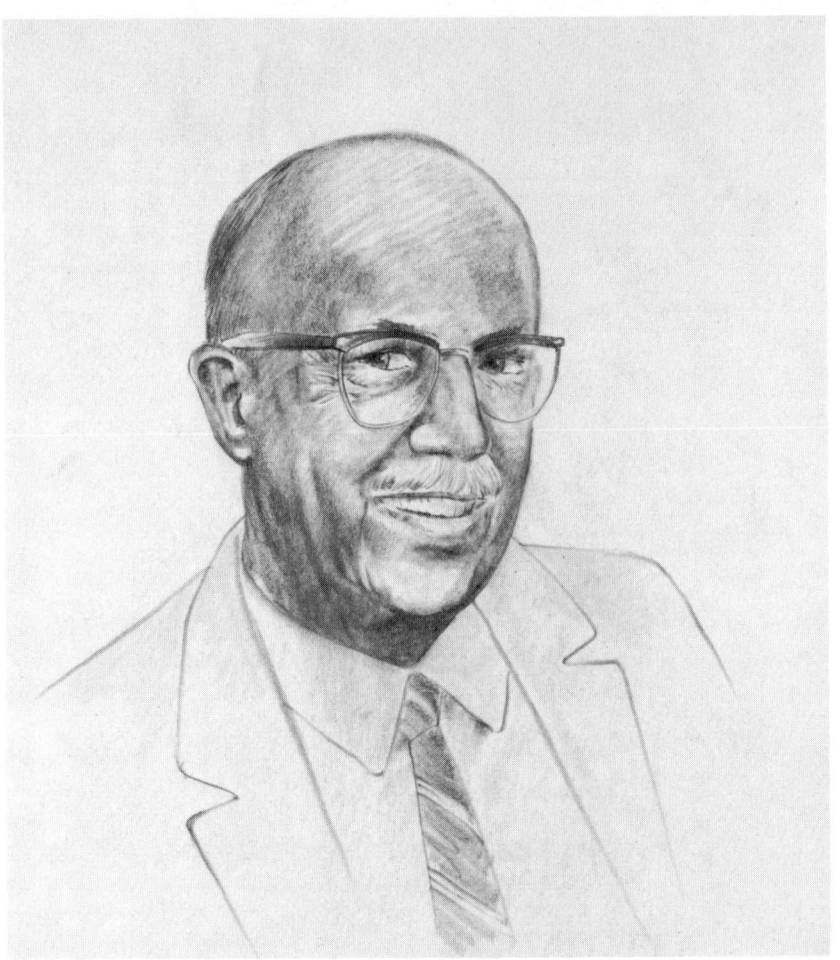

Richard H. Shyrock
PROFESSOR OF HISTORY OF MEDICINE

Dr. Shyrock was the distinguished William H. Welch Professor of the History of Medicine for many years. The work and the eras of many physicians—of yesterday, of several centuries ago, and of the distant past—were the things he meticulously searched out and brilliantly recorded. His philosophical observations regarding what has happened in medicine in the past gave new understanding to current trends and events and will help us predict what is likely to happen in the future.

With John Dresser Garrison he affirmed that "the history of medicine is, in fact, the history of humanity itself, with its ups and downs, its brave aspirations after truth and finality, its pathetic failures. The subject may be treated variously, as a pageant, an array of books, a procession of characters, a succession of theories, an exposition of human ineptitudes, or as the very bone and marrow of cultural history."

His scholarship was productive and enduring, in the very best traditions of this University. A mild but witty and jovial man, having great flair in expressing his strongly held convictions, he took keen interest in the historical aspects of disease, even of the protracted illness which finally befell him. Indomitable, emanating only the positive, it was a source of genuine satisfaction to him to challenge the "young doctors" who cared for him with an intriguing reflection upon some pertinent historical figure or incident of the past: "Do you know what Freud was really like ...?"

To challenge was his, and avid young minds were quick to recognize this. His life was enriched—as will be our present and our future—by what his keenly inquisitive intellect distilled from the past. He left a legacy to each of us, as all great scholars do.

1

A Systematic Approach to Differential Diagnosis

INTRODUCTION

Formerly, in the days when medical technology and treatment were not so advanced, it was not so essential that a physician be accurate in his diagnoses, and a brilliant diagnosis might have been regarded only as a display of clinical erudition. Today, however, with the availability of a wide variety of therapeutic agents and methods, many of which are highly specific in action, the greatest possible accuracy of diagnosis is essential to the future health and possibly even the life of the patient.

To ensure accuracy, the physician's analysis of all the clinical evidence must be methodical and disciplined, founded upon a highly organized *system* of approach to clinical problems, so that no diagnostic or therapeutic possibility is overlooked. This chapter is a discussion of one such system that has proved effective.

This proposed system of differential diagnosis is organized into five steps, as follows:

Step 1—Gather *all* of the clinical evidence.
Step 2—Organize the clinical evidence in a brief outline form in order to facilitate its analysis.
Step 3—Select from the outline one or more key features for detailed diagnostic analysis.
Step 4—List all of the various disorders capable of producing these key features.
Step 5—Select from these possibilities the one (or ones) that best explains the clinical evidence outlined in Step 2.

First Step—Gather All of the Clinical Evidence

The basic material with which the clinician works is the clinical evidence of the natural course of his patient's illness. He gathers this evidence from several sources, including the history, the physical examination, special studies (including x-rays), consultants' opinions, and continued observation of his patient. If the clinical evidence is not accurate, if it is incomplete, or if its implications are not fully appreciated, then only luck will produce a correct diagnosis.

Experience has repeatedly demonstrated the prime importance of the evidence obtained from a searching, meticulous physical examination and a detailed, analytical history. By no means can any of the newer "scientific techniques" supplant these. It is a good idea to regard with skepticism any evidence that doesn't fully jibe with information obtained from the primary techniques of history-taking and physical examination. Many able clinicians find it a sound practice to base their initial differential diagnosis only upon the clinical evidence that they have extracted from the history, physical examination, and routine examination of the blood and urine, subsequently reinterpreting this preliminary diagnosis as more information becomes available, either from special studies, or from the course of the disease itself. The physician who insists upon "having all of the studies back" before he will commit himself to a differential diagnosis will never become an expert diagnostician.

In gathering the clinical evidence, every precaution must be taken to make certain that it is factual. Examine the urine, blood smears, and x-rays yourself, and don't passively accept reported findings. If an operation was performed at another hospital, get the operative notes. If a biopsy was done, procure the histological sections and examine them together with your own pathologist. Challenge the validity of every previous report and statement of opinion. Be a skeptic until it is evident that the data you are working with are sound. Don't gulp down the so-called past "facts" of the patient's story like an oyster. Many such "facts" (and they may be key ones) won't stand up under critical analysis. For example, a young nurse was referred to us for treatment of "systemic lupus" because of a vague history of fatigue, malaise, arthralgias and myalgias. The patient had four young children and was working for her Ph.D. degree, in addition to holding her regular job. The referring physician reported positive LE cell preparations, as did our own laboratory at the time of admission. Because of skepticism about her story, we asked an expert to review all of the slides. None were found to be positive for LE cells; only erythrophagocytosis was present.

Second Step—Organize the Clinical Evidence in Brief Outline Form to Facilitate Its Analysis

Having reviewed all of the available clinical evidence, the physician should next sift out those facts that seem to him to be the most pertinent to the course of the patient's illness. These he lists in logical sequence. If the problem is at all complicated, the items should be arranged in a column according to decreasing significance. At times it is extremely difficult to know which data are essential and which are not, and it must be admitted that instances are not rare in which seemingly unimportant data are later found to contain the real clue. This is one of the intellectual challenges of clinical diagnosis. Only experience (and sometimes intuition!) helps one to "separate the wheat from the chaff." The physician should ask himself this question, "In terms of the total knowledge I now have of the natural history of this patient's illness, as well as the familiarity I have with similar illnesses, how likely is it that this particular fact is an essential part of this whole sequence of events?" The answer to this question will help to determine whether a particular item is retained or discarded, and whether it is given a high or a low priority.

Clearly, when such a list of clinical evidence has been completed, it must contain all of the major features of the patient's illness which call for explanation. It should be remembered that clinical diagnosis is not a one-shot affair, and as the physician's observation and study of a patient's illness advances, this list of pertinent facts will have to be revised repeatedly. Data considered of little or no import today may become of prime significance as new developments occur. The diagnostic approach must be constantly fluid and dynamic, never static.

In composing such a list of clinical evidence, lead off with such fundamentals as the patient's age, sex, and race, for these alone may have important differential diagnostic significance. Next, gather facts about the patient's personal life—his occupation, social status, habits. Then, add a notation about significant familial disorders. This should be followed by a succinct characterization of the general pattern of the natural course of the patient's illness. For example, has it been acute or chronic, persistent or episodic, progressive or stationary; associated or not associated with constitutional phenomena such as fever, weight loss, debility, and so forth; has it involved primarily one organ system, or several? An accurate characterization of the general pattern of a patient's illness may be of great aid in differential diagnoses. It can help distinguish, for example, among a number of disorders which typically follow a chronic, recurrent, episodic course, with involvement of several organ systems, such as systemic lupus erythematosus (SLE) and others of the so-called collagen groups, lymphomata, granulomatous infections, sarcoidosis, Whipple's disease, Mediterranean fever, enterocolitis, the dysproteinemic states, and some forms of leukemia. Then should be listed briefly the manner in which the various organ systems have been affected. This should be done chronologically. A brief summary of the pertinent laboratory results follows, and, finally, a notation about any drugs given, and the responses to any form of specific therapy.

When the list is done well, the physician will have, laid out clearly before him in the most succinct way, all the essential evidence with which his clinical analysis must deal. He will at least be aware of all the facts which his diagnosis must encompass. Unfortunately, some physicians impetuously begin their explanation of what has happened to their patient before they fully grasp exactly all that has happened to him. They may arrive at a differential diagnosis that fits most of the evidence beautifully, but which unfortunately leaves one or two essential knots untied. The perceptive, step by step analysis of all the clinical evidence, as recommended here, will prevent this from happening, for all the facts are spread out in tabular form, each demanding a reasonable, coordinated explanation.

Third Step—Select from the Outline One or More Key Features for Detailed Diagnostic Analysis

This step entails a reflective review of all the clinical evidence, with the specific purpose of selecting from the outline some particular feature or features a detailed analysis of which, the physician believes, will lead to a sound understanding of the entire course of events. This key feature will form the foundation of the observer's analysis, and upon and around it he will attempt to build a logical explanation of what is wrong with his patient. If such a basic feature is not selected for detailed analysis and the physician attempts a diffuse, generalized consideration of all the clinical evidence in an indiscriminate, unstructured manner, his thinking will become diffuse and haphazard, without point or direction. Ordered, logical analysis is possible only when some specific element or elements of the clinical evidence are analyzed in a methodical fashion. Examples of such elements might be the presence of hypochromic microcytic anemia, a mass in the region of the left kidney, uremia, migrating polyarthritis, and so forth.

An essential ingredient of accurate differential diagnosis is the ability to select such a feature or features wisely. To be able to do so consistently constitutes the art of diagnosis. If the wrong feature is selected, the wrong answer may be obtained, or, at the least, much time and effort may be wasted in fruitless analysis, leading only up blind alleys.

For this reason, adequate time should be spent in evaluating all the clinical evidence at hand to insure the selection of that feature which will most likely lead to a productive analysis. While the ability to select this feature with proficiency depends upon a number of factors, fundamental are knowledge of the natural courses of common (and some not so common) diseases and past clinical experiences.

If the illness is unusually complex, it is wise to carry out more than one such analysis of the clinical evidence, each based upon the selection of a different clinical feature. For example, in the case of an elderly white male patient with normocytic anemia, weight loss, low-grade fever, systolic murmur at the base, mild congestive heart failure, and renal insufficiency, with red blood cells, albumin, and casts in the urine, the data might be analyzed from the standpoints of congestive heart failure, renal insufficiency, or fever of unknown origin (FUO). If these separate analyses, based upon different clinical features, lead the observer to identical conclusions, his diagnosis is very likely

A SYSTEMATIC APPROACH TO DIFFERENTIAL DIAGNOSIS 193

to be correct. If the conclusions are disparate, the problem needs reevaluation.

The central feature selected for analysis may be derived from the history, the physical examination, or the information derived from laboratory tests, x-rays, or special procedures. Many physicians tend to lean heavily in favor of results derived from laboratory tests or x-rays when making their diagnoses. Often, however, this proves to be a less than wise selection, and it is usually more productive to build an hypothesis from a feature extracted from the history or physical examination.

In the process of selecting the clinical feature deemed most likely to lead to a profitable analysis, keep these characteristics in mind:

1. The feature in question should be *primary*, important, and significant, essential to the patient's illness, not a secondary effect. For example, if a patient has had a chronic fever for three months and during this time has also developed alopecia, among other occurrences, the feature to be selected for analysis would be chronic fever of unknown origin, not alopecia.

2. The feature must have *objective* validity. Also, it should be something which all observers agree is present, not something about which there is considerable debate and disagreement. For example, in the instance of the elderly male patient with the heart murmur, renal changes, and fever mentioned previously it would be erroneous to build one's "case" around the presence of enlargement of the spleen if there is considerable doubt as to whether or not the spleen is actually enlarged. Sometimes, however, it may be necessary to employ a particular subjective clinical feature as, for example, precordial pain or abdominal pain, because there may be no objective changes accompanying such complaints. If possible, one should strive to unite such a subjective feature with some objective alteration. Diagnoses derived entirely from analysis of subjective symptoms are more frequently incorrect than those obtained from analysis of objective data, for obvious reasons.

3. The feature should have a *broad* enough basis so that the observer can "think around it." That is to say, it should suggest grounds for logical consideration of a variety of possible disease mechanisms. On the other hand, it should not be so all-embracing that it will lead to a hopeless number of possible explanations. In the instance of the elderly male referred to previously selecting weight loss as the hub of one's thinking would probably lead to an excessively large number of possibilities, none of which would be very pointed in significance.

4. The clinical feature selected should be one with which the physician is *familiar* enough to know all of its common as well as its uncommon causes.

Fourth Step—List All the Various Disorders Capable of Producing These Key Features

The key feature or features for detailed analysis having thus been selected, the physician should then list in his mind (or better still, on a piece of paper!)

all of the various types of disorders, common as well as uncommon, that are capable of producing the particular clinical feature. It is important to emphasize here that this initial listing must be *all-inclusive*, not restricted to the problem of the specific patient under study. For to eliminate some types of disorders from the listing at this initial stage is to prejudge the diagnosis, and thus destroy the very system of logical, progressive, total analysis that one is attempting to develop. Elimination of some of the listed disease processes constitutes the next diagnostic step. However, it must be preceded by a listing of *all* possibilities, or diagnostic oversights will occur. It is surprising how frequently previously overlooked diagnostic considerations spring into one's mind as one lists total possibilities with this all-inclusive approach. Explanations hitherto ignored, or quickly disregarded, begin to take form and substance, and initial "obvious" answers start to seem less so.

Clearly, a major source of inaccuracy in diagnosis is failure to compose a list which contains *all* the disorders which can be related to the selected key features. As one's clinical knowledge and experience increase, one's list of possibilities grows larger. Frequently, the merit of a consultant is often tied in with his ability to add to this list. A clinician must learn through repeated practice to "computerize" his analyses, so that, when confronted with a particular clinical feature such as jaundice, he has prepared for himself an organized, workable way of thinking about it, in terms of knowing the types of disorders that are capable of inducing it. Complete, easily recalled, logically constructed categorizations of the causes of the common (and some uncommon) manifestations of disease are invaluable to him. Without them, diagnosis becomes a haphazard, helter-skelter guessing game, in which one flits from one fact and one possibility to another in a disorganized fashion.

For example, a patient presents with a very complicated, chronic illness associated with congestive heart failure. The clinician selects this feature of the patient's illness as the one about which he intends to build his clinical analysis. In doing so, he recalls and employs the categorization of the causes of congestive heart failure originally suggested by Dr. Louis Hamman, as follows:

1. Pericardial disease (constrictive or effusive).
2. Myocardial disease.
3. Endocardial disease.
4. Increased systemic pressure.
5. Increased pulmonic pressure.
6. Congenital disorders.
7. Disorders originating outside of the heart, but exactly imitating intrinsic cardiac disease (viz., mediastinal fibrosis).

In a similar fashion, as already indicated, a clinician must store in his mind well organized categorizations of the causes (common and uncommon) of other frequently encountered manifestations of disease, such as cyanosis, various types of anemia, clubbing of the extremities, precordial pain, shock, uremia, hypercalcemia, intestinal hemorrhage, polyarthritis, cerebral ischemia, splinter hemorrhages, and so forth.

A SYSTEMATIC APPROACH TO DIFFERENTIAL DIAGNOSIS 195

Having winnowed all the clinical evidence and selected from it a key feature for detailed analysis, and having prepared for himself and stored in his mind workable, time-tested categorizations of all the causes of that clinical feature, the clinician is in a sound position to start his clinical analysis, with the assurance that his initial differential diagnosis will at least be reasonable and complete.

Fifth Step—Select from These Possibilities the One (or Ones) That Best Explains the Clinical Evidence Outlined

Having listed in a logical fashion all the types of disorders which could possibly produce the key feature, the clinician is ready to take the final step toward a provisional diagnosis. This comprises an analytical review of the relative likelihood that each of the disorders listed could be playing a role in this particular patient's illness. This sorting out is based upon one's total knowledge of the patient, his history, physical examination, special studies, course, response to therapy, and whatever other information is available. One by one the observer first considers all the factors *favoring* the participation of each listed mechanism. He then considers the factors *opposing* each. The degree of likelihood and, hence, the priority given each mechanism will, of course, depend upon the weight of evidence marshaled for and against each.

Generally, several types of disorders can be quickly eliminated from the original list because they clearly don't fit the circumstances to any reasonable degree. The elimination of others may require much deeper reflection, and perhaps further observation and study. Ultimately one is left with one or more types of disorders which seem to most logically explain the main features of the patient's illness. These constitute the *provisional diagnosis*.

Using such a provisional diagnosis as a basis, one then develops a diagnostic plan of management for the patient, with the end in view of arriving at a final diagnosis in the most proficient way (see Section C, *Clinical Management*).

In rating the merits of each of the listed possible mechanisms, one should be influenced both by their statistical likelihood and by the therapeutic opportunities afforded. While all physicians on occasion are guilty of overlooking this, patients still are more likely to have common disorders than uncommon ones. Especially when dealing with very complex problems, the clinician often tends to lean toward selecting some unusual type of disease process, forgetting that, as in horse racing, statistical likelihood still pays off in clinical diagnosis. If the two most likely diagnostic possibilities are disseminated cancer or a disseminated granulomatous infection, one's main efforts should be directed towards the possibility that the patient has a disseminated infection, since the alternative is therapeutically hopeless.

SECTION D / CHAPTER 1

COMMON ERRORS

There are a number of errors in the approach to clinical diagnosis which physicians should guard against. The most common of all, and the most easily corrected, is the carrying out of an incomplete history and physical examination. Less easily corrected is misinterpretation of the clinical evidence so obtained. Another major source of error is impetuosity in concluding that some particular disease entity, which superficially explains the clinical problem, is present, instead of first logically considering *all* the mechanisms of disease which could possibly produce the clinical feature under consideration. For example, a 22 year old Negro male with a history of sore throats and vague joint pains entered the hospital in congestive heart failure. A low-pitched diastolic murmur was heard, originating at the aortic area and transmitting down the left sternal border. Because of this murmur and the history of joint pains and sore throat, the observers immediately jumped to the "obvious" conclusion of rheumatic heart disease with aortic insufficiency. No consideration was given to any of the other possible mechanisms for the production of an aortic diastolic murmur in such a situation. At operation done to repair the supposed incompetent valve, it was discovered that the patient actually had Marfan's disease with an aortic dissection. Retrospectively, attention was called to the fact that the patient was quite tall and slender, with long, tapering hands and feet. Clearly, lack of familiarity with all of the mechanisms of disease which may produce a particular clinical feature can lead to diagnostic mistakes. Here the necessity of keeping up-to-date with continuing medical advancements becomes evident. Still another source of error is lack of a logical, step-by-step analysis of *all* the pros and cons abstracted from the physician's total knowledge of the patient before proceeding to eliminate or include a particular disease mechanism. The physician must avoid being overly influenced by the pros or blinded by the cons. We must not force the data to fit any premature conclusion. We all have our "favorite diagnoses," and it is very easy to overuse them in attempting to explain poorly thought-through clinical problems. Although it is not easy to discipline ourselves to do this, we must learn not to substitute our hunches and intuitive feelings, and certainly not our prejudices, for a step-by-step judicial analysis of all of the clinical data. The correct diagnosis must supply a reasonable explanation for all the clinical data, not merely a part of it. If any of the clinical features originally listed by the physician as being integral parts of the patient's sickness are left unexplained, the provisional diagnosis is almost surely incorrect.

The clinician must carefully guard against overemphasis of some particular laboratory result, x-ray, or other piece of information, especially if it doesn't jibe with the clinical facts. As already emphasized, in the long run, information derived from clinical observation is more likely to have diagnostic meaning and validity than information obtained from some isolated laboratory procedure.

A clinical problem must be re-analyzed as new information is obtained. The diagnosis which initially seemed to fit the clinical data admirably may clearly be awry as new data are accumulated. This implies continuous re-questioning and re-examination of the patient as the illness unfolds. This also implies willingness to change one's mind as knowledge of the problem advances. A serious error is to become so wedded to some particular diagnosis that one is unwilling to abandon it when added information makes it evident that the original position is no longer tenable. Tenacious adherence to a weakening diagnostic position is sheer folly. Likewise, abandonment of a sound diagnostic view is unwise if this is prompted simply by results of some laboratory procedure or other data of questionable value.

We have already referred to failure of the observer to give proper weight to the statistical likelihood of the various possible diagnoses. A rare or "tricky" diagnosis sometimes has great intellectual or emotional appeal. Such diagnoses stand out in one's memory when they prove to be correct, but unfortunately the many failures of such an intuitive or sporting approach tend to be forgotten.

When dealing with a patient with a chronic illness, such as systemic lupus erythematosus, tuberculosis, or some type of neoplasm, a fatal trap to avoid is the assumption that whatever symptoms occur in such a patient are part and parcel of the basic disease; actually, they may result from some complicating illness or a totally unrelated disturbance. Thus, a patient with Hodgkin's disease may become jaundiced from silent gallstones, or he may acquire infectious hepatitis, as well as develop glandular enlargement at the porta hepatis. As one observes the progressive course of such chronic illnesses, one must adopt the habit of judging each clinical episode on its own merits, and analyze each new incident in a methodical fashion, taking nothing for granted.

By far the most common cause of inaccurate diagnosis is allowing *inadequate time*—first for completing a thorough history and physical examination, second for analyzing in a logical fashion selected features of the patient's illness, third for reviewing the history and physical examination and for re-evaluating the implications of whatever clinical evidence has been obtained thus far. Allowing inadequate time constitutes an inadequate approach to clinical diagnosis.

ILLUSTRATIVE EXAMPLE

In order to illustrate the application of this approach to differential diagnosis, let us briefly consider a relatively straightforward problem. A 26 year old white woman, mother of two children, was admitted to the hospital because of persistent low-grade fever, joint pains, and tender nodules in the skin of her lower legs.

Careful sifting of all of the clinical evidence gathered at the time of admission (Step 1) produced the following outline (Step 2) of the basic facts of the illness:

1. Female, white, 26 years old, mother of 2.
2. "Entirely well" in past.

3. No drugs or toxic exposures, no exposure to granulomatous infections.
4. Negative family history.
5. Illness began abruptly eight weeks prior to admission, with persistent evening fever to 101 degrees. No chills.
6. "Joint pains" actually were bilateral Achilles tendinitis and synovitis in both knees.
7. "Tender spots" actually were erythema nodosum.
8. On physical examination, patient didn't look ill and denied she felt at all constitutionally ill. Typical nodose lesions on legs.
9. Blood and urine normal except for increased sedimentation rate.

Step 3. Reviewing the clinical evidence thus outlined, several features could have been selected as the focal point of in-depth clinical analysis, as follows:
1. FUO.
2. Polyarthritis and tendinitis.
3. Erythema nodosum.

Erythema nodosum was chosen, as it seemed ideally suited to such an analysis.

Step 4. There are a wide variety of causes of erythema nodosum, which may be categorized as follows:
1. Drug reaction.
2. Granulomatous infections, including tuberculosis and histoplasmosis.
3. Chronic local infections.
4. Sarcoidosis.
5. Collagen vascular disturbances.
6. Crohn's disease and ulcerative colitis.
7. New growths (especially lymphomatous).
8. Dysproteinemic status.
9. Leukemia.
10. Unusual disorders, including Whipple's disease and Mediterranean fever.
11. Idiopathic.

Step 5. Brief analysis of the pros and cons of each of these listed possibilities against the background of the clinical evidence listed in Step 2 produced the following conclusions:
1. Drug reaction: Patient firmly denied taking any drugs despite closest questioning.
2. Granulomatous infections: These were high on list because of frequency of association with such a clinical presentation, and couldn't be discarded at this stage, but there was no history of exposure, and it would be peculiar for the patient to have felt "entirely well" despite other manifestations of an active process.
3. Local infection: No obvious evidence of such by history or physical examination.
4. Sarcoidosis: This is a common disease in young Baltimore women

presenting with joint pains and erythema nodosum. Typically there is not much of a constitutional reaction, in contrast to granulomatous infection or new growths. Tendinitis and synovitis common, as is low-grade, persistent fever. No strong cons.

5. Collagen vascular diseases: In a young female, SLE or rheumatoid arthritis (RA) are good bets. There was nothing to support other forms of arteritis. Somewhat against SLE is lack of any constitutional symptoms (malaise, and so forth) despite briskly active process elsewhere. The type of joint involvement is not typical of early RA.

6. Crohn's disease: This patient's manifestations may be the earliest features of enterocolitis, with little pointing to gut changes, but patient denies any gut symptoms whatsoever.

7. New growths: Right age for hidden lymphoma, but no enlargement of glands, liver, or spleen, and patient insists she doesn't feel unwell at all.

8. Dysproteinemic state: Uncommon, and the patient shows none of the usual manifestations of these, which are related to sludging of the blood and bleeding phenomena.

9. Leukemia: Peripheral blood cell counts were normal.

10. Unusual disorders: Whipple's disease is rare, particularly so in young females. Wrong racial background for Mediterranean fever.

11. Idiopathic. This offers no specific therapeutic approach.

Keeping these in mind, the most reasonable provisional diagnosis in these circumstances includes:

1. Sarcoidosis.
2. Granulomatous infection—statistically, the most likely is TBC or histoplasmosis in young females in this part of the country.
3. Collagen vascular disease: SLE?
4. Lymphoma.

Based upon this provisional differential diagnosis, the following studies were carried out: chest x-ray, skin tests for tuberculosis, serological studies for histoplasmosis, and LE (lupus erythematosus) cell smear. Chest film showed bilateral, symmetrical hilar adenopathy with enlarged paratracheal node, regarded as very suggestive of sarcoidosis. Skin tests were negative for TBC, as were the studies for SLE and histoplasmosis. The next diagnostic study was a punch biopsy of the liver, which disclosed hard tubercles, also considered compatible with sarcoidosis. The diagnosis seemed soundly arrived at and established on reasonable grounds.

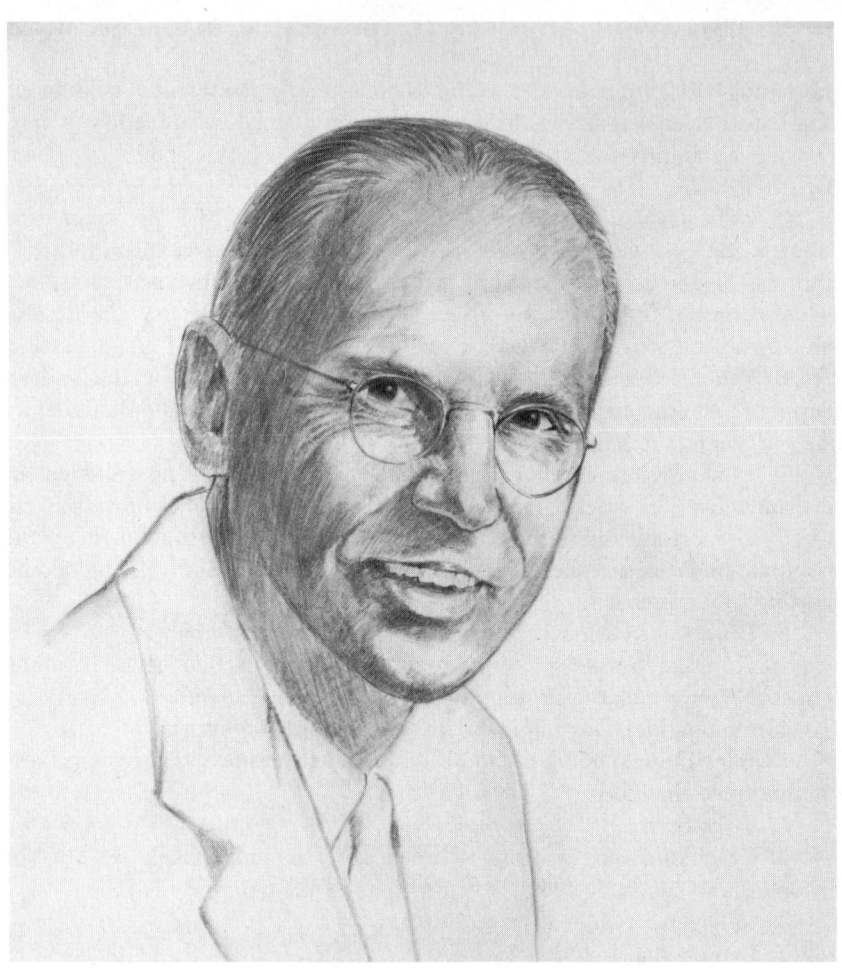

W. Barry Wood
PROFESSOR OF BACTERIOLOGY AND MEDICINE

Few men are given the superior endowments that were Dr. Wood's, and throughout his foreshortened career, he employed them so very effectively. A hero in sports, brilliant in scholarship, an eminent contributor to basic and clinical science, a vastly admired teacher and clinician, he was all this, and he put his talents to good use in ways that importantly aided others. His career could have come from a storybook; he was someone to admire and emulate. He was a person with a fine sense of timing, of piercing, balanced judgment, and of disciplined self-control. Whereas his life was crowded with honors of wide variety, he was modest and unassuming. Although very direct in expressing his opinions, he was sensitive to those of others. Whether one was a student, or subordinate, or confrere, it was a delight to be with Dr. Wood, because he was warm and understanding and had a lilting humor. He and his lovely wife, Mary Lee, made as perfect a pair as you are likely to encounter.

A man of legendary proportions, his accomplishments in widely differing areas will long be remembered and extolled by persons of very diverse interests. Those who follow sports will thrill to recall a great athlete in action; those he taught at any level will continue to be stimulated by his lucid teaching; those who benefited from his new understandings of bacteriological and clinical problems will continue to be grateful; all at Hopkins who felt and were affected by the incomparable qualities of this good man, and the devotion of his service, will realize that his memory can never be separated from what is best in this institution.

2

Problem-Oriented Diagnostic Discussions

A A PATIENT WITH HYPERCALCEMIA

THE CLINICAL PROBLEM

This 59 year old white hotel waiter was well until six weeks prior to hospital admission, when he developed weakness, fatigue, nausea, light-headedness, and vomiting, with progressive weight loss of 15 pounds. He had had a duodenal ulcer and renal calculi in the past. He smoked two packs of cigarettes daily, and at one time "drank too much."

Results of physical examination were unremarkable save for mental clouding and moderate liver enlargement. The significant laboratory findings were: serum urea nitrogen, 46 mg./100 ml.; creatinine, 2.2 mg./100 ml.; alkaline phosphatase elevated to 6 King-Armstrong units; calcium, 15.5 mg./100 ml.; phosphorus, 4.2 mg./100 ml.; total protein and albumin/globulin ratio, 6.3/3.6 g./100 ml.; sodium, 139 mEq./liter; potassium, 3.8 mEq./liter; chloride, 111 mEq./liter; carbon dioxide content, 17.5 mEq./liter; hematocrit, 30 percent. Chest x-ray revealed a fine accentuation of the markings, suggesting fibrosis. A rounded density was seen in the left apical area. Pyelograms and later an arteriogram indicated bilateral upper pole renal cysts.

The patient became progressively lethargic, was nauseated, and vomited a great deal. The serum calcium, varying between 12 and 15 gm., was controlled transiently with Mithramycin and there was temporary symptomatic improvement. An exploratory thoracotomy was done to determine the nature of the lesion in the left lung. Unfortunately, the patient died shortly afterward.

DISCUSSION OF THE PROBLEM

It seems clear-cut that the focal point of this patient's illness was a marked degree of hypercalcemia, manifested clinically by anorexia, nausea, vomiting, fatigue, lassitude, and mental confusion. It also appears that these clinical manifestations began rather abruptly, progressed rapidly in intensity, and became associated with a moderate degree of uremia. In other words, the patient appeared to be enduring what has been graphically described as a "hypercalcemic crisis."

There are a wide variety of different disease states which may become associated with hypercalcemia. I would categorize them as follows:

1. Diseases of the parathyroid gland, including adenoma, hyperplasia, and carcinoma.
2. Parathormone producing tumors, such as carcinoma of the lung.
3. Vitamin D intoxication.
4. The milk-alkali syndrome.
5. Sarcoidosis.
6. Involvement of bone by malignant tumors, including myeloma, leukemia, and lymphoma.
7. Chronic renal insufficiency leading to secondary hyperparathyroidism.
8. Other endocrine abnormalities, including hyperthyroidism.
9. Primary bone disease, such as Paget's.

Let us review each of these categories and try to determine which has the most statistical purtenance in this particular instance. There are several which can be readily eliminated.

Thus, none of the bone x-rays suggested the changes of Paget's disease. But for possible mild diabetes mellitus, there was no evidence of multiple endocrinopathy, including hyperthyroidism.

Although the studies which were carried out—in particular, the arteriogram—indicated bilateral cystic disease of the kidneys, it is very unlikely that chronic uremia resulting from these cysts could have produced hypercalcemia as a result of secondary hyperparathyroidism. In the first place, the patient's serum nitrogen had been normal in 1963, even following a gastrointestinal hemorrhage. Second, his serum phosphorus was never elevated; third, hypercalcemia of this degree is seldom encountered in uncomplicated renal insufficiency; and finally, prominent bone alterations generally accompany secondary hyperparathyroidism due to chronic renal insufficiency, and none were noted here.

This patient evidently had dyspeptic troubles from time to time, perhaps aggravated by overuse of alcohol, with some GI bleeding on occasion. He liked to drink milk. Could he have had the so-called milk-alkali syndrome?

It has been our experience that patients who progressively damage their kidneys by excessive intake of milk and alkaline powders are almost always totally oblivious to what they are doing. For they think, what in the world could be more harmless than milk and baking soda—especially since they make a miserably burning stomach feel so good so fast? Hence, unless one asks the right questions in the right way and in the right setting, the diagnosis of the milk-alkali syndrome is easily overlooked. This would be just such a setting. But we are informed that the only antacid the patient consumed was aluminum hydroxide. Even if this information is incorrect, however, the fact that this patient's urine was clear but for 2–3 RBC and WBC at the time he was uremic militates against this syndrome, for in this disorder appreciable abnormalities are usually observed in the urine by the time uremia appears.

Another cause of hypercalcemia associated with acute or chronic renal injury that is readily overlooked, if the history is inadequate, is Vitamin D intoxication. You may recall that just a few years ago the medical journals were filled with two-page blurbs in full color extolling the efficacy of Vitamin D preparations in the treatment of various forms of arthritis. "Does your patient have arthritis?" the headlines would ask—"then ertronize him!" they would advise. Dr. John Eager Howard and I, as long ago as 1942, first described a group of patients so treated who developed resultant hypercalcemia and permanent renal injury. It is important to remember that some physicians continue to treat various forms of arthritis with large doses of Vitamin D preparations. Almost always, patients presenting with hypercalcemia and renal injury stemming from Vitamin D intoxication deny that they are taking any drug which might be toxic—after all, Vitamin D is given to infants! Hence, pointed questions must be asked about Vitamin D therapy if such a patient has ever had any form of arthritis. This patient apparently did not.

Other causes of hypercalcemia are less readily eliminated in this diagnosis. The patient's symptoms developed acutely, as already mentioned, and he did not appear to be chronically or generally ill. He had had no bone pain. X-rays of the bones showed only mild, diffuse demineralization. The kind of anemia he developed was not the sort seen with bone marrow invasion by tumor. He did not have a thrombocytosis. No rouleaux formation of the RBCs was observed. The patient's peripheral blood smear was not peculiar. His serum protein levels were not grossly abnormal, and no protein whatever was found in the urine. These are all points diminishing the likelihood of hypercalcemia due to widespread involvement of bone by some malignant tumor.

On the other hand, he did have abnormal pyelograms. Instead of renal cysts could he have had a hypernephroma? The bilaterality of these changes, however, and—most important of all—the description of the renal arteriograms, make this type of malignancy highly unlikely.

What about the enlarged liver, which was tender, and the elevated alkaline phosphatase? The patient had drunk heavily in the past—why couldn't he have had a hepatoma, perhaps with widespread metastasis to the bones as well as to the left lung? Alternatively, might he not have had a primary carcinoma of the lung with metastases to the liver and to the bones?

The point to be established at this juncture is that if he did, indeed, have such a malignancy, it is unlikely that the attendant hypercalcemia could have been the result of widespread metastases to bones, for the reasons we have already outlined. On the other hand, we will consider very shortly an alternative mechanism by which such tumors could have accounted for the course of events noted here—namely, through the production of parathormone by the tumor.

The patient had had a cough for some 30 years. The lung fields are described as having finely accentuated markings, suggesting fibrosis. The liver was enlarged, and alkaline phosphatase levels were elevated. Why isn't sarcoidosis a good explanation for the course of events? Well, of course, he could have had active sarcoidosis, but he was white and 59 years of age. There was no history of implication of the uveal tract, the skin, the muscles, the joints, or the lymphoid tissues. No hilar lymphadenopathy was described. There was no increased serum gamma globulin. While we see a great many patients with sarcoid in the Negro population of Baltimore, I can't recall one who entered with the syndrome of "acute hypercalcemic crisis" so vividly portrayed here.

Therefore, at this juncture, we can only conclude, from a review of all of the causes of hypercalcemia, that in this patient the key abnormality must have been the result of excessive production of parathormone, either by the parathyroid gland itself, or by some malignant tumor. Differentiation of these two possibilities, tumor or parathyroid adenoma, is extremely difficult, for an obvious reason—namely, many of their accompanying alterations are common to both, dependent as they both are upon overproduction of parathormone. Sometimes, on purely clinical grounds, the differentiation is utterly impossible! Often one has to depend upon the setting, or upon collateral evidence. This, I believe, is the case here.

Clearly, a number of features of this patient's history point to a parathyroid adenoma, which is the most common abnormality of this endocrine gland, hyperplasia being less common, and carcinoma very rare. Thus, the patient is said to have had renal calculi 25 years ago. There is also mention in the system review of polyuria. We have already referred to the patient's past peptic problems, and, during this acute illness, a duodenal ulcer was thought to have been present. We have previously stressed the abrupt onset of his hypercalcemic crisis. Such episodes are part and parcel of the life story of parathyroid adenomas, although they are by no means restricted to them. I am struck by the description of a lacelike fibrotic process in the patient's lung fields. I recall a patient I discussed in a CPC at the Rhode Island Hospital many years ago. His lung fields had a similar appearance, and at post mortem calcium was found to be deposited in the pulmonary alveolar tissues, accounting for the x-ray changes. That patient had a parathyroid adenoma. While similar changes can, I'm certain, be seen in other hypercalcemic states, this finding is perhaps indicative of a hypercalcemic state of some standing. But, in fact, how much evidence do we have that this patient's hypercalcemia was indeed of long-standing duration? Certainly, the history of the renal stones and peptic troubles suggests a long-drawn-out process. On the other hand, the minor changes in the bone films do not. Unfortunately, the absence of significant abnormalities in the urine and lack of elevation of phosphorus levels in the presence of uremia are of no real aid in this regard, since we have seen patients hospitalized with uremia who apparently have had parathyroid adenomas for a number of years, and yet show few or no abnormalities in the urine.

It seems clear that the clinical evidence available is open to several interpretations; the history, and perhaps the changes in the lungs, points to long duration of the hypercalcemia, which would be most compatible with a parathyroid adenoma, while the modest bone changes, and perhaps the benignant urine, suggest a process of shorter duration, such as a malignant tumor.

We should discuss the point that the patient was somewhat acidotic on admission, his CO_2 being 17.5 mEq./liter. In patients with hypercalcemia, a finding of acidosis is said to favor a diagnosis of parathyroid adenoma, as contrasted with the alkalosis encountered in hypercalcemia resulting from bone involvement by tumor, but once the serum nitrogen is elevated, all bets are off, and this distinction is fallible. Besides, as already emphasized, we are trying to distinguish between two tumors, both of which produce parathormone, not between bone metastases and parathyroid adenoma.

We are left, then, with the coin lesion in the left apex. Its most important clinical features are these: it appeared de nouveau sometime after 1963 in a patient with a chronic cough who smoked two packs of cigarettes daily. Although it was located in an area in which granulomas are common, the burden of proof rests with anyone who says such a lesion in a 59 year old male patient is not a pulmonary carcinoma, and in particular, in this setting, an oat cell tumor, for these tumors are most commonly producers of parathormone and hypercalcemia. Perhaps, as previously indicated, liver enlargement was due to metastases from such a tumor, for they sometimes fill the liver before they appear anywhere else.

Here, then, we have the two most likely causes of this patient's malady: (1) oat cell carcinoma of the lung or (2) a parathyroid adenoma. It is a difficult choice to make. The acute onset of symptoms in a man who otherwise seemed well, the so-called "hypercalcemic crisis," plus the past history of renal stones and peptic disease, and the changes in the lung fields, are impelling arguments for a parathyroid adenoma.

However, we began this analysis by saying that we must select the possibility which has the greatest statistical likelihood. Parathyroid adenomata in males are not common. Carcinoma of the lung in 59 year old male patients with recently discovered silent coin lesions, who have smoked two packs of cigarettes daily for 30 years, and who have chronic cough, is very common.

Since either of these entities could have produced the hypercalcemic crisis and the related changes noted in this patient through the production of parathormone, I select as my final diagnosis the more common of the two—oat cell carcinoma of the lung.

POST MORTEM FINDINGS

Hypernephroma arising from both kidneys with metastases to lungs and liver. Hypercalcemia was secondary to parathormone production by this tumor.

REFERENCES

Anderson, E. G.: Non-metastatic syndromes associated with carcinoma of the bronchus. The endocrine syndromes. Hosp. Med. *1*:11, 1966.
Berger, L., and Sinkoh, M. W.: Systemic manifestations of hypernephroma, a review of 273 cases. Amer. J. Med. *22*:791, 1957.
Bower, B. F., and Gordon, G. S.: Hormonal effects of nonendocrine tumors. Ann. Rev. Med. *16*:83, 1965.
David, N. J., et al.: The diagnostic spectrum of hypercalcemia. Amer. J. Med. *33*:88, 1962.
Dent, C. E.: Some problems of hyperparathyroidism. Brit. Med. J. *2*:1495, 1962.
Endocrine abnormalities in bronchial carcinoma. Brit. Med. J. *3*:5, 1968.
Goldsmith, R. S.: Differential diagnosis of hypercalcemia. New Eng. J. Med. *74*:674, 1966.
Goldstein, R. A., et al.: Infrequency of hypercalcemia in sarcoidosis. Amer. J. Med. *51*:21, 1971.
Heinemann, H. O.: Metabolic alkalosis in patients with hypercalcemia. Metabolism *14*:1137, 1965.
Hobbs, C. B., and Miller, A. C.: Review of endocrine syndromes associated with tumors of nonendocrine origin. J. Clin. Path. *19*:119, 1966.
Howard, J. E.: Clinical disorders of calcium homeostasis. Medicine *42*:25, 1963.
Hyperparathyroidism—Symposium. Amer. J. Med. *50*:557, 1971.
Kielg, J. M.: Hypernephroma: The internist's tumor. Med. Clin. N. Amer. *50*:1067, 1966.
Klatskin, G., and Gordon, M.: Renal complications of sarcoidosis and their relationship to hypercalcemia, with report of 2 cases simulating hyperparathyroidism. Amer. J. Med. *15*:84, 1953.
Knowles, J. H., and Smith, L. H., Jr.: Extrapulmonary manifestations of bronchogenic carcinoma. New Eng. J. Med. *262*:505, 1960.
Lipsett, M. G., Odell, W. D., Rosenberg, L. E., and Waldman, T. A.: Humoral syndromes associated with nonendocrine tumors. Ann. Intern. Med. *61*:733, 1964.
Longcope, W. T. and Frieman, D. G.: Review of sarcoidosis. Medicine *31*:1, 1952.
Margolis, S., and Homcy, C.: Systemic manifestation of hepatoma. Medicine *51*:381, 1972.
McMillan, D. E., and Freeman, R. B.: The milk-alkali syndrome: A study of the acute disorder with comments on the development of the chronic condition. Medicine *44*:485, 1965.
Moggia, F. M., et al.: Hypercalcemia associated with neoplastic disease. Ann. Intern. Med. *73*:281, 1970.
Myers, W. P., Tashima, C. K., and Rothschild, E. O.: Endocrine syndromes associated with nonendocrine neoplasms. Med. Clin. N. Amer. *50*:763, 1966.
Odell, W. D.: Hyperparathyroidism. *In* Williams' Textbook of Endocrinology. 4th ed. Robert H. Williams (Ed.). Philadelphia, W. B. Saunders Company, 1968, p. 922.
Pedersen, K. O.: Coexistent sarcoidosis and hyperparathyroidism. Acta Med. Scand. *182*:781, 1967.
Raisz, L. G.: The diagnosis of hyperparathyroidism. New Eng. J. Med. *285*:1006, 1971.
Randall, R. E., Jr., et al.: The milk-alkali syndrome. Arch. Intern. Med. *107*:163, 1961.
Stroh, C. A., and Nugent, C. A.: Laboratory tests in the diagnosis of hyperparathyroidism in hypercalcemic patients. Ann. Int. Med. *68*:188, 1968.
Thomas, W. C., Jr., Wiswek, J. G., Connor, T. B., and Howard, J. E.: Hypercalcemic crisis due to hyperparathyroidism. Amer. J. Med. *24*:229, 1958.
Tumulty, P. A., and Howard, J. E.: Irradiated ergosterol poisoning. JAMA *119*:233, 1942.
Underdahl, L. E., et al.: Multiple endocrine adenomas: report of 8 cases in which the parathyroids, pituitary and pancreatic islets were involved. J. Clin. Endocrinol. *13*:20, 1953.
Wilder, W. T., Frame, B., and Hambrick, W. W.: Peptic ulcer in primary hyperparathyroidism: an analysis of 52 cases. Ann. Intern. Med. *55*:885, 1961.

B A PATIENT WITH MULTIPLE PULMONARY EMBOLI

THE CLINICAL PROBLEM

This 60 year old Negro laborer, who had drunk heavily in the past and had been treated for syphilis, developed a cough, tightness in the chest and progressive dyspnea on exertion eight weeks prior to hospital admission. He rapidly became so short of breath he could walk but a few steps. His heartbeat became rapid and a tight, constricting sensation developed in his lower chest and upper abdomen. He lost 14 pounds. In the chest clinic, he was found to have a greatly enlarged, tender liver, and splenomegaly. X-ray of the chest was clear. The hematocrit value was 44 ml./100 ml., and the white blood cell count was 5800 per cu. mm. The urine was clear. The bromsulphalein (BSP) retention was 30 percent. Alkaline phosphatase levels were elevated to 24 King-Armstrong units and the bilirubin value was 1.4 mg./100 ml. Transaminases were normal, as was the standard test for syphilis (STS).

The patient was admitted for further studies. Punch biopsy of the liver was unsatisfactory. The liver scan showed some areas of decreased radioactive uptake, particularly in the posterior-lateral portions of the right lobe. The lung scan was suggestive of pulmonary emboli, as was the arteriogram. An inferior vena caval ligation was performed, but shortly thereafter the patient developed pulmonary edema and died.

DISCUSSION OF THE PROBLEM

In summary, the patient was an elderly Negro male who had been an excessively heavy drinker for many years, until saved by the grace of religion. In addition, he had been plagued by a chronic urinary tract infection, and had had syphilis. Otherwise he had enjoyed good health until abruptly becoming short of breath, and this progressed so rapidly that he could scarcely move about without becoming acutely breathless. In spite of this marked degree of exertional dyspnea, there were no signs whatever of congestive heart failure, and the chest x-rays remained quite clear.

He lost appreciable weight, and on entry into the hospital had had fever. Also, he was constantly made uncomfortable by a peculiar tight, distended, overfilled, cinchlike sensation involving both the lower chest and the upper abdomen. He felt sated as soon as he had begun to eat. The liver was discovered to be greatly enlarged, firm, and nodular.

It would seem profitable to consider in some detail the three basic features of this patient's illness (exertional dyspnea, upper abdominal fullness, and fever with weight loss) and explore their possible relationships.

While this patient was not a lucid "historian," and we would like to have more details than are at hand, his account of tightness and fullness and overdistention in the upper abdomen and lower chest, as though a rope were being cinched about his middle, is typical of the discomfort of which patients complain when the liver capsule is being rapidly stretched by increasing distention of the liver, by either congestive heart failure, tumor, infection, or some infiltrative process. The true significance of this frequently occurring symptom complex is easily misinterpreted. For example, elderly persons who are developing congestive heart failure may mistakenly be considered to have some sort of primary intra-abdominal disease because of the prominence of such complaints and a concomitant dearth of classical evidences of congestive heart failure.

In this particular instance, congestive heart failure appears to be eliminated by the absence of venous congestion or edema. Furthermore, the liver was described as being hard and nodular, and the liver scan showed changes which would not be explained on the basis of congestive heart failure.

Next to congestive heart failure, the most common cause of such symptoms associated with an enlarged liver is some type of rapidly growing malignant tumor. There are obviously compelling reasons to suspect such an occurrence here, including the firmness and nodularity of the surface of the liver, the weight loss and fever, the appearance of the scan, and the liver function tests. As you will recall, the BSP retention was very significantly elevated, and alkaline phosphatase less so, although the remaining tests of liver function were essentially normal. This is a common pattern of tumors spreading within the liver.

If the patient had had a malignant tumor within his liver, and it seems entirely likely that he had, where was its point of origin?

There are several likely sites in such a setting as this. The patient was becoming progressively constipated, so carcinoma of the colon is suspect. But on the other hand, the stools were guaiac negative and the barium enema results were normal. The flatulence, dyspepsia, and sensation of rapid filling of the stomach of which he complained makes one think of a malignancy of the stomach, but again the gastrointestinal x-rays showed no abnormalities. The chronic urinary infections should lead one to question the possibility of a carcinoma of the bladder or prostate, tumors which occasionally fill up the liver very rapidly without making themselves evident elsewhere, but the patient was examined and cystoscoped by urologists, who found no sign of such tumors.

There are several reasons for considering carcinoma of the pancreas. First, the patient was a chronic alcoholic. Second, the feeling of epigastric fullness and the distention of which he complained are typical of pancreatic carcinoma. Third, his spleen was enlarged. As you may well know, carcinomas do not usually metastasize to the spleen (although they *may*), and even when the liver is diffusely involved by metastatic tumor, the spleen usually doesn't become enlarged (although it *may*). On the other hand, in carcinoma of the pancreas, it is not unusual for the spleen to become enlarged as a result of blockage of the splenic veins by tumor extension. Fourth, as we shall shortly discuss, the patient probably had pulmonary emboli, and while any neoplasm may be associated with pulmonary embolism, statistically speaking pancreatic carcinoma is associated with pulmonary embolism with very high frequency.

Clearly, we cannot dismiss the possibility of a pancreatic neoplasm. On the other hand, the GI series failed to show any of the x-ray changes sometimes present in pancreatic carcinoma, nor did the patient have pain in the back, ascites, significant jaundice, or a systolic bruit in the left upper quadrant of the abdomen, all common—although unfortunately inconstant—presentations of pancreatic carcinoma. Hence, while we can't exclude the diagnosis of carcinoma of the pancreas, we won't embrace it either.

Many of the considerations just reviewed apply to the possibility of some other type of retroperitoneal tumor, such as a sarcoma or lymphoma; in particular the presence of an enlarged spleen.

While such a tumor can't be excluded on the basis of the information given here, and although it would well explain the fever and pulmonary emboli, there is another type of new growth which affords a more pertinent explanation of the facts of this patient's illness. For we must not forget that he had been an alcoholic of considerable capacity, and that the biopsy of his liver showed some scarring, though granted it wasn't much of a biopsy. His hands were described as showing suggestive evidence of "liver palms." His spleen was enlarged. Do not all of these little points favor the possibility that this patient may have had well compensated hepatic cirrhosis of long standing? And, if so, could this not have led to the development of carcinoma of the liver?

Most certainly it could have, and, in fact, I believe it did, for his story is so typical of advancing carcinoma of the liver. The rapid enlargement of the liver, the pronounced degree of distending discomfort which he endured, the sepsis-like febrile course, and the high BSP retention and alkaline phosphatase level despite only mild hyperbilirubinemia are all points that are characteristic of the way primary hepatic carcinoma behaves.

Before turning to a consideration of the other main complaint, exertional dyspnea, we should mention three additional causes of painful enlargement of the liver. First, it should be recalled that metastatic carcinoma of the lung may produce rapid and massive enlargement of the liver in the complete absence of any other suggestion of such a tumor, and in fact, even in the presence of a clear x-ray of the chest. Carcinoma of the lung is, of course, statistically a common cause of pulmonary embolism associated with tumor. All we can say here is that nothing was seen in this patient's chest x-rays to indicate such a tumor.

The patient had had syphilis, and the description of a greatly enlarged, nodular liver should bring to mind the question of syphilis of the liver, but we are assured that he had been treated adequately for syphilis.

So far as liver abscess is concerned, the proportions and consistency of this patient's liver would be somewhat unusual for such a lesion, and there was a dearth of constitutional symptoms, such as malaise, sweats, chills, muscular aching, and so forth, which are frequent accompaniments of multiple liver abscesses.

We turn now to the most prominent and somewhat unusual component of this patient's illness, namely, the fact that despite the absence of evidence of both congestive heart failure and changes in the lung fields by x-ray, the patient was intolerably short of breath even on very mild exertion.

In our experience, there aren't a great number of conditions which produce severe exertional dyspnea in the absence of heart failure or of visible alterations in the lung fields. The following mechanisms come immediately to mind in this regard:

1. A large pericardial effusion, but clearly such was not present here.
2. A large mediastinal mass with compression, but again this clearly was not present.
3. A pronounced degree of emphysema, also not existent here.
4. Asthma, which was not noted here.
5. Pneumothorax, not seen here.
6. Diffuse cystic disease of the lungs. One must be careful in excluding this entity, because it may be present with few or none of the expected alterations in the chest films. As a matter of fact, the presence of cystic disease may become evident only after a patient develops a pneumonitis, the honeycombing then becoming clearly obvious. But at the age of 60 one would not expect cystic disease to appear from out of the blue in an individual previously free of pulmonary sickness.
7. Some type of diffuse fibrotic disease. Sometimes such a process may be present in its early stages and manifest few or no abnormalities in the x-rays or on physical examination. Thus, we have seen patients with early scleroderma of the lungs of the fibrotic type who were quite short of breath but whose chest films remained clear, despite the discovery at post mortem examination of a considerable degree of fibrosis. The same can be said for a wide variety of the processes producing the so-called alveolo-capillary block syndrome. However, for such processes to be present in association with the degree of disability clinically manifested by this patient, and yet to have consistently clear lung fields, would be somewhat unusual, I believe. In addition, we have the advantage of the information obtained from the special pulmonary studies which were carried out.
8. One cause of rapidly advancing exertional dyspnea to be considered in the setting of an elderly patient with fever and weight loss would be lymphangitic spread of a tumor, either primary within the lungs, or secondary. Sometimes such infiltrating tumors are quite silent, in terms of both physical and x-ray alterations. We have already stressed the likelihood of a malignant process here, including bronchogenic carcinoma.
9. Still another good likelihood in the elderly, febrile male would be miliary tuberculosis, and here the telltale changes in the lung fields may be long in appearing, or even absent.

10. Some process affecting the pulmonary vascular bed, including embolism of various etiologies and occlusive and thrombotic processes. For example, an intense degree of dyspnea is encountered in fat emboli to the lungs, despite clear lung fields. Likewise, patients with scleroderma of the lungs, polyarteritis nodosa and, rarely, lupus, may have diffuse pulmonary arteritis with occlusion so extensive that marked exertional dyspnea results, the lung fields remaining clear all the while.

Certainly we have little reason to postulate the existence of some sort of a pulmonary arteritic process, such as scleroderma, SLE, or Wegener's granulomatosis. In an elderly male with fever and weight loss, one should, of course, consider polyarteritis nodosa, but the greatly enlarged, nodular liver would be difficult to explain on this basis, nor were there evidences of a diffuse arteritis in other organ structures. A pronounced eosinophilia, not present here, is a common finding in association with pulmonary arteritis.

We are, therefore, left with the likelihood that this patient has multiple pulmonary emboli. There are many clinical points indicating the likelihood of embolism, including the following: (1) As just stressed, the sudden onset of marked exertional dyspnea in an individual with clear lung fields, a normal heart, and no previous pulmonary troubles. (2) The sudden onset of severe dyspnea in a person who has features suggesting the possible presence of a new growth, in this instance, weight loss, fever, and an enlarged, nodular liver.

In this regard, there are certain clinical situations in which pulmonary embolism occurs so commonly that any type of acute pulmonary incident should raise the suspicion of a possible embolism. These include:

1. Any debilitating disorder.
2. Any new growth, including leukemia.
3. Any systemic infection.
4. The presence of significant vascular disease, whether arterial or venous (here is included diabetes).
5. The collagen disorders.
6. Conditions leading to increased sludging or viscosity of the blood, such as dehydration, polycythemia, or dysproteinemia.
7. Processes inducing venous stasis, whether localized or generalized, such as heart failure or large fibroids of the uterus.
8. Hepatic cirrhosis.
9. Severe degrees of anemia or anoxia.
10. Immobilization, such as may occur in the Guillain-Barré syndrome, or many other chronic, debilitating diseases, or in feeble elderly persons.
11. The administration of certain drugs, including perhaps oral contraceptives, and the overzealous use of diuretics to older individuals in hot, sweaty weather.
12. So-called toxic states, such as uremia or acidosis.
13. Prolonged hypotension.

One might surmise from this list that pulmonary embolism is much more of a problem for the medical man than for the surgeon, with whom postoperative embolism is historically associated, and most assuredly embolism is the bête noire of the internist. It is unfortunate that often he isn't aware of this, and that so frequently pulmonary embolism is only discovered at post mortem examination, to the consternation of the physician who says, "I can't understand it, the patient was doing so well!"

In many such instances, the patient might not have been regarded as "doing so well" if more attention and proper evaluation had been given to the following:

1. Unexplained changes in pulse, respiratory rate and temperature, even though of minor degree.
2. Episodes of anxiety and restlessness.
3. Sudden dizziness, syncope, or seizures.
4. Vague tightness, fullness, or discomfort in the chest.
5. Episodes of asthma, or sudden dyspnea, even if short-lived.
6. "Coronary" pain.
7. A paroxysmal tachycardia or arrhythmia.
8. Development or increase in congestive failure.
9. Appearance of a gallop rhythm or of a tender liver edge.
10. Patches of pneumonitis or of atelectasis.
11. Unexplained onset of cough.
12. Unexplained persistent fever.

It is interesting that this patient's episodes of shortness of breath were interpreted by one of the staff members caring for him as possibly being psychogenic in origin. The basis for this conclusion, I'm sure, was the absence of readily blamed organic changes. So often this is the type of clinical analysis which leads so many patients to die "unexpectedly" of pulmonary embolism.

In addition to the general setting of this patient's illness, which was certainly a fertile one for the genesis of pulmonary emboli, we have other clinical points, including: (1) the recurrent nature of the episodes of severe dyspnea, cough, and tachycardia; (2) the times when he would feel faint and lightheaded; (3) the transient pleural rub heard over the right chest; (4) the loud P_2; (5) the prominent right ventricular impulse; and (6) the systolic murmur heard along the left sternal border with inspiration, perhaps originating within the affected pulmonary vessels.

We come finally, therefore, to the conclusion that this patient had some sort of a malignant tumor widely involving his liver, and that in this classic setting for embolism, multiple pulmonary emboli ensued. For the reasons already presented in detail, it seems most reasonable to conclude that this patient, who had consumed so much alcohol for so long a time, probably had cirrhosis of the liver, and that this condition was ultimately joined by the development of hepatic carcinoma. Obviously, carcinoma of the pancreas or a lymphomatous tumor cannot be excluded, but, for the reasons given, hepatic carcinoma fits the data more logically.

The pulmonary emboli may have arisen in the peripheral or pelvic veins or in the hepatic veins and the vena cava. The sudden death following vena caval ligation may indicate that there was seeding of the lungs with emboli both from a site above the point of ligation of the vena cava and from the hepatic veins themselves.

Several patients with hepatic carcinoma who died as the result of embolism of large masses of tumor tissue—as well as of the usual thrombus material—into their pulmonary vascular bed have been described. The conclusion seems reasonable that this is a similar occurrence of hepatic carcinoma with tumor embolization to the lungs.

POST MORTEM FINDINGS

Cirrhosis of the liver. Hepatoma. Multiple pulmonary emboli, consisting of masses of tumor cells and thrombi.

REFERENCES

Carcinoma of the Liver

Alpert, M. E., Uriel, J., and deNechaud, B.: Alpha-1 fetoglobulin in the diagnosis of human hepatoma. New Eng. J. Med. 278:984, 1968.
Fensten, L. F., and Klatskin, G.: Manifestation of metastatic tumors of the liver. Amer. J. Med. 31:238, 1961.
Hughes, E. S. R., et al.: Systolic liver murmurs in primary carcinoma of the liver. Med. J. Aust. 1:569, 1969.
MacDonald, R. A.: Primary carcinoma of the liver. A clinicopathologic study of 108 cases. Arch. Intern. Med. 99:226, 1957.
Moseley, R. V.: Primary malignant tumors of the liver. A review of 47 cases. Surgery 61:674, 1967.
San Jose, D., et al.: Primary carcinoma of the liver. Amer. J. Digest. Dis. 10:657, 1965.
Walter, E. P., Hanauer, F. A., and Kent, D. C.: Primary liver carcinoma in young men. Amer. J. Med. Sci. 252:675, 1966.
Yesner, R., and Conn, H. O.: Liver function tests and needle biopsy in diagnosis of metastatic carcinoma of liver. Ann. Intern. Med. 59:62, 1963.

Carcinoma of the Pancreas

Bouchier, I. A. D.: Cancer of the pancreas. Brit. Med. J. 3:169, 1968.
Burch, G. E., and Ansari, A.: Chronic alcoholism and carcinoma of the pancreas. Arch. Intern. Med. 122:273, 1968.
Fras, I., et al.: Mental symptoms as an aid in early diagnosis of carcinoma of the pancreas. Gastroenterology 55:191, 1968.
Gullick, H. D.: Carcinoma of the pancreas. A review and critical study of 100 cases. Medicine 38:47, 1959.
Serebro, H. H.: A diagnostic sign of carcinoma of the pancreas. Lancet 1:85, 1965.
Smith, P. E., et al.: An analysis of 600 patients with carcinoma of the pancreas. Surg. Gynec. Obstet. 124:1288, 1967.

Pulmonary Embolization

DeVita, V. T., Trufilla, N. P., Blackman, H. H., and Ticktin, H. E.: Pulmonary manifestations of primary hepatic carcinoma. Amer. J. Med. Sci. 250:428, 1965.
McDonald, I. G., et al.: Major pulmonary embolism: A correlation of clinical findings, haemodynamics, pulmonary angiography and pathologic physiology. Brit. Heart J. 34:356, 1972.
Parmley, J. R., et al.: Clinically deceptive massive pulmonary embolism. Chest 58:15, 1970.
Story, P. B., and Goldstein, W.: Pulmonary embolization from primary hepatic carcinoma. Arch. Intern. Med. 110:262, 1962.
Winterbauer, R., et al.: The incidence and clinical significance of tumor embolization to the lungs. Amer. J. Med. 45:271, 1968.

Retroperitoneal Tumors

Melicon, M. M.: Primary tumors of the retroperitoneum; clinicopathologic analysis of 162 cases; review of the literature and tables of classification. J. Int. Coll. Surg. *19*:401, 1953.

Syphilis of the Liver

Shapiro, E., and Weiner, H.: The diagnosis of tertiary syphilis of the liver 25 years after McCrae. Amer. J. Med. Sci. *22*:494, 1951.

C A PATIENT WITH PERSISTENT FEVER AND MALAISE AFTER CARDIAC SURGERY

THE CLINICAL PROBLEM

A 62 year old white male, a Professor of Chemistry, was admitted because of a rash, fever, malaise, and hematuria which appeared $3\frac{1}{2}$ months after aortic valve replacement with a Starr-Edwards prosthesis, performed because of aortic stenosis and coronary insufficiency. Following the operation, the patient failed to thrive, having episodes of low-grade fever and complaining of anorexia, malaise, fatigue, and weight loss, for which no obvious causes could be found. Blood cultures were sterile. Liver function studies showed only very mild abnormalities, not regarded as significant. Shortly after discharge the patient was found to have some peculiar monocytes in his peripheral smear and was thought to be suffering from a mild case of "pump fever," but this seemed to subside quickly. He was maintained on Coumadin throughout. Prior to admission, gross hematuria was noted, and the prothrombin time was increased to 83 seconds. On the night of admission, he was found totally unresponsive and died shortly thereafter.

DISCUSSION OF THE PROBLEM

The basic elements of this patient's problem seem to be quite straightforward. He was 62 years old, and because of increasing severity of angina pectoris, which was considered to be related to his calcific aortic stenosis, the aortic valve was replaced by a Starr-Edwards prosthesis, which distinctly improved his cardiovascular status. Unfortunately, within a matter of several weeks postoperatively, he became unwell with fever, malaise, a petechial rash, and hematuria.

Admitted to the hospital for study of these matters, death came unexpectedly like a thief in the night. At 3:00 A.M., when a nurse checked his vital signs, his condition seemed satisfactory, but when she next visited him at 7:00 A.M., he was totally unresponsive and soon expired.

PART C / PERSISTENT FEVER AND MALAISE

Before considering his terminal illness, we might briefly comment about his calcific aortic stenosis, which caused his difficulty in the first place. What was its etiology? As you well know, there are unsolved mysteries about the genesis of calcific aortic stenosis. The pat answer I was given in medical school, that in most instances this valvular abnormality stems from rheumatic fever, no longer satisfies. Thus, while this patient had no history of rheumatic fever, there was a family history of diabetes and of degenerative vascular disease. In some instances, these factors may be of significance in the development of aortic stenosis. In addition, the patient had a family history of congenital heart disease, and in some cases bicuspid aortic valves may become stenotic. I simply want to emphasize what we don't know about the etiology of calcific aortic stenosis, and to stress that it has a spectrum of causes. In the present setting, and in the absence of any evidence of mitral disease, it seems more likely that congenital or metabolic factors, not rheumatic fever, were causal.

Unfortunately, a significant number of patients who have a Starr-Edwards valve replacement subsequently develop infectious endocarditis. We use the expression "infectious endocarditis" rather than the time-honored term "bacterial endocarditis" because, with increasing frequency, the causative organisms are found to be not bacteria, but fungi and, less often, rickettsia. Surely, the reasons for suspecting infectious endocarditis in this instance are several and are very impelling. Thus, fever and malaise very commonly are the sole indications of postsurgical endocarditis, the "classical" manifestations of endocarditis, including clubbing, splenomegaly, and so forth, being absent. What makes the clinician's problem exceedingly hard is that after cardiac surgery so many other likely causes of fever and malaise are at hand. These include:

1. Pneumonitis.
2. Atelectasis.
3. Pulmonary emboli.
4. Drug reactions.
5. Urinary tract infection.
6. Phlebitis.
7. Wound infection.
8. The use of intravenous catheters.
9. Hepatitis, resulting from either virus or halothane.
10. Postpericardiotomy syndrome.
11. Pump fever.
12. Serum sickness.
13. Hypersensitivity angiitis.

Thus, this patient's initial episode of fever was attributed to infectious mononucleosis. While I would be leery of this diagnosis in a man of 62 years, he probably did have so-called "pump fever," now believed to be caused by the cytomegalovirus. Enlargement of lymph nodes, lymphocytosis, and atypical lymphocytes in the blood smear, all observed in this patient, are some of its characteristics. These infections generally begin a number of weeks postoperatively and persist for several weeks. While they are usually benign, death has been associated with severe instances, and their course may become protracted. Could this have happened here?

Another, but less likely, explanation for that first episode of fever could have been a hepatitis, for he received transfusions and halothane anesthesia. It now seems clear that the cytomegalovirus, as well as the usual viral agents, may produce a hepatitis. While his liver function was essentially normal when subsequently studied, a latent process can't be excluded.

In any event, the fever and malaise persisted without satisfactory explanation several weeks after the usual accompaniments of "pump fever" had gone. When the patient was re-admitted to the hospital, a diastolic murmur, not heard previously postoperatively, was present. The appearance of such a diastolic murmur would be compatible with leakage around the footings of a Starr-Edwards valve or with failure of the valve ball to seal properly, common happenings when they become infected. We must be circumspect, however, in our interpretation of the significance of this diastolic murmur, for such murmurs commonly appear after prosthetic replacement, even in the absence of infection or of clotting, sometimes for quite obscure reasons. Clearly, while a key piece of evidence, it must be interpreted with care.

The manner in which the patient's unanticipated death took place is indicative of a massive cerebrovascular incident, occurring as it did with dramatic suddenness, unresponsiveness, and stertorous breathing. Surely, the evidence pointing to infective endocarditis terminating with a cerebrovascular accident is very strong indeed.

But, was this his total problem? I think not. There were several indications of a generalized hemorrhagic process, including bleeding from the nasopharynx and trachea, the petechiae, the hematuria, and the rapid drop in the hematocrit reading from 29 to 22 ml./100 ml. What could have produced it?

The obvious answer is over-dosage of the anticoagulant he was taking. His prothrombin time was greatly prolonged. Hematuria without other alterations of renal function, as was noted here, is so often the very earliest manifestation of anticoagulant over-dosage that patients on anticoagulants should be instructed to examine their urine. It is possible, as already mentioned, that the patient's liver function may have been somewhat impaired by the halothane anesthesia or by a latent transfusion hepatitis, and thus enhanced the action of Coumadin, despite the results of the liver function tests. But let us not be content with the most obvious explanation for the bleeding phenomena, and overlook the fact that a certain percentage of patients become sick and die owing to considerably less than obvious causes.

Could the patient have had a consumption coagulopathy leading to intervascular clotting, with plugging of small vessels and diffuse hemorrhage? This could explain several of the main events here, obviously. Keep in mind that we have already postulated a blood stream infection, which is one of the inducers of a consumption coagulopathy, particularly when caused by gram-negative organisms. Unfortunately, such organisms have now become not infrequent causes of endocarditis following the implantation of cardiac prostheses, perhaps resulting from the prophylactic use of broad spectrum antibiotics, as was done here. Also, this patient's prostate was said to be greatly enlarged and nodular. Could all of his other troubles have become compounded by the unrecognized development of prostatic cancer? Among other neoplasms, prostatic cancer may be associated with a hypercoagulable state, as you well know. But, the clinical evidence rules out these possibilities, for the platelet count was normal, which would be highly unusual in a consumption coagulopathy. Also, while the patient was anemic, his blood smears showed none of the fragmentation of the red cells so characteristically produced when they are buffeted about in their passage through partially occluded vessels, a sequela of intravascular clotting.

Could he have had some other type of disease of the blood vessels, eventuating in diffuse bleeding and thrombosis? The three possibilities that come immediately to mind are (1) an arteritis; (2) thrombotic thrombocytopenic purpura; and (3) amyloidosis.

Thrombotic thrombocytopenic purpura seems excluded by several items, including the absence of splenomegaly, a low platelet count, renal insufficiency, and fragmented RBCs. While this disorder may occur without one or more of these classical accompaniments, not to find any of them would be too much. A major manifestation of amyloidosis is bleeding, into the skin or elsewhere, and it should always be considered in these circumstances, despite its unusualness. However, the intracutaneous bleeding of amyloidosis generally is first seen around hair follicles, and about the eyes and the neck, not as described here. Besides, this would be an unusual setting for amyloidosis, and there were no obvious deposits in the soft tissues, no protein in the urine, and no neurological changes, so common in generalized amyloidosis. Finally, the tempo of this illness was too fast for this process.

The possibility of a diffuse arteritis deserves more consideration, however, since the patient was a 62 year old male who had recently been given a wide variety of drugs, including several antibiotics, and had also received blood transfusions. So the stage was set for the potential development of a hypersensitivity angiitis. Unexplained, intermittent fever, malaise, hematuria, petechiae, and a cerebrovascular accident are common hallmarks of any form of arteritis. On the other hand, the patient had never had joint or muscle pains, neuropathy or abdominal pain, leukocytosis or eosinophilia. Hematuria in the absence of any other evidence of renal injury would be unusual in an arteritis. Nor, finally, would an arteritis explain one of the key pieces of clinical evidence here—already highlighted—the development of a diastolic murmur not previously detected.

The conclusion seems reasonable, therefore, that the course of the patient's primary illness became complicated by bleeding secondary to Coumadin over-dosage, perhaps associated with latent hepatitis, viral or halothane induced.

If, indeed, he had endocarditis, when did he acquire it, at the time of the operation, or later?

This is impossible to answer, but I suspect that it was acquired in the hospital, and that its inception was hidden under cover of the prophylactic antibiotics he received, for he began to have persistent fever and malaise so soon after his departure from the hospital, his symptoms continuing and growing worse, even after his apparent recovery from "pump fever."

What was the likely responsible organism? Admittedly, again, we cannot be sure, but we can speculate, and in planning treatment for such a patient, accurate speculation is a must, unless one is fortunate enough to have isolated the organism, which was not the case here. At least 37 species of organisms may cause such infections. The most common is the staphylococcus, either S. *aureus* or S. *albus*. The relatively mild nature of the patient's course is unlike the usual fulminant progress of staphylococcal endocarditis, though we must not forget that in about 15 percent of instances of staphylococcal endocarditis, the course is surprisingly benign, resembling that of *Streptococcus viridans*. However, this is usually an easily cultured organism, and the two cultures taken were both negative. Gram-negative organisms are now not infrequent causes of postoperative endocarditis, as already indicated. Undoubtedly a urinary catheter was employed postoperatively. Could the enlarged prostate gland have harbored a focus of gram-negative bacteria? When no organisms are cultured with ordinary media, one should consider the possible presence of such organisms as:

1. Bacteroides.
2. Various L forms, perhaps resulting from prophylactic antibiotics.
3. Various fungi, including *Candida* and *Histoplasma*.
4. The rickettsia of Q fever.
5. The gonococcus.
6. Diphtheroids.

In addition, we must consider the possibility of other organisms having fastidious requirements for culture media. In this case, Q fever is suggested by the extensive purpuric eruption in the hands and legs. While this infection is being reported more and more frequently in this country (particularly in patients exposed to sheep and cattle and their products), and we must be on the lookout for it, we have never recognized an instance of it in this hospital. Still, perhaps this is our first! The diagnosis is made by appropriate serological studies, which were not done here. In fungal endocarditis, very large and succulent vegetations grow on the affected valve. These may disclose their presence in two ways:

1. By blocking valve orifices, and in the case of Starr-Edwards valves, by plugging them up.

2. By releasing very large emboli which cause blockage of major peripheral arteries. In this instance, the prosthesis was not plugged because one could still hear the ball bouncing. The only indication of a massive embolus was the terminal event.

In summary, I don't think the evidence points to a staphylococcal endocarditis, nor, if the infection began early, to a *viridans* streptococcal infection, for the prophylactic antibiotics the patient was given should have prevented this. The fact that the valve was still functioning, and the absence of embolism to major peripheral vessels, reduce somewhat the likelihood of fungal endocarditis. We are left with the prospect of a wide variety of other organisms, many of them resistant to penicillin therapy, and some, unhappily, to any form of therapy.

In conclusion, I believe that this patient acquired an infective endocarditis postoperatively, at the footings of the Starr-Edwards valve. His abrupt death no doubt resulted from a massive cerebrovascular accident. It seems likely that two factors interplayed in causing this:

1. The marked prolongation of the prothrombin time, which no doubt also contributed to the hematuria and perhaps also the petechial eruption.
2. The infective endocarditis.

Anticoagulants were long ago eliminated from the management of patients with endocarditis for the very reason that they tended to convert minor cerebral and other vascular accidents into major and sometimes catastrophic episodes, such as I believe took place here. In endocarditis, a cerebrovascular accident may result from either an embolus or a focal vasculitis, sometimes with mycotic aneurysm formation, the course of either of which may be made more grave by anticoagulants.

It should be made clear that the clinical evidence we are given permits a different explanation for this course of events than the one I have espoused, but one which seems less reasonable to me. Thus, it is possible that he did not have infective endocarditis at all, and that the persistent postoperative fever and malaise were the result of unusually prolonged cytomegalovirus infection, the terminal event being a massive intracerebral hemorrhage secondary to an interplay of Coumadin over-dosage and a chronic hepatitis. However, the characteristic manifestations of "pump fever" had long vanished, and yet he continued to have fever and to become progressively more ill. Finally, therapeutic opportunities make the diagnosis of endocarditis a must.

POST MORTEM FINDINGS

Hepatitis and myocarditis due to prolonged cytomegalovirus infection. Massive intracerebral hemorrhage secondary to hypoprothrombinemia. No evidence of infective endocarditis.

REFERENCES

Infective Endocarditis

Braniff, B. A., Shumway, N. E., and Harrison, D. C.: Valve replacement in active bacterial endocarditis. New Eng. J. Med. 276:1467, 1967.

Cooper, E. S., et al.: Pitfalls in diagnosis of bacterial endocarditis. A review of 159 patients with 96 autopsied. Arch. Intern. Med. *118:*55, 1966.
Cummings, V., et al.: Subacute endocarditis in older age group. JAMA *172:*137, 1960.
Finland, M., and Barnes, M. W.: Changing etiology of bacterial endocarditis in the antibacterial era. Ann. Intern. Med. *72:*341, 1970.
Fraser, R. S., Rossall, R. E., and Dvorkin, J.: Bacterial endocarditis after open heart surgery. Canad. Med. Ass. J. *96:*1551, 1967.
Geraci, J. E., et al.: Endocarditis caused by coagulase-negative staphylococci. Mayo Clin. Proc. *43:*420, 1968.
Grist, N. R.: Q fever endocarditis. Amer. Heart J. *75:*846, 1968.
Hampton, J. R., and Harrison, M. J. G.: Sterile blood cultures in bacterial endocarditis. Quart. J. Med. *36:*167, 1967.
Kay, J. H., et al.: Surgical treatment of *Candida* endocarditis. JAMA *203:*621, 1968.
Laurence, T., et al.: *Aspergillus* infection of prosthetic aortic valve. Chest *60:*406, 1971.
Lerner, P. I., and Weinstein, L.: Infective endocarditis in the antibiotic era. New Eng. J. Med. *274:*199, 259, 323, 388; 1966.
Okies, J. E., et al.: Endocarditis after cardiac valvular replacement. Chest *59:*198, 1971.
Q fever endocarditis. Proc. Roy. Soc. Med. *63:*282, 1970.
Rabinovich, S., Smith, I. M., and January, L. E.: The changing pattern of bacterial endocarditis. Med. Clin. N. Amer. *52:*1091, 1968.
Roberts, W. C., and Bachbinder, N. A.: Right-sided valvular infective endocarditis. Amer. J. Med. *53:*7, 1972.
Shaffer, R. B., and Hall, W. T.: Bacterial endocarditis following open heart surgery. Amer. J. Cardiol. *25:*602, 1970.
Tompsett, R.: Bacterial endocarditis. Changes in the clinical spectrum. Arch. Intern. Med. *119:* 329, 1967.

Cytomegalovirus Infection

Armstrong, D., et al.: Cytomegalovirus infections with viremia following renal transplantation. Arch. Intern. Med. *127:*111, 1971.
Caul, E. O., et al.: Cytomegalovirus infections after open heart surgery. Lancet *1:*777, 1971.
Hanshaw, J. B.: Clinical significance of cytomegalovirus infection. Postgrad. Med. J. *35:*472, 1964.
Lang, D. J.: Cytomegalovirus infection and the postperfusion syndrome. New Eng. J. Med. *280:*1145, 1969.
Lang, D. J., Scolnick, E., and Willerson, J.: Association of cytomegalovirus infection with the postperfusion syndrome. New Eng. J. Med. *278:*1147, 1968.
Reyman, T. A.: Postperfusion syndrome. A review and report of 21 cases. Amer. Heart J. *72:*116, 1966.
Uricchio, J. J.: The postcommissurotomy (postpericardiotomy) syndrome. Amer. J. Cardiol. *12:*436, 1963.
Wilson, R. S. E.: Cytomegalovirus myocarditis. Brit. Heart J. *34:*865, 1972.

Disseminated Intravascular Coagulation

Corrigan, J. J.: Changes in blood coagulation system associated with septicemia. New Eng. J. Med. *279:*851, 1968.
Marden, V. J., et al.: Detection of serum fibrinogen and fibrin products. Amer. J. Med. *51:*71, 1971.
Merskey, C., et al.: The defibrination syndrome: Clinical features and laboratory diagnosis. Brit. J. Haemat. *13:*528, 1967.
Pitney, W. R.: Disseminated intravascular coagulation. Seminars Hemat. *8:*65, 1971.
Yoshikawa, G., et al.: Infection and disseminated intravascular coagulation. Medicine *50:*237, 1971.

Microangiopathic Anemia

Brain, M. C.: Microangiopathic hemolytic anemia. New Eng. J. Med. *281:*833, 1969.

Thrombotic Thrombocytopenic Purpura

Amorosi, E. L., and Ultmann, J. E.: Thrombotic thrombocytopenic purpura: report of 16 cases and review of literature. Medicine *45:*139, 1966.
Umlas, J., and Kaiser, J.: Thrombohemolytic thrombocytopenic purpura (TTP); a disease or a syndrome? Amer. J. Med. *49:*723, 1970.

Aortic Stenosis

Roberts, W. C.: Anatomically isolated aortic valvular disease: the case against its being of rheumatic etiology. Amer. J. Med. *49:*151, 1970.

Roberts, W. C.: The structure of the aortic valve in clinically isolated aortic stenosis. A study of 162 autopsy patients over 15 years of age. Circulation *42:*91, 1970.

Immune Disorders

Brandt, K., Cathcart, E. S., and Cohen, A. S.: A clinical analysis of the course and prognosis of forty-two patients with amyloidosis. Amer. J. Med. *44:*955, 1963.

Christian, C. L.: Amyloidosis. New Eng. J. Med. *280:*878, 1969.

Christian, C. L.: Immune complex disease. New Eng. J. Med. *280:*878, 1969.

McCombs, R. P.: Systemic "allergic" vasculitis. Clinical and pathological relationships. JAMA *194:*1059, 1965.

D A PATIENT WITH FULMINANT PNEUMOCOCCAL PNEUMONIA

THE CLINICAL PROBLEM

This patient was a severe, chronic alcoholic, 62 years old. He had paid many visits to the Accident Room in an intoxicated state, and it was noted that his nutritional state was becoming progressively worse. It was thought that he had hepatic cirrhosis. He was said to have had three episodes of pneumonia in the past, and these were associated with a chronic, productive cough.

Three weeks before admission, his chronic cough worsened. Nine days before admission, he became acutely ill, with worsening of the cough, fever, chills, and pain in the right chest. He became so ill he fell off a bar stool and was immediately admitted to the hospital in a semicomatose state. At the time of admission, he was found to be wasted and icteric. There were signs of right upper lobe, right middle lobe, and right lower lobe pneumonia. He was breathing rapidly and with effort. The heart was fibrillating at a fast rate. The liver was enlarged. There were no focal neurological changes, but the patient was very uncooperative. The WBC count was 9500 cu. mm., with shift to left. Pneumococcus was cultured from the sputum and blood. A lumbar puncture was normal. The patient was given 600,000 units of penicillin IV on admission and 600,000 units twice daily. He seemed to be improving slowly, but upon returning from the EEG lab, he suddenly became short of breath, cyanotic, and convulsed, then died.

DISCUSSION OF THE PROBLEM

It seems to me that at the very outset it is reasonable for us to make certain assumptions and even to come to certain conclusions about this patient and the nature of his illness. In the first place, the history indicates that he was an alcoholic of considerable capacity. Second, his state of nutrition appears to have been inadequate. Third, as a result of the combination of the foregoing two factors, it is likely that he had cirrhosis of the liver. Fourth, the history of chronic cough and repeated episodes of so-called pneumonia associated with pleurisy indicate that he may have had some type of chronic architectural disorder of the lungs, such as bronchiectasis. Fifth, when he entered the hospital, the evidence indicated that he had a pulmonary infection due to the pneumococcus, and this was associated with a pneumococcal bacteremia.

Further, when the patient entered the hospital, he was very seriously ill, and it could have been predicted that he would not sustain his infection well, and that his chances of either succumbing to it, or of developing some serious complication, were exceedingly grave, despite the best use of the most effective antibiotics.

As emphasized by Dr. Robert Austrian, pneumococcal pneumonia continues to be a potentially fatal infection, in spite of the availability of effective antibacterial agents, and there is a group of patients who do not fare well, even when given maximal therapy.

The key to the optimal management of pneumococcal infections is the ability to recognize this particular group of patients at the very outset, to intensify therapy appropriately, and also to anticipate serious complications and appreciate the threat of death unless each exigency is satisfactorily met. Sadly, too often patients with pneumococcal pneumonia are handled in a routine, blasé fashion, as though a cure is always secured when an order is given for antibiotics.

The essential points to be reviewed in evaluating the potential severity of an episode of pneumococcal pneumonia are these:

1. The patient's age.
2. General nutrition.
3. Use of alcohol.
4. General health, with particular reference to the status of the heart, the kidneys and, very important, the liver.
5. The presence of any disorder, in which host defenses may be abnormal, such as SLE, myeloma, or leukemia.
6. A history of previous pulmonary disease.
7. The duration of the pneumonitis prior to commencement of specific therapy.
8. The number of lobes involved.
9. The level of the WBC count.
10. Persistence of bacteremia.
11. Quality of breathing.
12. Mental status.
13. Evidence of shock of any degree.
14. Any degree of jaundice.
15. Heart failure.

16. The type of pneumococcus (type 3, for example, has an appreciably greater mortality and complication rate).

These are the critical points to be evaluated immediately in each patient *before* a plan of management has been evolved.

Now let us take these clinical features, which we regard as accurate indicants of the severity of a pneumococcal pulmonary infection, and see how they apply to this patient. First, there was a background of chronic alcoholism and malnutrition. Second, there was a clinical suspicion of cirrhosis of the liver, as indicated by the presence of multiple spider angiomata, an enlarged liver, and some degree of bilirubin retention. Third, while we cannot be certain of the exact time relationships, the history indicates that he entered the hospital as late as the eighth day of his acute illness. Fourth, the right middle, right upper, and a part of the right lower lobe appeared to have been involved in this process. Fifth, even after the eighth day of his illness, he was still suffering from persistent bacteremia. Sixth, the white blood cell count was 9000. Seventh, he was mildly jaundiced. Eighth, he was cyanotic and his respirations are repeatedly described as labored. Ninth, at the time of his admission to the ward, his blood pressure was slightly depressed, and he had a marked cardiac arrhythmia and a rapid auricular fibrillation. Tenth, there was persistent clouding of his sensorium, as demonstrated by constant mumbling, climbing in and out of bed, removing I.V. fluid tubes, and so forth.

In other words, our analysis of these indicants of severity of infection tells us that this patient had at least 10 strikes against him, and hence his outlook for recovery was in serious doubt, even though antibiotics and other therapy had been given to him in an optimum manner.

It is of the utmost importance to realize that even when pneumococcal infections of the lungs are treated with antibiotics, patients with a significant number of such strikes against them will show increased morbidity and mortality rates, and for this reason one cannot afford to be cookbookish in the treatment of this type of patient. The program of therapy must be designed to meet the estimated degree of severity of the infection. Dr. Thomas Van Metre demonstrated this fact in an admirable study which he carried out when he was with me at St. Louis University. It is frequently a fatal error for the patient when the physician tries to guess how sick he is by simply making a rapid survey of his general status.

Instead, one must meticulously analyze the patient's status and determine how many of these critical factors are present, before an accurate estimate of the severity of the patient's illness can be made and appropriate measures applied to meet it. It is clear from the record, therefore, that this patient was extremely ill from the very outset, and that it should have been anticipated that the outcome might be an unfortunate one, as it subsequently proved to be.

Why did this patient fail to continue to respond to the penicillin therapy, since he did seem to have a satisfactory initial response, insofar as the temperature and pulse had returned to the normal range by the second hospital day?

Those who were responsible for his care felt that he was getting over the hump. Second, what was the ultimate cause of his death?

In the past, I have found it helpful to consider the possible causes of failure in the treatment of pulmonary infections under the following five categories:

1. Failure due to inadequate resistance to infection on the part of the patient.

2. Failure due to the use of an ineffective antibiotic, or use of the antibiotic in inadequate dosage, or inability of the antibiotic to penetrate the infected tissue, such as a loculated abscess, and so forth.

3. Failure due to the development of some complication which is a *direct* result of the infectious process.

4. Failure due to the development of some complication which is an *indirect* result of the infectious process.

5. Failure due to some *associated disease process*, such as cirrhosis, heart failure, and so forth.

Certainly there is every reason to conclude that this patient's resistance to infection may well have been considerably less than sufficient, what with the long history of chronic alcoholism, malnutrition, and possible cirrhosis of the liver.

One might argue whether or not this patient, who had 10 serious strikes against him at the time of admission, was initially given a large enough dose of penicillin, but since this is a debatable point, I will not pursue it.

Can we be certain that there was not some other organism present, in addition to the pneumococcus, against which he was not receiving adequate antibiotic treatment? Several possibilities come to mind in this respect. We all know that the Friedlander's bacillus commonly produces pneumonia in debilitated alcoholics, and that when it does, the type of course which this patient ran is not an unusual one. On the other hand, no Friedlander's bacilli were observed in the examination of the sputum or in the blood cultures, nor was the description of the sputum which this patient produced that of the usual glary, thick, mucoid material which is characteristic of Friedlander's infections—although it is not always present, to be sure. A complicating staphylococcal or streptococcal infection would also have to be considered, but, once again, examination of the sputum did not disclose these organisms. However, it should be stressed that examination of the sputum is very often misleading in these circumstances. As already emphasized, this patient was thought to have had a chronic pulmonary infection, dating back several years, and an infection due to a yeast or fungus should be mentioned. In particular, I would mention a pulmonary infection due to the *Cryptococcus*, and I refer to this because we have seen one or two such infections in the recent past and also because of the mumbling disorientation and confusion which this patient manifested. This sort of clinical picture is not unusual in *Cryptococcus* infections of the brain. However, this is a somewhat unusual type of infection, and the spinal fluid findings were unremarkable.

In addition, there is one complicating infection that deserves to be placed high on the list of possibilities, and that is tuberculosis. At least two or three times a year we see patients come in with what appears to be an uncomplicated pneumococcal pneumonia; initially they respond very satisfactorily to penicillin, but ultimately they succumb to what is later discovered to be associated tuberculosis. Not rarely, tuberculosis seems to become disseminated under the influence of the pneumococcal infection. There are a number of features of this patient's history which make us seriously consider the possibility of associated tuberculosis. In the first place, he seems to have been sick for a number of weeks before the onset of his acute illness. He had a chronic cough with heavy sputum production, suggesting bronchiectasis, yet at the time of this admission the inflammatory process seemed to be confined to the right upper lobe, the lower portions of the lung fields being clear. As you well know, the most common cause of upper lobe bronchiectasis is tuberculosis. The enlarged, tender liver and the patient's mental reaction, his intense cyanosis without significant sounds being heard in the lung fields, the progressive failure to respond to penicillin therapy, the dense lesion in the right upper lobe—all these features could be explained by disseminated tuberculosis complicating the pneumococcal infection.

Even though penicillin is given in large doese, therapeutic failure is sometimes due, as already indicated, to inability of the antibiotic agent to reach some infected focus, which keeps the infection extant. Could such a localized area of infection have existed here? To begin with, I am very much struck by the very dense and somewhat rounded and circumscribed character of the lesion seen in this patient's right upper lung field, and over this area the breath sounds are said to have been markedly suppressed. One wonders whether an empyema could have been present there. Second, although we see no fluid air level anywhere in these x-rays, it is still possible that a large lung abscess or cystic cavity may have been hidden beneath this diffuse inflammatory reaction. Third, the patient's liver was very tender and enlarged, and he was mildly jaundiced. It is possible therefore that the liver may have contained one or more abscesses. Fourth, the patient's heart was fibrillating rapidly, which brings to mind the question of bacterial endocarditis or pericarditis, and finally, his disordered mental behavior. The flattening of the right side of his face, the irregularity of the pupils, and the terminal convulsive episode involving the left side of the body raise the question of the possibility of a brain abscess. Localized infection in any one of these areas might have prevented the treatment he received from being effective.

In considering some additional complications which might have resulted directly from the infection which he had, other possibilities come to mind. According to this patient's clinical chart, he appeared to be getting along fairly well until he was sent to the EEG laboratory, where he is described as becoming rather suddenly in need of suctioning. When he returned to the ward he was deeply cyanotic, his extremities were cold, and there were scattered rales throughout the left chest, which heretofore had been clear.

At that juncture, did he experience rupture of a large abscess or cystic cavity, thereby spreading the infection throughout the remaining lung fields? Or could an empyema cavity have ruptured? Or might he have vomited and aspirated? Or, finally, could he have had cerebral damage due to the rupture of a mycotic aneurysm, or of a brain abscess, with the development of a meningitis which was not recognized?

As far as indirect complications of his infection are concerned, he was very dehydrated on admission, and the possibility of a cerebral thrombosis would have to be considered. Again, we suspect that he had cirrhosis of the liver and under the impetus of this infection he might have gone into hepatic insufficiency. It is interesting that no blood sugar determinations were ever made, although it is well recognized that disordered behavior in patients with diffuse liver disease is sometimes due to hypoglycemia. Finally, sudden death might have been due to a pulmonary embolus.

There are two associated diseases, in addition to tuberculosis, which I think deserve particular mention as possible accompaniments of this patient's pneumococcal infection. Either of them might have resulted in the failure of penicillin to work effectively, and both could have caused the death of the patient. We have already discussed the possibility of an associated tuberculous infection, and we won't labor this point any further. Obviously, in a 62 year old male who has had a chronic cough for a number of weeks, who has been weak, easily fatigued, and losing weight, and who is admitted with pulmonary infection, bronchogenic carcinoma deserves one of the very highest places on anyone's list of possibilities. Again and again we see patients enter the hospital with what appears to be a primary, uncomplicated pneumococcal pneumonia, only to find subsequently that the pneumonia is overriding bronchogenic carcinoma. We don't have to emphasize bronchogenic carcinoma as being an excellent bet here. When the radiologists first saw this patient's films they mentioned the fact that the rounded contour of the lesion suggested the presence of some type of a tumor. Again, the patient's disordered mental behavior is the sort of thing which is commonly seen when the brain becomes seeded by bronchogenic carcinoma, as it often does. The enlargement of the liver could have been due to hepatic metastases. It is indeed hard to exclude carcinoma of the lung.

When the patient arrived on the ward, he was fibrillating at a very rapid rate. In addition, he had a questionable lid lag and on two occasions he was described as having a peculiar stare. Also, he was jaundiced and mentally he was constantly out in left field. He was malnourished, weak, and had lost a lot of weight. Despite the fact that the thyroid was not thought to be enlarged, we must not fail to seriously consider the fact that hyperthyroidism might have been associated with this pneumococcal infection. As you well know, elderly individuals may have hyperthyroidism without any significant enlargement of the thyroid gland. Furthermore, it is a well-known fact that a thyroid storm is often precipitated by the inception of pulmonary and other acute infectious processes. Perhaps that is what happened here.

Thus, when we analyze this patient's course in terms of the five categories of factors that are often responsible for unsatisfactory therapeutic response and death of patients with pulmonary infections, we are left with a very wide variety of possible factors to explain what happened to this patient.

We come then, at last, to the stage where we begin putting together these various considerations. The finding of the pneumococcus in the patient's sputum and in his blood on two occasions led me to conclude that he must have had a pneumococcal pneumonia involving the right middle and upper lobes and a portion of the right lower lobe. In view of the 10 strikes against him, which we have already described in some detail, it is perfectly possible that the pneumococcal infection per se was of adequate severity to account for all the changes observed in this patient, including inability of the penicillin to save him. There is little to suggest bacterial endocarditis or a pericarditis, and the clear spinal fluid is reasonable grounds for excluding meningitis. For the same reason, a brain abscess is not too likely, in addition to the fact that there were no focal signs and the convulsions occurred at a time when the patient was in shock and nearly dead. The rather abrupt way in which the patient became cyanotic and critically ill, requiring suction, following return from the EEG laboratory, suggests that he may have had a lung abscess, cyst, or empyema which precipitously emptied. The history of repeated pulmonary infections and episodes of pneumonia with pleurisy extending back several years prior to the onset of the present illness obviously points to some type of architectural abnormality of the lungs, such as bronchiectasis or cystic disease. The fact that this episode of pneumonia occurred in the upper lung field rather than the lower might favor cystic disease, as opposed to bronchiectasis, unless the bronchiectasis was secondary to chronic fibrotic tuberculosis. The history of chronic alcoholism, inadequate nutritional intake, the spider angiomata, jaundice, and the enlarged liver all point to the existence of cirrhosis of the liver, which would adequately explain why the patient handled this infection so poorly. The fact that this patient was ill in a progressive manner for an indeterminate number of weeks before the acute episode began and that he continued to be ill, ultimately to die, even after penicillin therapy was initially and temporarily effective, seems to me to point to the presence of some associated disease state—in particular, either carcinoma or tuberculosis. The fact that the patient's pulmonary symptoms had existed for a number of years and were confined to the right upper lung field, in addition to the fact that it offers therapeutic opportunities, makes me select tuberculosis as the more likely diagnosis of the two. While latent hyperthyroidism is suggested for the reasons I have mentioned, it also should be emphasized because of its specific therapeutic implications. But there was no enlargement of the thyroid gland whatever, and perhaps even more significant is the fact that the auricular fibrillation responded rather satisfactorily to moderate digitalization. This is not usually the case in auricular fibrillation due to severe hyperthyroidism. I don't see how one can reasonably go any farther with diagnostic speculations with the data we have at hand.

POST MORTEM FINDINGS

At autopsy, pneumonia of some standing was found in all lobes of the right lung. Occasional gram-positive diplococci could be seen in the sections. There was striking inflammatory involvement of the pulmonary arteries and veins, with thrombosis and huge areas of necrosis (resembling infarct) showing abscess formation. In addition, there was an extensive acute glomerulonephritis of the type frequently associated with severe bacterial infections, and several glomeruli contained fibrin thrombi. The whole picture was considered to be best explained by a pneumococcal infection in an alcoholic whose resistance was poor.

REFERENCES

Alexander, W. D., et al.: Emotion and nonspecific infection as possible etiologic factors in Grave's disease. Lancet 2:196, 1968.
American Thoracic Society: Fungal infections of the lungs. Amer. Rev. Resp. Dis. 87:784, 1963.
Barrett, R. J., et al.: Primary carcinoma of the lung. Experience with 1312 patients. J. Thoracic Cardiovasc. Surg. 46:292, 1963.
Butler, W. T., Alling, D. W., Spickard, A., et al.: Diagnostic and prognostic value of clinical and laboratory findings in cryptococcal meningitis. New Eng. J. Med. 270:59, 1964.
Cohen, M. L., and Weiss, E. B.: *Pneumocystis carinii* pneumonia—Review. Chest 60:195, 1971.
Dowling, H. F., and Lepper, M. H.: The effect of antibiotics on the fatality rate and incidence of complications in pneumococcic pneumonia. Amer. J. Med. Sci. 222:396, 1951.
Ferguson, T. B., and Burford, T. H.: The changing pattern of pulmonary suppuration. Surgical implications. Dis. Chest 53:396, 1968.
Fiala, M.: A study of the combined role of viruses, mycoplasmas and bacteria in adult pneumonia. Amer. J. Med. Sci. 257:44, 1969.
Gherman, C. R., and Simon, H. J.: Pneumonia complicating severe underlying disease: a current appraisal of transthoracic lung puncture. Dis. Chest 48:297, 1965.
Goldstein, E., Daly, A. K., and Seamans, C.: *Haemophilus influenzae* as cause of adult pneumonia. Ann. Intern. Med. 66:35, 1967.
Hinshaw, H. C., and Garland, L. H.: Diseases of the Chest. 3rd ed. Philadelphia, W. B. Saunders Company, 1969.
Hoffman, N. R., and Preston, F. S., Jr.: Friedlander's pneumonia. Dis. Chest 53:481, 1968.
Magbar, S. H.: Thyrotoxic storm. New Eng. J. Med. 274:1252, 1966.
Manfredi, F., Daly, W. J., and Behnke, R. H.: Clinical observations of acute Friedlander's pneumonia. Ann. Intern. Med. 58:642, 1963.
Meyers, B. R., et al: Current patterns of infection in multiple myeloma. Amer. J. Med. 52:87, 1972.
Morrow, G. W., et al: Infectious pneumonia, a continuing problem in diagnosis and management. Proc. Staff Meeting Mayo Clin. 37:151, 1962.
Ochsner, A., Jr., and Ochsner, A.: Cancer of the lung; recognition and management. Surg. Clin. N. Amer. 46:144, 1966.
Pinner, M.: Pulmonary Tuberculosis in the Adult: Its Fundamental Aspects. 2nd ed. Springfield, Ill., Charles C Thomas, 1951.
Rich, A. R.: The Pathology of Tuberculosis. 2nd ed. Springfield, Ill., Charles C Thomas, 1951.
Rosen, P., Armstrong, D., and Ramos, C.: *Pneumocystis carinii* pneumonia. Study of 20 patients with neoplasms. Amer. J. Med. 53:428, 1972.
Rubin, P., et al.: Bronchogenic carcinoma. JAMA 195:653, 1966.
Stead, W. W., et al.: The clinical spectrum of primary tuberculosis in adults. Confusion with reinfection in the pathogenesis of chronic tuberculosis. Ann. Intern. Med. 68:731, 1968.
Shulman, J. A., Phillips, L. A., and Petersdorf, R. G.: Errors and hazards in the diagnosis and treatment of bacterial pneumonias. Ann Intern. Med. 62:41, 1965.

Sullivan, R. J., et al.: Adult pneumonia in a general hospital. Arch. Intern. Med. *139*:935, 1972.
Utz, J. P.: The spectrum of opportunistic fungus infections. Lab. Invest. *11*:1018, 1962.
VanMetre, T. E.: Pneumococcal pneumonia treated with antibiotics; the prognostic significance of certain clinical findings. New Eng. J. Med. *251:* 1048, 1954.
Waldstein, S. S., Slodki, S. J., Kaganiec, I., and Bronsky, D.: A clinical study of thyroid storm. Ann. Intern. Med. *52:*626, 1960.
Witt, R. L., and Hamburger, M.: The nature and treatment of pneumococcal pneumonia. Med. Clin. N. Amer. *47:*1257, 1963.
Young, A. C., et al.: Aspergillosis; the spectrum of the disease in 98 patients. Medicine *49:*147, 1970.

E A PATIENT WITH A LIVER ABSCESS

THE CLINICAL PROBLEM

This 31 year old white single male was admitted on October 6 complaining of shortness of breath of several days' duration. The patient was so extremely ill on admission that his history had to be obtained from members of the family. The patient was apparently in good health until the previous July, when he had had an illness which was called "virus pneumonia." He appeared to have never completely recovered from this illness: he continued to lose weight and become easily fatigued. About three weeks before admission he was examined by a doctor because of epileptic seizures, from which he had been suffering since birth. After the examination, the doctor told the parents that the patient had heart trouble and also that there was fluid in his abdomen. The patient seemed to get along fairly well but for mild ankle edema and night sweats until a few days before admission, when he became so markedly short of breath that he could not walk upstairs. He developed pain in the right side of his chest. He was found by his mother gasping for breath, and covered with perspiration. He was therefore brought to the accident room and admitted to the hospital. The history revealed that the patient had had convulsions since he was a baby, and he had never been to school because of mental deficiency, spending his time working about the house.

Physical examination revealed the following: pulse, 135; respirations, 40; temperature, 99.8 degrees; blood pressure not obtainable. The patient appeared to be critically ill, in severe respiratory distress, and had the facies and demeanor characteristic of mental deficiency. He was very poorly nourished and very pale, but not jaundiced. There was a marked tachycardia. The heart was thought to be markedly enlarged to the left, dullness appearing in the anterior axillary line. There were no unusual heart sounds. There appeared to be a large effusion at the right lung base and a few scattered rales. The abdomen was greatly distended, with a prominent venous pattern. The liver was greatly enlarged, extending down to the umbilicus. Its surface was very hard. The spleen was not felt. There was a two- to three-plus bilateral pitting edema of the ankles. The arterial pulsations of the wrists and ankles could not be felt, and the brachial pulses were weak. Neurological examination did not show any unusual results.

Course in the Hospital

The admission white cell count was 93,300/cu. mm., with 17 percent neutrophilic myelocytes, 15 percent juvenile neutrophils, 26 percent stab cells, 29 percent segmented neutrophils, 4 percent lymphoblasts, 9 percent lymphocytes. Hemoglobin, 13 grams/100 ml. Hematocrit, 36 ml./100 ml.; RBC, 5.5 million/cu. mm. No urine was obtained for examination. The ECG showed a sinus tachycardia. The serological test for syphilis was negative. On admission, it was thought that the patient was in severe congestive heart failure, and he was given intravenous digitoxin. Venous pressure, however, was only 13 centimeters of water. A few hours after admission, the patient suddenly stopped breathing and died. We are told that a large liver abscess was found at post mortem.

DISCUSSION OF THE PROBLEM

While being informed that some type of liver abscess was found at post mortem, we are given no other details, and there are a number of related problems to which we do not know the answer. These we will now consider—namely, (1) What was the etiology of this abscess? (2) What was the nature of the terminal event, associated as it was with profound respiratory distress, shock, and an unusual blood picture?

In general, there are two kinds of liver abscesses: (1) those resulting from amebic infection, and (2) those stemming from pyogenic infection. Both of these in turn may be either single or multiple.

The existence of either type of liver abscess is a relatively uncommon occurrence. In some areas, amebic abscess occurs about three times as frequently as pyogenic abscess, while in other areas the incidence is reversed. For reasons not clear, both types of abscesses occur much more frequently in males than in females. This is particularly true of amebic disease, in which the incidence is 75 to 95 percent male. Generally, young adults in their 20's to 40's are most frequently affected. The mistake is often made in clinical diagnosis of regarding the liver as affected by a single abscess, whereas post mortem examination subsequently often reveals multiple areas of involvement. Multiple small abscesses may coalesce to form one or more large abscesses. Where the present patient is concerned, it is important to emphasize that solitary large pyogenic abscesses are rare. The right lobe of the liver is much more commonly affected than is the left lobe by both types of abscesses, as was observed in this patient. This is because the superior mesenteric vein drains principally to the right lobe of the liver, while the left lobe is fed by the inferior mesenteric and splenic veins. In amebic infections, infestation occurs more often in the right colon, which is drained by the superior mesenteric vein, than in the left colon, and appendicitis is one of the more common causes of secondary pyogenic abscess.

Abscess of the liver may be produced in five general ways:

1. By spread to the liver of a contiguous process, such as a ruptured peptic ulcer.
2. By an ascending infection from the biliary ducts.
3. By dissemination through the portal venous system.
4. By systemic arterial infection (sepsis).
5. By trauma.

The organisms usually responsible are streptococci, staphylococci, coliform organisms, and bacteroides. Rarely, various fungi and actinomycosis are causal. Not at all infrequently, for obscure reasons, the pus removed from pyogenic abscesses is sterile, even though the patient was untreated. In amebic abscess, the amebae commonly are found not in the abscess material but rather in its fibrous walls. After an abscess has been evacuated, however, the organisms appear in the drainage fluid. This may be a result of their need for O_2 in order to survive. Since amebae are usually not found in the pus, and since this material may be sterile in pyogenic abscess, it may be difficult or impossible to ascertain the specific nature of a liver abscess even at operation. However, the appearance of the fluid evacuated from an amebic abscess may be helpful in this regard. It has been described in a variety of ways: (1) Like chocolate sauce; (2) like anchovy paste (to cocktail set); (3) liver paste (to less imaginative); (4) crushed strawberries; (5) wine dregs (to elderly successful practitioners).

If an amebic abscess becomes secondarily infected, the character of the abscess material, as well as the clinical course, may be markedly altered. There is considerable debate regarding the frequency with which secondary infection occurs in amebiasis. Some say 20 percent, while others maintain that secondary infection is unusual until after external drainage is achieved.

While the point of origin of a pyogenic abscess may be obvious, not infrequently the source of the infection may be completely hidden, and the conclusion may be reached that it is a primary abscess. Such cryptogenic abscesses have had a 17 to 50 percent incidence. Failure to localize any primary source of infection in this patient, therefore, doesn't exclude a pyogenic abscess. Furthermore, it would not be surprising for a mentally deficient person such as this patient to have had acute appendicitis which went unrecognized.

Amebic abscess is often also of obscure origin, for fully 30 to 50 percent of patients with amebic abscess have no dysenteric symptoms, and amebae are found in the stools of only one third of such patients. The absence of enteric manifestations in this patient is, therefore, of no diagnostic importance.

This patient's illness began with an episode which was called pneumonia, and subsequently he became very fatigued and weak, lost weight, and had night sweats. Such nonspecific symptoms are often the earliest manifestations of liver abscess, and they may be of minimal intensity for a prolonged period of time. Furthermore, in early stages, the symptoms of liver abscess not infrequently mimic those of a pneumonitis resulting from involvement of the right diaphragm and the collection of fluid in the right pleural space.

The findings described in this patient, of an enlarged liver and elevation of the right diaphragm associated with an effusion at the right base and compression of the right lung, are those very commonly observed in either type of liver abscess. It is important to emphasize, however, that early in the course of liver abscess, fever may be the sole abnormality.

Note that for a period of 3 to 4 months during which we suspect that this patient had a liver abscess, he did not appear to be very ill to his family. In this regard, solitary abscess of the liver, particularly if amebic in origin, may have a very insidious and benign initial course. This is in contrast to multiple pyogenic abscesses in which the manifestations tend to be more outspoken. For a long period of time, a thick walled amebic abscess may do little more to the patient than take up space.

In contrasting the usual features of amebic abscess with the pyogenic sort, these statements can be made:

1. A large, single abscess is more likely to be amebic than pyogenic.
2. In amebic disease, there is no obvious source of a pyogenic infection such as appendicitis, gallbladder disease, etc.
3. Amebic abscess occurs in a somewhat younger group than pyogenic abscess.
4. The pus from an amebic abscess is characteristic, if no secondary infection is present.
5. In amebic abscess, the clinical course tends to be less acute and more bland than in the pyogenic variety.
    a. The onset is more insidious.
    b. Fever is slightly or moderately increased.
    c. Chills are rare.
    d. The white blood cell count is lower, on average, with not so marked a shift to the left. However, amebiasis may become associated with a marked leukocytosis if there is a secondary infection or if some complication occurs.

Furthermore, in amebiasis there is a greater tendency for the production of changes at the right lung base than in pyogenic infection. Such changes may be pleuritis, sympathetic effusion, pneumonitis, ruptured pleura, and lung abscess.

In view of these considerations, it would seem most likely that this patient's liver abscess was due to an amebic infection, in view of:

1. The insidious onset.
2. The bland course initially.
3. The absence of any obvious focal pyogenic infection.

4. The marked enlargement of the liver, indicating a solitary or numerous very large abscesses.

5. Finally, the prominent changes at the right lung base.

There are, nevertheless, some points favoring pyogenic infection—namely, the suggestion that ascites was present, and the unusual leukocytosis with a profound shift to the left.

Ascites is unusual in uncomplicated amebic abscess. Its presence suggests the possibility of thrombosis of the portal vein, one of the common causes of which is suppuration associated with appendicitis. We have already indicated that this unfortunate patient could well have had an undetected ruptured appendix.

Certainly, the degree of leukocytosis with shift to the left in the differential count reported here is never seen in amebiasis unless there is secondary infection or some other complication, and even then it would be unusual. As a matter of fact, this leukemoid picture would be equally uncommon in uncomplicated pyogenic abscess.

It seems evident that some dramatic event must have precipitated the profound state of shock in which this patient was found by his mother, which was associated with extreme dyspnea and pleural pain in the right chest and the leukemoid changes.

The commonest complication of amebic abscess is rupture into an adjoining structure or cavity. Such occurrences are usually manifested by a sudden dramatic change in the patient's status and the development of shock and leukocytosis. The degree of dyspnea manifested by this patient and the signs at the right base make rupture into the right pleural space a likely possibility, and one which we can't exclude. However, there are others—the abscess might have ruptured into the pericardial sac, with resultant cardiac tamponade, but this is partially excluded by the absence of signs of increased venous pressure.

When Dr. George Edwards, the resident physician, saw this patient, he suggested that the leukemoid picture may have resulted from rupture of the abscess into the hepatic vein or the inferior vena cava. This is a rare occurrence, but I think it likely here.

As we have indicated, this patient was said to have ascites, and there was a prominent venous pattern, edema, and a huge liver. All of these features indicate that the abscess may well have ruptured into the venous system of the liver or inferior vena cava, resulting in the leukemoid reaction. Finally, there may well have been massive pulmonary infarctions arising from the affected cava.

PATHOLOGICAL FINDINGS

Amebic abscess of the liver with rupture into the right pleural space, the pericardium, the hepatic veins, and the inferior vena cava. Multiple pulmonary emboli.

REFERENCES

Liver Abscess

Berke, J., and Pecora, C.: Diagnostic problems of pyogenic hepatic abscess. Amer. J. Surg. *111*:678, 1966.
Butler, T. J., and McCarthy, C. F.: Pyogenic liver abscess. Gut *10*:389, 1969.
Cain, G. D., Moore, P., Jr., and Patterson, M.: A ten year review of amebic abscess of the liver. Amer. J. Digest. Dis. *13*:709, 1968.
Cronin, K.: Pyogenic abscess of the liver. Gut *2*:53, 1961.
Joseph, W. L., Kahn, A. M., and Longmire, W. P., Jr.: Pyogenic liver abscess: changing patterns in approach. Amer. J. Surg. *115*:63, 1968.
Keefer, C. S.: Liver abscess: Review of 85 cases. New Eng. J. Med. *211*:21, 1934.
Lamont, N. M., and Pooler, N. R.: Hepatic amebiasis. Quart. J. Med. *27*:389, 1958.
Millekin, N. T., and Stryker, H. B., Jr.: Suppurative pylethrombophlebitis and multiple liver abscesses following acute appendicitis; report of case with recovery. New Eng. J. Med. *244*:52, 1951.
Ochsner, A., DeBakey, M., and Murray, S.: Pyogenic abscess of liver. II. Analysis of 47 cases with review of literature. Amer. J. Surg. *40*:292, 1938.
Pyrtek, C. J., and Bartus, S. A.: Hepatic pyemia. New Eng. J. Med. *272*:551, 1965.
Sabbaj, L., et al.: Anaerobic pyogenic liver abscess. Ann. Intern. Med. *77*:629, 1972.
Sherman, J. D., and Robbins, S. L.: Changing trends in the casuistics of hepatic abscess. Amer. J. Med. *28*:943, 1960.
Turriel, F. L., and Burnham, J. R.: Hepatic amebiasis. Report of 100 cases. Amer. J. Surg. *111*:424, 1966.

Leukemoid Reaction

Heck, F. J., and Hall, B. E.: Leukemoid reactions of myeloid type. JAMA *112*:95, 1939.
Hill, J. M., and Duncan, C. N.: Leukemoid reactions. Amer. J. Med. Sci. *201*:847, 1941.
Krumbhaar, E. B.: Leukemoid blood pictures in various clinical conditions. Amer. J. Med. Sci. *172*:519, 1926.
Meyer, L. M., and Botter, S. D.: Leukemoid reaction in malignancy. Amer. J. Clin. Path. *12*:218, 1942.
Schmidt, D. M., et al.: Granulocytic leukemoid reactions associated with malignant disease. Calif. Med. *99*:24, 1963.

F A PATIENT SUFFERING SUDDEN DEATH

THE CLINICAL PROBLEM

This 23 year old student priest was admitted as an emergency patient, so acutely ill that only a fragmentary story could be obtained. Apparently, he suddenly became dizzy and collapsed while on his way to visit a patient. He was largely unresponsive for one to two minutes when first observed. He then revived and was able to talk. He coughed several times without production of sputum. His color was pale and his skin was drenched in sweat. Just before he was placed in bed he vomited a large amount of recently eaten food. No blood was noted. He was in no pain at this time. As soon as the patient had been put to bed, he began complaining that he could not breathe, and it was noted that his lips and nail beds were deeply cyanotic. At this

PART F / A PATIENT SUFFERING SUDDEN DEATH

time a brief bit of information was obtained from the patient to the effect that he had been seeing one of the local physicians for stomach trouble, characterized as a "nervous stomach." An ECG and GI series had been normal.

On physical examination the patient, a healthy appearing young white male, was seen to be in extreme distress. He was drenched in sweat, with very cyanotic lips and nail beds, and was restless and very agitated, thrashing about and complaining that he could not breathe. His color was not improved by giving oxygen. When first examined, there was a fairly strong pulse (rate about 76 to 80) felt in the right wrist, but soon thereafter this pulse was unobtainable. Respiratory rate was 30 and respirations were very deep. Blood pressure could not be obtained. There was no evidence of weight loss, and no indication of trauma about the head. Neck was supple. Chest was symmetrical and resonant throughout. Breath sounds were normal in all areas. The airway was patent. The heart was not enlarged, and the heart rhythm was regular but the rate was slow. The sounds were of good quality when first heard, but later were very slow and very faint. No murmurs were heard. The peripheral pulses, except for the right radial, were not felt. The abdomen was flat, and there was no tenderness, rigidity, or spasm. No palpable organs or masses were found. Bowel sounds were hypoactive, but normal in quality. Extremities were not remarkable; there was no clubbing and no edema of the legs. On neurological examination, no gross evidence of neurological deficit was found.

Oxygen was given by nasal catheter, but there was no improvement in cyanosis. The patient continued to cry out that he could not get enough air in spite of free air movement into the lungs. He began to complain of pain across the upper abdomen, which he could not characterize, although apparently it was quite severe, and he stated that it seemed to be interfering with his breathing. He also said that he had never had such pain before. He expressed the opinion that he was dying. Despite all measures, his shock did not abate and he died in an hour.

DISCUSSION OF THE PROBLEM

While death is always the harbinger of sorrow, there are many times when its arrival can be gracefully accepted as the anticipated termination of a long, full life. There are still other times when death is embraced almost eagerly, as it brings peace and surcease from suffering to the individual with an incurable disability. But death is deeply resented when it strikes a vigorous youth in the bloom of health, as it did here, and only faith can force a graceful acceptance. It seems to me that all of the mystery and pathos of death are acutely felt in this story of a seemingly healthy 23 year old man, smitten as he ascends the steps of a hospital to visit a sick friend. It is a tale which produces an introspective pause, and throughout it is the theme, "I will come like a thief in the night, and you shall not know the day nor the hour." Surely this is death in its most fearsome guise. This is *sudden* death.

The expression "sudden death" is one which requires definition. It means something more than merely a quick or abrupt death—there must be an element of surprise at its arrival. For example, an elderly male who has had increasingly severe angina pectoris for three years, associated with congestive heart failure, and who abruptly becomes acutely ill and dies in heart failure cannot be said to have had a sudden death, for in such circumstances death must have been anticipated from the very inception of the condition. The element of surprise is lacking. Hence we define sudden death as death which comes both quickly and *unexpectedly*. The question which then naturally arises is "How quickly is sudden?" If a 15 year old boy previously in good health falls to the street in deep coma, but lingers in this state for three days before death intervenes, can his death be called sudden? Clearly no definite restrictions can be placed upon the time intervals within which death must occur for it to be sudden. Death need not be instantaneous, yet it cannot be too long delayed. Still, we cannot afford to be too precise in our definition—death is sudden if it comes reasonably quickly under circumstances in which its immediate arrival is unexpected.

When confronted by such a problem of sudden death as this, the clinician is sometimes faced with insuperable diagnostic difficulties. This is because the two principal clinical tools with which he works, namely the facts of the history and the physical examination, are often inadequate because of the emergent course of the illness which may have ended in death before all the significant facts in the matter are known or appreciated. Furthermore, even the pathologist may be at a loss to explain the cause of death in such circumstances, although he may not always admit it. This is because death not infrequently is caused by changes in function rather than alterations in structure.

In general, there are three general categories of causes of sudden death:
1. Sudden death due to violence.
2. Sudden death due to poisoning.
3. Sudden death due to natural causes.

It seems apparent from the circumstances that we are not dealing with a violent death, and I know of no toxic material which would produce the changes noted here. This would seem to be a natural death, though an untimely one.

Now a sudden natural death is almost always due to some acute disorder arising somewhere within the circulatory apparatus. For example, in a group of 700 cases of sudden natural death, fully 91 percent were due to circulatory accidents of some sort. Such circulatory abnormalities can be grouped as follows:

1. Sudden alteration of the contractility of the heart muscle, resulting in stoppage of the heart, or abnormal beating.
2. Hemorrhage.

3. Embolism and thrombosis.

It is difficult to quantitate accurately the incidence of occurrence of these various mechanisms, but it has been estimated as follows: (1) Abnormal heart action, 71 percent; (2) hemorrhage, 23 percent; (3) embolism and thrombosis, 5 percent.

In addition to these more common causes of sudden death, there are a wide variety of unusual and sometimes bizarre etiologies, and as already mentioned, there is a small but significant group of people who die suddenly, and no underlying cause is ever found.

Let us now see how these categories of causes apply to this particular patient's demise.

Stoppage of the heart is far and away the most common cause of sudden death, occurring three times more frequently than any other single cause, and so we shall consider it first. It can be said with reasonable assurance that if an adult in perfect health suddenly falls dead, the chances are overwhelmingly in favor of coronary occlusion. This is particularly true if death is instantaneous. There are certain features of this history which suggest the patient may have had such a coronary occlusion. There is the history of "indigestion" in the past, for which he sought the advice of a local physician, and we know that time and again the symptoms of coronary insufficiency are mistaken for some type of digestive disturbance. Again, the severe, terrifying pain in the upper abdomen that was described could have arisen from myocardial infarction, and the shock, restlessness, and anxiety are all typical features of such an event.

However, there are a number of elements in this history which exclude such a possible cause of death. In the first place, the patient was only 23. While it is true that as a result of experience during the past war we now recognize that coronary heart disease may occur at a much younger age than previously recognized, and myocardial infarction is not a rare happening in persons 30 to 40 years of age, it would still be somewhat unusual for a youth of 23 to die as a result of coronary occlusion. This is especially true in this situation, in which the patient is known to have had normal blood pressure and a normal ECG and negative cardiac history just a few months prior to his death. Furthermore, it is of some significance that his pain made its appearance after the onset of shock, and did not precede the inception of vascular collapse, which is usually the course of events in myocardial infarctions. Most important of all in excluding coronary occlusion is the presence of a marked degree of dyspnea and intense cyanosis, in the absence of significant cardiac failure. There is no basis for severe dyspnea and cyanosis in myocardial infarction unless the patient is in cardiac failure, which does not appear to have been the case here.

Could he have had a Stokes-Adams attack? These, as you well know, are acute periods of cerebral ischemia resulting from a precipitous fall in cardiac output, secondary to sudden asystole of the heart muscle, or the sudden onset of some type of abnormal rapid heart action. Such attacks generally occur in association with some type of myocardial or endocardial disease. Against this possibility once more is the age of the patient, and the absence of hypertension or other cardiac abnormality when examined a few months previously, and the dearth of signs of intrinsic heart disease at the time of admission. Also of great importance are the repeated statements in the chart that the patient's heart was beating both slowly and regularly, and finally, unless such an attack had precipitated heart failure, it offers no explanation for the intense dyspnea and cyanosis manifested, since as already noted, there was no significant heart failure.

Now let us turn to a consideration of the possibility of some type of hemorrhagic catastrophe.

Such a hemorrhage might have originated in a variety of areas of the body, and we will consider each in turn.

1. A hemorrhage within the substance of the brain is excluded by the complete lack of abnormal neuromuscular function. Furthermore, this type of hemorrhage does not usually result in death quite so rapidly as in this circumstance. The same may be said of hemorrhage into the subarachnoid space, and an additional point against this latter was the absence of rigidity of the neck. In addition, dyspnea and cyanosis of a marked degree are not found in intracranial hemorrhage, unless there is some associated phenomenon, such as obstruction of the air passages, atelectatic pneumonia or depression of the respiratory reflex, and the clinical notes state clearly that in this patient breathing was rapid, deep, and free, and that the lungs were quite clear. Finally, the severe abdominal pain could not be explained by such an event.

2. Hemorrhage within the lungs is excluded by the failure to cough blood, the negative physical examination of the chest, the persistently slow pulse, and the severe abdominal pain which was a predominant part of the picture.

3. Hemorrhage from a ruptured aneurysm of the aorta is not so readily excluded. Such an aneurysm could have been either one of two types, saccular or dissecting. When such aneurysms rupture, they frequently empty into nearby structures, such as the vena cava, the pulmonary artery, the bronchi, the pleural cavity, or the retroperitoneal or abdominal spaces.

Ruptured aneurysms are not uncommonly the cause of obscure, sudden death. Again, a characteristic feature of such events is the development of profound shock associated with the onset of excruciating pain, such as was present here. In addition, the heart sounds are described as becoming progressively more and more faint until finally they were inaudible shortly before death, and this is exactly the course of events during the terminal stages of dissecting aneurysm or rupture of the aorta, as bleeding occurs into the pericardial cavity. Such intrapericardial bleeding, with the development of cardiac tamponade, is very commonly the final event in such circumstances. Cyanosis and dyspnea may be present in this situation, in the absence of heart failure.

While this possibility merits serious attention, there are a number of excluding factors. At the age of 23, aneurysm resulting either from arteriosclerosis or syphilis would be most unusual. Furthermore, hypertension is very commonly present in dissecting aneurysm, and no hypertension was seen here. A few months prior to this final event, the patient was considered in good health by his local physician. Obviously, we cannot positively exclude some type of latent congenital abnormality of the aorta which could have led to this catastrophe. Furthermore, the excruciating pain made its appearance after the onset of shock, and the reverse is usually true in dissecting aneurysm, which is characteristically ushered in by the dramatic onset of pain. Moreover, this pain is more often first felt in the neck and back and shoulders, rather than in the abdomen, as in this instance. In addition, no murmurs were heard over the heart or vessels, and very often murmurs are noted when an aneurysm is present. Against the possibility of rupture into the pericardium with the production of cardiac tamponade is the persistence of a slow heart beat and the absence of venous enlargement in the neck, as well as the failure to demonstrate cardiac enlargement. In cardiac tamponade, the progressive development of tachycardia and venous engorgement are classical features. The absence of venous engorgement also excludes the possibility of rupture into the vena cava, and the clear lung fields eliminate rupture into that area. Massive bleeding into the chest or abdomen seems most unlikely in view of the failure of the patient to develop a significant tachycardia despite the profound shock. Rupture of an abdominal aneurysm is also excluded by the absence of rigidity or tenderness of the abdomen. The marked degree of dyspnea and cyanosis would be out of place in such a situation.

The past history of indigestion suggests the recurrence of a peptic ulcer with massive GI bleeding, but this type of hemorrhage rarely results in such a precipitous death. Furthermore, there was neither hematemesis nor melena, and the excruciating pain would be hard to account for, as would also be the lack of tachycardia and the presence of marked dyspnea and cyanosis.

We come then to the clinical consideration that this patient's sudden death was the result of an acute embolic or thrombotic occurrence. Such an occlusive episode might have involved arteries in the lung, brain, or heart, for it is involvement of these structures which generally results in sudden death. We have already given reasons why we do not think that acute injury to the heart or brain caused this patient's death. So we now turn to pulmonary embolism. As a matter of fact, next to coronary occlusion, acute occlusion of the pulmonary vascular bed is most frequently responsible for a sudden death that occurs either instantaneously or within a short span of time.

It seems to us entirely likely that this patient's death was the result of a massive pulmonary embolism. The whole picture fits this likelihood. The initial spell of syncope and the subsequent vascular collapse is explained by the block imposed in the lesser circulation by the embolus, and the subsequent fall in cardiac output. The marked hunger for air and the intense cyanosis, associated with extreme anxiety, restlessness, and premonitions of death, are all typical of massive pulmonary embolism. There are a variety of explanations offered for the subsequent development of the severe, deep pain in the upper abdomen and lower chest. Acute coronary insufficiency, acute congestion of the liver, and pleuritis may all play a role in the inception of this pain. There are only two features in this present situation which cast doubt upon this diagnosis of embolism—the absence of tachycardia and the absence of venous distention. The former might be explained on the basis of vagal discharge, which is said to occur with acute occlusion of the pulmonary arteries. In any event, I don't believe these peculiarities should discourage us from a diagnosis which so well fits the bill in all other respects.

If, indeed, the patient had a pulmonary embolus, where was its origin? Not infrequently, such emboli arise from an unrecognized source. It is not too well understood that venous thrombosis in the peripheral vessels may follow a seemingly trivial accident which may be entirely disregarded by the patient. Such may have been true here.

On the other hand, we do know that for several months the patient was bothered by indigestion to the point that a GI series was carried out. This raises the possibility that the patient may have had some sort of latent intra-abdominal or systemic disease which could have become associated with the formation of venous thrombosis, including pancreatitis or carcinoma of the pancreas, and, in this age group, a latent lymphoma or sarcoma.

Other systemic conditions to be considered would be a primary blood disorder or a collagen-vascular disease.

I don't believe we can intelligently do more than speculate as to the source of this pulmonary embolus, and additional speculation would seem profitless. At this age, a lymphoma would seem most likely, with pancreatic disease next.

POST MORTEM FINDINGS

Massive acute pulmonary embolism. Retroperitoneal lymphosarcoma.

REFERENCES

Sudden Death

Croce, L., Noseda, V., Bertelli, A., and Bossi, E.: Sudden and unexpected death from heart disease: Epidemiologic, anatomical and physiopathologic aspects. A study of 1047 cases. Cardiologia 37:331, 1960.

Engel, G. L.: Sudden and rapid death during psychological stress. Ann. Intern. Med. 74:771, 1971.

Green, J. R., Jr., et al.: Sudden unexpected death in three generations. Arch. Intern. Med. 124:359, 1969.

Hamman, L. A.: Sudden death. Bull. Johns Hopkins Hosp. 55:387, 1934.

Helpern, M.: Sudden and unexpected natural death. Trans. Assoc. Life Insurance Med. Dir. Amer. 31:131, 1947.

Helpern, M., and Rabson, S. M.: Sudden and unexpected natural death—general considerations and statistics. New York J. Med. 45:1197, 1945.

Kuller, L., Lilienfeld, A., and Fisher, R.: An epidemiological study of sudden and unexpected deaths in adults. Medicine 46:341, 1967.

Paul, O., and Schatz, M.: On sudden death. Circulation 43:7, 1971.

Simpson, K.: Pathology of sudden death. Ann. Roy. Coll. Surg. Eng. 2:18, 1948.
Sudden death in young adults [editorial]. JAMA 203:138, 1968.

Pulmonary Embolism

McDonald, I. G., et al.: Major pulmonary embolism, a correlation of clinical findings, haemodynamics, pulmonary angiography and pathologic physiology. Brit. Heart J. 34:356, 1972.
Murray, J. F.: The pathogenesis, diagnosis and treatment of pulmonary embolus. Calif. Med. 114:36, 1971.
Parmley, L. F.: Clinically deceptive massive pulmonary embolism. Chest 58:15, 1970.
Ratnoff, O. D., and Breckenridge, R. T.: Pulmonary embolism and unexpected death in supposedly normal persons. New Eng. J. Med. 270:298, 1964.

Cardiac Arrhythmias

Hoffman, B. F., and Cranefield, P. F.: The physiologic basis of cardiac arrhythmias. Amer. J. Med. 37:670, 1964.
Watanabe, Y., and Dreifus, L. S.: Newer concepts in the genesis of cardiac arrhythmias. Amer. Heart J. 76:114, 1968.
Wolf, S.: Central autonomic influences in cardiac rate and rhythm. Mod. Concepts Cardiovas. Dis. 38:29, 1969.

Pericardial Effusion

Morgan, B. C., et al.: The effect of blood volume in venous pressure in cardiac tamponade. J. Thor. Cardiovasc. Surg. 51:575, 1966.
Spodick, D. H.: Acute pericarditis. New York, Gruen & Stratton, 1959.

Coronary Artery Disease

Kannel, W. B., and Feinleib, M.: Natural history of angina pectoris in the Framingham study. Amer. J. Cardiol. 29:154, 1972.
Oberman, A., et al.: Natural history of coronary artery disease. Bull. N. Y. Acad. Med. 48:1109, 1972.

Dissecting Aortic Aneurysm

Baer, S., and Goldburg, H. C.: The varied clinical syndromes produced by dissecting aneurysms. Amer. Heart J. 35:198, 1948.
Fomor, J. J., et al.: Aneurysms of the aorta—a review. Ann. Surg. 165:557, 1967.
Hirst, A. E., Jr., Johns, V. F., Jr., and Kima, S. W., Jr.: Dissecting aneurysms of the aorta—505 cases. Medicine 37:217, 1958.
Lindsay, J., Jr., and Hurst, J. W.: Clinical features and prognosis in dissecting aneurysms of the aorta. Circulation 35:880, 1967.
Prokop, E. K., Palmer, R. F., and Wheat, M. W., Jr.: Hydrodynamic forces in dissecting aneurysms. Circulation 38(Suppl. VI):159, 1968.
Wheat, M. W., Jr., Harris, P. D., Malm, J. R., Kaiser, G., Bowman, F. O., and Palmer, R. F.: Acute dissecting aneurysms of the aorta. J. Thor. Cardiovasc. Surg. 58:344, 1969.

Lymphosarcoma

Rosenberg, S. A., Diamond, H. D., Jaslowitz, B., and Carver, L. F.: Lymphosarcoma: A review of 1269 cases. Medicine 40:31, 1961.

G A PATIENT WITH A MEDIASTINAL MASS

THE CLINICAL PROBLEM

A 58 year old white bar owner was admitted because of pain in his chest of three months' duration and hoarseness of two weeks' standing. A sister had died of tuberculosis. Five years prior to admission he had had a small hemoptysis following a heavy paroxysm of cough. He was advised to stop smoking. He was found to have mild diabetes mellitus, which he never bothered to adjust to.

Three months prior to admission the patient noted the onset of a burning substernal pain, associated with vague sensations of pressure in the chest, and a boring pain over the postthoracic spine. The pain worsened at night and he would sit up to obtain relief. Two weeks prior to admission he lost his voice and couldn't speak above a whisper. He next found it difficult to swallow solid food. A chest film was taken and revealed a mediastinal mass, and he was admitted to the hospital. He had lost 30 pounds since his first symptom appeared. At times he felt feverish, and had had night sweats. Just prior to admission he had suffered a transitory blindness and diplopia.

On admission, his temperature was 101 degrees, but subsequently it became normal. The patient looked acutely and chronically ill. He spoke in a whisper. His peripheral arterial pulses were equal. There were firm subcutaneous nodules scattered over the forearms. The neck veins were distended. The patient was fibrillating. The lungs were clear. The liver was five fingerbreadths below the right costal margin. The spleen was not felt. The neurological examination was normal. The STS was negative. Hematocrit value was 44 ml/100 ml. The white blood cell count was 9,500 cu. mm., with slight shift to left. The urine was clear.

Punch biopsy of the liver showed nodular cirrhosis. The left arytenoid did not move when the patient was laryngoscoped. At fluoroscopic examination, a large mass which seemed to pulsate very slightly, was seen extending from the right upper mediastinum. The mass appeared to lie primarily in the middle and anterior portions of the upper mediastinum. The lung fields were essentially clear. The heart was at the upper limits of normal size. An arteriogram indicated that the mass was probably not of vascular origin.

After these studies, the patient was taken to the general operating room for an exploratory thoracotomy. We are not told of the findings.

DISCUSSION OF THE PROBLEM

Our concern is not the circumstances surrounding this patient's subsequent death, but rather the nature of the mediastinal mass for which he was sent to surgery.

We believe it important to note that it is often very difficult, and frequently impossible, to determine on clinical grounds alone the true nature of a mediastinal mass. I am aware of no symptom or physical sign which is unfailingly helpful in this regard. Furthermore, special diagnostic procedures may lead to false interpretations. Even the surgeon at the operating table may be misled by his eyes and his hands. We are well acquainted with instances in which attempts have been made to wire solid tumors. The mistakes when vascular tumors were incised are recalled even more vividly. Chronic inflammatory tissue in the chest may have the consistency and appearance of neoplasm. So we commence our differential diagnosis filled with respect for the fact that we may be attempting the impossible.

It is helpful to consider the etiology of masses presenting in the mediastinum under three headings, according to (1) vascular origin, (2) infectious origin, and (3) neoplastic origin.

Tuberculosis and other granulomatous processes, of course, may produce such alterations, and there were features of this patient's illness which suggest it. In the first place, there was a history of tuberculosis in the family, and the patient was a diabetic. We know that tuberculosis is a common and frequently unsuspected complication of diabetes. Furthermore, there was a three months' history of recurrent fever, sweats, weight loss and weakness, and, in the background, an episode of unexplained hemoptysis. One x-ray was read as showing a rim of calcium around the edge of this mass, a finding not uncommon with a tuberculous or other inflammatory lesion.

However, there are compelling reasons why tuberculosis or some other granulomatous process would seem unlikely. As far as the episode of hemoptysis is concerned, it should be recalled that throughout that entire period the patient gave no indication of having an active pulmonary infection, though he was not entirely well. Sweats and fever, of course, are not trademarks solely of infectious disorders, being common in neoplastic processes as well. Aneurysms may produce similar manifestations by preventing proper pulmonary drainage. Furthermore, this patient had no significant elevation of temperature while hospitalized, and the white blood cell count failed to show the changes sometimes observed in tuberculosis or other infectious diseases. Perhaps the strongest point against a granulomatous infection is the clinical course of his illness. Rather abruptly, without antecedent symptoms, the patient began to complain of unremitting, deep, boring chest pain, which continued to be the predominant symptom of his illness. There was no clinical evidence whatever of concomitant inflammatory involvement of the lung parenchyma, the pleura, pericardium, or adjacent skeletal structures. This would seem a peculiar course of events for tuberculosis, in which one would expect more patent evidences of infection, with some indications of involvement of lung parenchyma, serous surfaces, or skeletal structures. Severe, constant, boring pain in the chest must be most unusual in tuberculous mediastinal lymphadenitis. A final point is the fact that the patient's diabetes remained mild throughout. In the face of a spreading infection, it might be expected to increase in severity, but it did not.

In addition to tuberculosis, other infectious processes have to be considered, such as chronic lung abscess or a loculated empyema, but these can be eliminated for similar reasons.

There are, indeed, features of this patient's illness which suggest that he might have had an aneurysm of the thoracic aorta. He was of an age at which such lesions often become manifest. The manner in which his symptoms unfolded followed the classical pattern of aneurysm, in which pain in the chest is one of the earliest features, followed shortly by hoarseness, difficulty in swallowing, and venous obstruction. As already noted, pain was the most prominent and earliest evidence of this patient's illness, and the boring, deep, constant pain which he described under his sternum and between his shoulders is the sort often produced by aneurysms.

On the other hand, there are valid reasons for ruling out the presence of an aneurysm. In the first place, there was no history of syphilis, and the STS was negative. A spinal fluid examination made shortly before admission was also negative for syphilis. Furthermore, the patient presented none of the usual physical manifestations of aneurysm, such as external expansile pulsations, tracheal deviation and tug, thrills and murmurs, diastolic shock at the aortic area, a ringing second aortic sound, or alteration in the peripheral arterial pulsations. It should be made clear, however, that such findings are not at all constant, and that many aneurysms of the thoracic aorta are clinically silent. This is more true of aneurysms of the descending aorta than of those of the ascending or transverse portions.

If this was a silent aneurysm on physical examination, it was likewise silent when studied by special techniques, for no significant pulsation could be observed by fluoroscopy or kymography, and the mass failed to fill when Diodrast was injected. None of these points is, of course, conclusive in excluding aneurysm. If an aneurysmal sac is well filled with laminated clot it may neither pulsate nor fill with radio-opaque material. As a matter of fact, a solid tumor lying against a vigorously pulsating artery may pulsate much more actively than a clot filled aneurysm. However, the absence of any physical signs of aneurysm, in addition to failure to demonstrate filling or pulsation, cannot be ignored, as they are strong points against the likelihood of aneurysm. An additional point is the failure to show bone erosion of the spine or sternum, although this may not occur until late in the process. This is only a minor point, as pain may be severe in aneurysm without demonstrable bone erosion occurring. Perhaps the firmest argument against aneurysm was the very marked degree of weight loss and debility which he manifested, and the absence of significant dyspnea. Weight loss and debility are generally mild in aneurysm, and do not become pronounced unless the individual is incapacitated by pain, inability to swallow, or heart failure. On the other hand, dyspnea is a very prominent symptom of aneurysm, considered secondary in importance to pain. It would, therefore, seem unlikely that an aneurysm accounted for this mass.

It is our belief that the mass was neoplastic in nature. The patient was of an age at which such things occur. The kind of pain he suffered is frequently observed in mediastinal new growths. Difficulty in swallowing and hoarseness may be produced by encroachment upon the esophagus and involvement of the recurrent laryngeal nerve. The marked degree of weight loss and debility are typical of neoplasms. Recurrent sweats and feverishness are common accompaniments of intrathoracic neoplasms. Finally, neoplasm offers a convenient explanation for the hard subcutaneous nodules and the enlarged, firm liver noted during the course of his illness.

Before turning to a discussion of the type of neoplasm likely to have been responsible for this tumor, we wish to emphasize that in distinguishing the possible causes of this mass, we have not stressed the involvement of the left recurrent laryngeal nerve as a differential point, because this nerve may be involved by any of these types of disorders.

There are a wide variety of tumors, both benign and malignant, which make their appearance in the mediastinum. Common are bronchogenic, thyroid, thymus, dermoid, neurogenic, and pericardial tumors; lymphoma; teratoma; fibroma; lipoma; sarcoma; and metastatic carcinoma.

In view of the pronounced degree of weight loss and debility exhibited by this patient, it seems highly unlikely that the mass was a benign tumor, and hence we shall focus our attention upon the malignant varieties. It is true that benign tumors in the mediastinum may be associated with considerable evidences of malnutrition, if pressure upon the esophagus has been of a degree and duration to interfere significantly with nourishment, but such does not appear to have been the case in this instance.

Nor will we consider neurogenic tumors, for these generally, although not always, lie in the posterior mediastinum, an area clearly not the site of origin of the tumor under discussion. We shall also discard the possibility that this might have been a metastatic process, for this is not the way metastatic tissue usually makes its appearance in the chest. It would be unusual to find metastatic tumor in the guise of a single large mediastinal mass, with clear lung parenchyma. There is, however, at least one important exception to this general statement: testicular tumors not infrequently appear as primary mediastinal tumors. This patient's genitalia were described as normal.

We must certainly consider the possibility that this might have been a thyroid tumor.

The manifestations of intrathoracic goiter may be of two types: (1) toxic symptoms, and (2) pressure phenomenon. The latter has been stressed in the diagnosis of intrathoracic goiter. The brunt of the pressure is exerted on the trachea, which is commonly deviated and compressed, at times markedly so. This compression of the trachea leads to prominent respiratory symptoms, such as dyspnea, audible wheezing, spells of suffocation, particularly on reclining, and cyanosis. The voice may be husky, owing to involvement of the recurrent laryngeal nerve. In addition, there is often distention of neck veins. It has been emphasized frequently that in the majority of instances of substernal thyroid, a mass can be felt at the anterior root of the neck. This is an important point.

As far as this patient is concerned, the only possible indications of hyperthyroidism were weight loss and auricular fibrillation, and there are ample other possible explanations for the presence of these. The absence of a palpable mass at the base of the neck and the dearth of indications of tracheal distortion and compression make such a tumor unlikely.

Could this have been a tumor of the thymus gland? Tumors involving the thymus are not common. Symmens has reported an incidence of 0.14 percent in 17,000 autopsies at the Bellevue Hospital. One of their extraordinary features is a tendency to infiltrate adjacent structures, such as the heart, pericardium, pleura, bronchi, and pulmonary parenchyma.

The presence of thymus tumors provides a remarkable illustration of the adaptability of the surrounding tissues in accommodating themselves to a foreign invader. Early symptoms are absent, even when the tumor has reached large proportions. Almost invariably the symptoms, which are traced almost entirely to pressure, manifest themselves suddenly. It is evident that when the limit of accommodation is reached, symptoms suddenly appear. The outstanding sign of thymus tumors is dyspnea, which at times becomes extreme. Difficulty in swallowing and a choking sensation are also common. Cough, expectoration and blood spitting, and substernal pain and aphonia are also observed. The most prominent physical signs are those indicating pressure—namely, cyanosis, edema of face and extremities, and venous distention. At times a tumor mass may be seen or felt at the base of the neck. Frequently there is increased retromanubrial dullness.

A striking feature of our patient's course was the absence of significant dyspnea or other indications of interference with respiratory exchange. Indications of pressure, while present, were not prominent. The absence of such symptoms, and the rarity of thymic tumors, makes this condition unlikely in our patient.

Dermoids and teratomata may lie dormant within the chest for many years, and become obtrusive only in later life. Common causes for sudden enlargement of these tumors are: (1) hemorrhage, (2) infection, and (3) malignant change. About 10 to 12 percent are believed to undergo malignant transformation. Most of these growths make themselves felt in adolescence or early adult life; it is unusual for them to become clinically evident late in life. In one series of 174 cases, only 13 were observed in the 50 to 60 year old age group.

The symptoms of dermoids and teratomata may be considered to result from three mechanisms: (1) pressure upon adjacent structures, (2) formation of bronchial fistulae, and (3) development of infections. Of these, symptoms stemming from pressure are by far the most common and the most pronounced. Cough is the most prevalent individual symptom, and dyspnea runs a close second. These symptoms are often modified with change in position of the patient. Pain is another frequent complaint. It may be localized in the pleura, lie deep within the chest, or extend to shoulders and arms. Sometimes it mimics angina. Engorgement of the neck veins, edema of the face, and cyanosis, pupillary changes, and hoarseness are other manifestations of pressure. The formation of a bronchial fistula becomes evident when the patient begins to cough blood, and characteristically the sputum contains hairs and peculiar fatty, greasy particles. It should be pointed out that a bronchial connection may exist for many years without an infection occurring within the cyst.

Could this patient have had such a tumor, which lay dormant for many years, suddenly undergoing malignant change and becoming evident? Could the spell of hemoptysis which he had had in the preceding five years have resulted from a fistulous connection? This is an interesting possibility but an unlikely one. As already indicated, these tumors are rare under any circumstances, and are particularly unusual after the age of 45. Again, the most pronounced and earliest symptoms are those resulting from pressure. As we have already emphasized, indications of increased mediastinal pressure were only mild in our patient. There is no history of coughing up hairs or other peculiar debris.

It appears that we have narrowed our considerations to a differentiation between bronchogenic carcinoma and Hodgkin's disease or one of the other lymphomas. Here the going becomes very hard, indeed, because not infrequently it is impossible to distinguish one from the other on clinical grounds. As Dr. Longcope has pointed out, in about 10 percent of patients with Hodgkin's disease, the process is restricted entirely to the mediastinum. The superior mediastinal glands and the tracheal nodes tend to be involved to a greater extent than the posterior mediastinal or periaortic glands. It is, therefore, easy to understand why mediastinal Hodgkin's disease is often mistaken for aneurysm and bronchogenic carcinoma.

The symptoms and signs produced by a mediastinal lymphoma are those resulting mainly from pressure upon surrounding structures, and hence have no specificity.

At this juncture it would be well to analyze carefully the symptoms presented by our patient. Conspicuous were very marked and constant pain, weight loss, and debility. On the other hand, he had only slight cough and mild dyspnea, orthopnea, and venous distention. It seems to us to be a fair assumption that mediastinal Hodgkin's disease, consisting as it does of a collection of more or less discrete nodular masses, could be expected to produce pressure symptoms to a greater extent than a diffusely infiltrating tumor, such as certain forms of bronchogenic carcinoma. While not wishing to push this point too far, it appears to us that the mild degree of pressure symptoms evidenced by this patient suggests that he had an infiltrating bronchogenic carcinoma rather than a conglomerate solid mass of tumor. In addition, other factors add weight to this impression. Constant, unremitting, deep, boring pain—our patient's outstanding symptom—would be most unusual in a lymphoma. It is said that the pain observed in bronchogenic carcinoma is more continuous than in any other intrathoracic disease, except possibly aortic aneurysm with bone destruction. Such constant pain in the chest, in the absence of an aneurysm or metastases from some other source than the lungs, is considered by some to be almost diagnostic of bronchogenic carcinoma. Again, as pointed out by Dr. Longcope, when Hodgkin's disease of the mediastinum is present, there is usually also an accompanying enlargement of the supraclavicular lymph nodes. No significant swelling of peripheral glands was noted in this patient. Also, not infrequently mediastinal Hodgkin's disease will spread into the lung parenchyma, which did not take place here. Finally, splenic enlargement occurs in 60 to 80 percent of patients with this disease, and again none was noted here.

While it is a difficult choice, it seems to me most probable that our patient had a bronchogenic carcinoma infiltrating the mediastinum. In general, there are considered to be three cellular types of this tumor: (1) adenocarcinoma, (2) squamous cell carcinoma, and (3) undifferentiated round or oat cell carcinoma. It is this latter type, the round or oat cell carcinoma, which has a predilection for spreading to the mediastinum, not infrequently producing what seems to be primary mediastinal tumor, often confused with Hodgkin's disease. Instead of spreading into the bronchus, and thus producing the usual irritative and obstructive manifestations of cough, infection, atelectasis, or emphysema, the tumor may spread outside the bronchus, spilling over into and filling the mediastinum. Such is the picture we have of the tumor before us now.

There are a few other observations to be made. The round cell type of bronchogenic carcinoma has a great tendency to produce distant metastases. It seems likely that the subcutaneous nodules which the patient had were metastatic. Also, at peritoneoscopic examination, the observation was made that the right lobe of the liver was considerably larger than the left. Despite the pathological diagnosis of cirrhosis made from the punch biopsy, one must yet consider metastatic carcinoma, in the face of the unilobar enlargement of the liver. Finally, on hospital admission the patient was noted to be profoundly weak, and his blood pressure, which had been elevated considerably in the past, was reduced to 130/80. As metastatic involvement of the adrenals is common in bronchogenic carcinoma, the possibility of a mild degree of hypoadrenalism comes to mind. The visual difficulties which occurred shortly before admission might indicate metastases to the brain, as well, so common in all forms of bronchogenic carcinoma.

POST MORTEM FINDINGS

Bronchogenic carcinoma, oat cell type, with mediastinal metastases, and metastases to brain, subcutaneous tissues, adrenals, and liver. Arteriosclerotic heart disease with auricular fibrillation. Diabetes mellitus. Laennec's cirrhosis.

REFERENCES

Barke, W. A., et al.: Hodgkin's disease of the mediastinum. Ann. Thor. Surg. 3:287, 1967.
Boyd, L. J.: Study of 4000 reported cases of aneurysm of the thoracic aorta. Am. J. Med. Sci. 168:654, 1924.
Brewer, D., and Dolley, A.: Tumors of the mediastinum. Ann. Rev. Tuberculosis 60:419, 1949.
Godgson, C. L., et al.: Bilateral hilar adenopathy. Its significance and management. Ann. Intern. Med. 43:83, 1955.
Gray, S. J., Olson, T. E., and Manrique, J.: Hematemesis and melena. Med. Clin. N. Amer. 41:1327, 1957.
Hinshaw, H. C., and Garland, L. H.: Bronchogenic carcinoma. In Diseases of the Chest. 3rd ed. Philadelphia, W. B. Saunders Company, 1969.
Jones, E. B.: Saccular aneurysms of the thoracic aorta: A clinical study of 633 cases. Ann. Intern. Med. 12:624, 1938.

Joseph, W. L., Murray, J. F., and Mulder, D. G.: Mediastinal tumors—problems in diagnosis. Dis. Chest 50:150, 1966.
Kurohara, S. S., et al.: Testicular tumors. Cancer 20:1089, 1967.
Lagos, T. Z., et al.: Primary mediastinal seminoma. Chest 71:575, 1959.
Lindskog, G. E.: Benign mediastinal tumors. New Eng. J. Med. 244:250, 1951.
Mark, J. B. D.: Ectopic mediastinal thyroid—features in diagnosis. Dis. Chest 45:412, 1964.
Meyer, K. K., and Ochsner, J. L.: Intrathoracic neurogenic tumors. Surg. Clin. N. Amer. 46:1427, 1966.
Moore, S. W., and Cole, D. R.: Primary malignant neoplasms of the lungs. Ann. Surg. 141:457, 1955.
Morrison, I. M.: Tumors and cysts of the mediastinum. Thorax 13:294, 1958.
Ochsner, J. L., and Ochsner, S. F.: Congenital cysts of the mediastinum—20 year experience with 42 cases. Ann. Surg. 163:909, 1966.
Oldham, H. N., and Sabiston, D. C., Jr.: Primary tumors and cysts of the mediastinum. Lesions presenting as cardiovascular abnormalities. Arch. Surg. 96:71, 1968.
Oosterwijk, W., and Swierenga, J.: Neurogenic tumors with an intrathoracic localization. Thorax 23:374, 1968.
Rosenberg, R. R., et al.: Intrathoracic lipomas. Chest 60:507, 1971.
Sabiston, D., and Scott, H. W.: Primary neoplasms and cysts of the mediastinum. Ann. Surg. 136:777, 1952.
Schuman, B. M.: Mediastinal lipomatosis complicating steroid therapy of regional enteritis. Gastroenterology 61:244, 1971.
Sellors, T. H., Thackray, A. L., and Thomsen, A. D.: Tumors of the thymus: A review of 88 cases. Thorax 22:193, 1967.
Thomas, V., et al.: Diagnosis of mediastinal tumors. Chest 59:324, 1971.
Wilkins, E. W., Jr.: Cases of thymoma at the Massachusetts General Hospital. J. Thor. Cardiovasc. Surg. 52:322, 1966.

H A PATIENT WITH OBSCURE GASTROINTESTINAL HEMORRHAGE

THE CLINICAL PROBLEM

This 55 year old Negro male was admitted for the first time on April 23, 1965, because of melena and hematemesis.

Past history showed many traumatic injuries, including numerous fractures and lacerations. The patient had been unemployed for long periods of time and had a sociopathic personality. Since the 1920's, he had been a heavy drinker, imbibing approximately one pint of whiskey or a quart of wine per day. From August 1964 to March 1965 he was followed in the Medical Clinic for mild hypertension, which was thought to be essential. He was treated with Serpasil (0.25 mg. BID) and phenobarbital (32 mg. BID). Except for occasional crampy abdominal pains and an ill defined substernal discomfort, questionably relieved by ingestion of food, the patient was well until the day of admission, when he experienced the sudden passing of six black, diarrheal stools, followed by two episodes of hematemesis, the latter described as "dark blood and clots." This was followed by two episodes of vomiting of bright red blood. He presented himself to the Emergency Department and was admitted to the hospital.

The patient denied the presence of any other symptoms or that he had been drinking more heavily than usual. The only additional medication he had been taking was an occasional aspirin.

The patient was a well developed, apparently well nourished middle aged Negro male in no acute distress. Temperature was 99 degrees; pulse, 96 (supine), 126 (sitting); blood pressure, 176/100 (supine). Positive physical findings included many well healed scars, pallor of the left disc with decreased vision in the left eye, and mild cardiomegaly with a Grade II/VI systolic ejection murmur. The abdominal examination was remarkable only for a slight protuberance. Bowel sounds were active and there were no masses or tenderness. Pertinent negative findings were the absence of stigmata of chronic liver disease or significant wasting of muscle mass.

Other findings included: hematocrit 38 ml./100 ml.; WBC, 4000/cu. mm.; stool guaiac, 4+; urine unremarkable; serum urea nitrogen, 20 mg./100 ml.; sodium, 149 mEq./liter; potassium, 3.7 mEq./liter; bilirubin, less than 0.8 mg./100 ml.; amylase, 150 Somogyi units/100 ml.; prothrombin time, greater than 65 percent; bromsulphalein, 9 percent. Chest x-ray showed the cardiac configuration of hypertensive disease and a right lower lobe infiltrate. Esophagoscopy and gastroscopy were attempted but were not successful. Upper GI series was of poor quality because of the presence of fluid in the stomach, but results did not show the presence of an esophageal lesion; the only remarkable finding was evidence of mild duodenal spasm.

The patient was treated with iced saline gastric lavage, atropine, and fluid and blood replacement. Over the course of the first 12 hours, he received six units of whole blood. However, because he continued to have bright red bleeding via nasogastric tube, 18 hours after admission he was brought to the general operating room for an exploratory laparotomy. He died shortly thereafter.

DISCUSSION OF THE PROBLEM

The accurate diagnosis and proper management of obscure hemorrhage from the GI tract are always most difficult matters, as they were here. Unfortunately, the final outcome of such obscure bleeding is frequently lamentable—as it was here, the patient having succumbed on the fourth hospital day.

There are, of course, a myriad of causes of hemorrhage from the GI tract, some common, some rare, and this plethora is one of the reasons why the accurate pinpointing of the source of hemorrhage may be so hard to achieve. Frequently, only "luck" turns up the right answer.

Furthermore, often the information derived from the history and physical examination, as well as from the laboratory tests and x-rays, is either so vague or so nonspecific that it is of little or no diagnostic value, just as it was in this instance.

From the standpoint of clinical management, the physician frequently finds himself ensnared in a trap which has two sharp teeth. On the one hand, he is most anxious to allow enough time to pass to afford adequate opportunity for localizing the point of origin of the bleeding—if possible—and, through conservative means, to stop the hemorrhage. The physician wants to be conservative, to take his time, not to be pushed or hurried, to give the clinical problem an opportunity to fully mature. An exploratory laparotomy, in particular if done "flying blind," is a course of action the anxiously observing physician is loath to pursue, as he worriedly watches the hour-to-hour progress of his bleeding patient.

On the other hand, the physician is uncomfortably aware of the fact that as he waits and watches, and the bleeding continues, the optimal opportunity for an exploratory operation may be passing, and he may be frittering away the patient's best opportunity for recovery. He becomes fearful that his instinctive desires for a conservative solution to the patient's bleeding problem may, as time passes, ultimately be setting the stage for an even more hazardous surgical approach to it. Continued hemorrhage renders the patient a less and less good candidate for an operation. Such problems try men's souls!

Clearly, management problems of this type become somewhat less precarious if the site of the bleeding can be localized clinically, so that the most effective conservative treatment can be instituted. Should that prove unavailing, at least a blind operative approach can be avoided.

In such challenging circumstances, one must scour every vestige of clinical evidence afforded by the history, the physical examination, and whatever ancillary information is available, in an effort to discover clues which, hopefully, may give some specificity to a devastating phenomenon that all too commonly is thoroughly nonspecific in its manifestations.

In truth, such a scouring of this patient's clinical course produces slim pickings indeed, but in a way this is good, for it makes this patient's illness typical and everyday, and separates it from those rare and seldom seen cases, sometimes reserved for CPC discussions.

The clinical evidence which seems to me to be most pertinent in this problem is as follows:

1. 55 year old Negro male.

2. Unemployed chronic alcoholic who had suffered many injuries.

3. He was highly nervous and had been in a state hospital for the mentally ill.

4. He was known to have hypertension, and on occasion, in the outpatient department, the possibility of syphilitic aortitis had been raised.

5. He took aspirin and Serpasil.

6. He had complained of vague epigastric discomfort, as well as of cramping lower abdominal pains.

7. His bleeding apparently began suddenly, was massive, and was associated with both the vomiting of bright blood with clots and the passage of blood per rectum.

8. The bleeding episode was painless and the patient did not go into shock.

9. The physical examination showed nothing to point to the origin of the bleeding.

10. The white blood cell count at the time of admission was 4000/cu. mm.

Let us now see to what diagnosis pursuit of these various pieces of information leads us.

The fact that the patient suddenly vomited a large quantity of bright red blood with clots almost surely means that the origin of his hemorrhage must have been either the esophagus, stomach, or duodenum; much less often, however, this type of hemorrhage may actually originate in the upper jejunum.

The fact that the patient was a chronic alcoholic, almost constantly on relief and perhaps not well nourished, brings one to suspect bleeding produced by one of the following three general mechanisms:

1. Cirrhosis of the liver with bleeding from (a) esophageal varices, (b) esophagitis, (c) peptic ulcer, or (d) gastritis, the latter two accompanying cirrhosis in some 10 to 15 percent of instances.

2. Pancreatitis, or carcinoma of the pancreas.

3. Rupture of the esophagus, the so-called Mallory-Weiss syndrome.

Let us consider each of these possibilities, in brief.

While this patient was certainly a perfect candidate for cirrhosis of the liver, and he well may have had it to some degree, the evidence is against his having any scarring of the liver severe enough to result in portal hypertension and esophageal varices. Thus:

1. There were no stigmata of cirrhosis or portal hypertension noted on the physical examination.

2. The x-rays of the esophagus failed to show varices.

3. Despite a massive hemorrhage, the bromsulphalein (BSP) was only 9 percent, the bilirubin content only 0.8 mg./100 ml., and the prothrombin time 65 per cent. It has been shown that absence of significant BSP retention indicates that hepatic disease of sufficient severity to cause portal hypertension is not present.

While esophageal varices can be excluded, a duodenal or gastric ulcer cannot, nor can gastritis or esophagitis. From a purely statistical standpoint, a peptic ulcer and gastritis are by far the most common causes of the kind of bleeding which occurred here. In this setting, not infrequently peptic ulceration and gastritis occur simultaneously. It is important to note this fact, because in such a case the demonstration of a peptic ulcer does not necessarily mean that the site of the patient's active bleeding has been located: he may actually be hemorrhaging from a gastritis. Alternatively, the reverse situation could occur.

This patient was described as being highly nervous and tense, he drank excessively, his nutrition must have been poor, he complained of epigastric distress vaguely related to eating, and the unsatisfactory GI series was said to show duodenal spasm. Clearly, peptic ulcer and gastritis remain excellent possibilities.

The fact that he took aspirin and Serpasil is additional reason for suspecting a gastritis, since both of these agents, together with an enlarging list of other medications, are capable of inciting gastritis and hemorrhage.

While it is perhaps a moot question at this time whether or not chronic gastritis or esophagitis may lead to the development of carcinoma, there is some evidence that it may, and we have seen such lesions appear in just this setting. With the meager information we have here, we cannot exclude such an occurrence; we can only point out that prior to the sudden onset of the hemorrhage the patient is said to have been as well as he ever was, and there was no history of weight loss or of localizing symptoms or signs. In addition, from a statistical standpoint, massive bleeding such as occurred here is more often seen in benign than in malignant ulceration. Only 5 to 10 percent of gastric malignancies bleed severely initially.

Whereas he was the kind of man who might well develop pancreatic disease, what with his alcoholism and poor nutrition, and whereas pancreatitis as well as carcinoma of the pancreas is capable of inducing gastrointestinal bleeding, the type of profuse hemorrhage noted here would be uncommon, occult bleeding or melena being much more usual in these pancreatic disorders than hematemesis. Again, he is said to have been well, the bleeding was painless, the abdominal examination was unremarkable, and the amylase reading was normal.

The absence of any indications of a mediastinitis or of an inflammatory process in the pleural spaces seems to exclude a rupture of the esophagus, which, incidentally, is not usually associated with massive hemorrhage. These points do not, however, exclude a vertical laceration of the gastroesophageal junction, which is not accompanied by mediastinitis, and which characteristically is associated with severe, intractable and often exsanguinating hemorrhage. This so-called Mallory-Weiss syndrome probably occurs more often than it is detected. It is frequently, but not always, seen in chronic alcoholics, often in association with (1) chronic gastritis, (2) peptic ulcer, (3) gallbladder disease, (4) pancreatitis, and (5) cirrhosis of the liver. This lesion is difficult to demonstrate by x-ray, and it may even be missed at gastrotomy. From a management standpoint, the Mallory-Weiss syndrome may be overlooked at exploratory laparotomy, and the usual partial gastrectomy which is sometimes done in an effort to control hemorrhage from site unknown may fail to include this lesion because of its anatomic location. For this reason, it should always be considered when a patient continues to bleed following such a procedure. The etiology of this syndrome is not known, but it is often related to gastritis and violent vomiting.

Clearly, such a process has pertinence in these present circumstances. It might be argued that we have no history of violent retching here, but this patient was not a completely reliable witness. It should be noted that gastroscopy had to be discontinued because he became too uncooperative. Finally, a review of the Boston City Hospital experience with the Mallory-Weiss syndrome will show that often there was no definite history of profound retching preceding the hemorrhage.

The patient was known to have had hypertension for several years. This brings to mind two other possible mechanisms leading to massive gastrointestinal bleeding: (1) an aneurysm, and (2) an acute arteritis.

There is little evidence to support either of these. As for aneurysm, there was no pain, no shock, no alteration in the peripheral pulses, no abdominal masses, no murmurs, and no leukocytosis or hematuria. As for an active arteritis, the patient had been known to have hypertension for many years, and yet all during this period there was nothing whatever to indicate a progressive, poly-organ system disease. Against the possibility of an acute, fulminant arteritis is the fact, already stressed, that he is said to have been as well as usual until the sudden hemorrhage.

The patient's personality, the tremors, the visual impairment, and the questionable presence of an aortic diastolic murmur suggested by one observer, raise the question of syphilis and of gumma of the stomach. However, gummas are unusual, they generally do not bleed massively, and the patient's STS was negative.

While the description we are given of this patient's chronic abdominal distress is devoid of needed details, we still should not ignore its diagnostic potentials. You will recall it was of two types: (1) an epigastric burning, perhaps related to eating, and (2) a *cramping* lower abdominal pain.

The epigastric burning is, of course, suggestive of the conditions we have already mentioned as being likely: peptic ulcer, gastritis, esophagitis, pancreatitis. There is another condition which should always be considered in accompaniment with these, since it may exactly mimic them, and this is a diverticulum of the duodenum or jejunum. These may ulcerate and bleed massively. The failure of the GI series to demonstrate such a lesion would seem to exclude this possibility, even though the examination left much to be desired.

Cramping pains always suggest spasm of a smooth muscle viscus, and in these particular circumstances one might think of a tumor of the duodenum or upper jejunum (such as a leiomyoma, leiosarcoma, or carcinoid), or of a hemangioma, which could intermittently cause obstruction and undergo hemorrhage. But these are unusual abnormalities, they cause melena more often than hematemesis, and again the x-rays showed no gross intraluminal lesion.

The unique situation in which gallstones may produce cramping pain and subsequently hemorrhage as the result of penetration into the gut we will dismiss mainly because it is unique! But it should be given consideration, nonetheless. Careful scrutiny of a flat film of the abdomen may show telltale gas patterns outlining some of the biliary ducts, and establish the diagnosis.

The last clue we will pursue, and it is the faintest of the lot, is the fact that on a single occasion the WBC count was only 4000/cu. mm. Now, generally, in association with a brisk hemorrhage, there is a mild to moderate leukocytosis, in the range of 12,000 to 15,000/cu. mm. Could the count of only 4000 indicate some type of poisoning, a blood dyscrasia, or a disseminated infection or neoplasm?

Once again we return to the information given that he was well until he started to hemorrhage. Certainly, there was no collateral evidence in the history, physical examination, or laboratory studies to support any of these possibilities.

Before turning to our final considerations, we must not fail to mention a vascular telangiectasis. Special mention was made of the absence of such mucocutaneous lesions when the patient's admission physical examination was described. Failure to find such lesions in the skin or mucous membranes does not, of course, exclude their presence, for they may all be hidden from view or be excessively hard to find. There was an oft-quoted patient of Dr. James Bordley who was admitted repeatedly because of recurrent GI hemorrhages. Finally, the nature of the bleeding was discovered when a single vascular lesion was seen high in the nasopharynx when the patient was pharyngoscoped. The moral is clear: if there is a question of telangiectasis, search meticulously all viewable mucocutaneous surfaces by whatever means available.

After observing this patient for several hours, and giving him several pints of blood, the decision was made that the site of the bleeding could not be ascertained by conservative means, nor the hemorrhage halted, and he was transferred to surgery for an exploratory laparotomy. He died two days later. About these events we know nothing, for the pertinent pages have all been removed from the chart. Hence, from here on we shall have to abandon deductive reasoning and turn to our "male intuition."

As already emphasized, the decision to perform a blind exploratory laparotomy upon a patient severely hemorrhaging from an obscure cause is made with reluctance. In an effort to make this decision less demanding of the physician's intellectual and emotional resources, a variety of clinical criteria have been evolved. For example, one is advised to operate after so many hours of observation, or after so many pints of blood have been given, or when the patient's age, pulse, hematocrit, and blood pressure fall within certain prescribed ranges. These attempts to simplify a very complicated problem, and to supplant magical numbers and formulae for meticulous observation and experienced clinical judgment are to be thoroughly abhorred. In my opinion, they have caused a number of patients to be operated upon who would have fared better if handled conservatively.

You may have read in a biographical sketch of Mr. Chris Kraft, the man who was Flight Director for the first astronauts, and who made all the critical decisions governing their flights. He is quoted as saying, "One of the basic maxims of space travel is this: If you don't *clearly* know what to do, don't do anything." This advice is sound in dealing with critical medical problems as well.

Is it possible that the mode of this patient's postoperative death could shed light upon the nature of the lesion which caused him to hemorrhage? It is worth speculating upon. There are several possibilities.

1. Perhaps the stress of the exploratory operation was too much for his heart and liver, both of which were abnormal to begin with, especially with

the added deleterious effects of the severe hemorrhage. But his liver function was reasonably good, he was not in heart failure and had never been in shock, and he should therefore have been able to withstand the stresses of an uncomplicated exploratory operation.

2. Death on the second postoperative day was too early to succumb from the usual type of postoperative infection—or from a pulmonary embolism, for that matter.

3. Perhaps, in addition to a hemorrhaging ulcer, the ulcer had also perforated. It should be stressed that perforation occurs simultaneously with hemorrhage more often than many suppose, and it may be obscure and overlooked. Or, perhaps the patient had a fulminant pancreatitis. But, as we have already noted, there was no clinical or other evidence to support either of these possibilities.

4. Perhaps, when the surgeon opened the abdomen, he found some major abnormality, such as a rupturing aneurysm, which he attempted to repair under unfavorable circumstances. But we have already considered the possible presence of such a lesion, and have excluded it as being unlikely.

5. It seems much more likely to me, therefore, that the patient died, not of the operation per se or of some complication directly related to its performance, but rather as a result of the fact that the true site of the hemorrhage was never detected or adequately corrected, and that the patient continued to bleed after the operation was completed.

In conclusion, it seems to us most likely that this patient, a chronic alcoholic with chronic dyspepsia, had persistent gastritis, perhaps associated with peptic disease as well. In addition, it is likely he also had, as an acute event, the Mallory-Weiss syndrome. We suspect that at exploratory laparotomy a subtotal gastrectomy was performed in an effort to halt the bleeding, but that, unfortunately, the true site of bleeding was not included in the tissue removed. We believe the patient's subsequent death was the product of persistent bleeding, either from an undetected tear at the esophagogastric junction, or from bleeding points remaining in the unresected gastric or duodenal mucosa. The Mallory-Weiss syndrome seems the most plausible explanation.

POST MORTEM FINDINGS

Acute hemorrhagic, phlegmonous gastritis. Fatty liver. Pulmonary congestion, edema, and atelectasis. Marked left ventricular and mild right ventricular hypertrophy. Myocardial fibrosis. Arteriolonephrosclerosis. Arteriosclerotic cardiovascular disease.

REFERENCES

Baum, S., Nusbaum, M., Clearfield, H. R., Kuroda, K., and Tumen, H. J.: Angiography in the diagnosis of gastrointestinal bleeding. Arch. Intern. Med. 119:16–24, 1967.

Bean, W. B.: Enteric bleeding in rare conditions with diagnostic lesions of the skin and mucous membrane. Gastroenterology 2:807, 1958.
Brick, I. B., and Jeghers, H. J.: Gastrointestinal hemorrhages (excluding peptic ulcer and esophageal varices). New Eng. J. Med. 253:458, 1955.
Cope, J. R.: Haemobilia as a cause of gastrointestinal hemorrhage. Scand. J. Gastroent. 3:285, 1968.
Flatley, F. J., Atwell, M. E., and McEvoy, R. K. Pseudoxanthoma elasticum with gastric hemorrhage. Arch. Intern. Med. 112:352, 1963.
Haller, J. D., et al.: Massive upper gastrointestinal hemorrhage due to pancreatitis. Arch. Surg. 93:867, 1966.
Halpern, M., Turner, A. F., and Citron, B. F.: Hereditary hemorrhagic telangiectasia. Radiology 90:1143, 1968.
Hinchey, E. J., et al.: Postemetic gastroesophageal laceration with hemorrhage. Surg. Gynec. Obstet. 126:324, 1968.
Hislop, I. G., et al.: The natural history of hemorrhage from esophageal varices. Lancet 1:945, 1966.
Holmes, K. D.: Mallory-Weiss syndrome. Review of 20 cases and literature review. Ann. Surg. 164:811, 1966.
Larmi, T. K. I.: Hemobilia associated with cholycystitis, postcholecystectomy conditions and trauma. Ann. Surg. 163:373, 1966.
McHardy, G., Bechtold, J. E., and McHardy, R. J.: Hemorrhage from primary disease of the small intestine; review of the literature and analysis of 216 cases. Gastroenterology 28:17, 1955.
Merigan, T. C., et al.: Gastrointestinal bleeding with cirrhosis: a study of 172 episodes in 158 patients. New Eng. J. Med. 263:579, 1960.
Netterville, R. E., Hardy, J. D., and Martin, R. S., Jr.: Small bowel hemorrhage. Ann. Surg. 167:949, 1968.
Ostermiller, W. Joergenson, E. J., and Weibel, L.: A clinical review of tumors of the small bowel. Amer. J. Surg. 111:403, 1966.
Ottinger, L. W., and Austin, W. G.: A study of 136 patients with mesenteric infarction. Surg. Gynec. Obstet. 124:251, 1967.
Palmer, E.: Vigorous diagnostic approach to upper GI hemorrhage. JAMA 207:1477, 1969.
Patterson, M., Forman, S., Weeden, K., and Zonana, E.: Fatal gastrointestinal bleeding. JAMA 175:19, 1961.
Quinn, W. C.: Gross hemorrhage from presumed diverticular disease of the colon: Results of treatment in 103 patients. Ann. Surg. 153:851, 1961.
Souliotis, P. T., Pettgrew, A. H., and Chamberlain, J. W.: Traumatic haemobilia. New Eng. J. Med. 268:565, 1963.
Stone, H. B.: Large hemorrhages from the bowel of obscure origin. Maryland Med. J. 1:555, 1952.
Thompson, C. E. R., Ashurst, P. M., and Butler, T. J.: Survey of haemorrhagic erosive gastritis. Brit. Med. J. 3:283, 1968.
Thorsen, W. B., Jr., et al.: Aspirin injury to the gastric mucosa. Arch. Intern. Med. 121:499, 1968.
Volman, H. B., et al.: Lesions associated with gastrointestinal hemorrhage in aspirin intake. Brit. Med. J. 11:661, 1968.
Wilson, D. E., and Chalmers, T. C.: Management of emergencies: XI. Acute hemorrhage from the upper gastrointestinal tract. New Eng. J. Med. 274:1368, 1966.

I A PATIENT WITH CHEST PAIN, SEVERE VENOUS IN-FLOW BLOCK AND CORONARY ARTERY DISEASE

THE CLINICAL PROBLEM

This 48 year old white male, a government materials inspector, suddenly slumped from his chair to the floor while at work and was taken by ambulance to another hospital, where he was pronounced dead on arrival.

At the age of 32, in 1947, the patient had had a transient episode of cramping substernal and anterior chest pain, with radiation into both arms and generalized weakness. He was treated with brief rest and medication in the accident room of another hospital, obtaining complete relief. He was first admitted to this hospital in 1954 with a similar, more severe episode, in which there occurred a subsequent transient rise in the sedimentation rate and ECG findings compatible with an anterolateral myocardial infarction of indeterminate age. After discharge in four weeks, he was felt to be excitable and nervous, and was started on long-term sedation and tranquilization. He had intermittent angina postprandially and on exertion, and was again admitted to the hospital in 1956 with a severe episode. His blood pressure was 110/90, cholesterol level was 258 mg./100 ml., and on the basis of suggestive ECG changes and the lack of definite evidence for infarction, the patient was felt to have had an episode of severe coronary insufficiency. He was bothered less by angina after discharge, but he was readmitted to the hospital in 1958 with severe precordial pain which awakened him from sleep, in shock, and with impending pulmonary edema. The electrocardiogram did not reveal infarction, but the WBC count, the erythrocyte sedimentation rate and the transaminase level were elevated. He was given supportive therapy, and digitalis and anticoagulants were administered. He was given quinidine temporarily for premature ventricular contractions. His fourth hospital admission was in 1959, after six weeks of attacks of paroxysmal nocturnal dyspnea and episodes of "seizing" in the epigastrium, flushing of the face and neck (felt as if all his blood had rushed to his head), and shortness of breath, which was precipitated by emotion, relieved by sitting, standing, yawning, or sneezing, and which lasted 10 to 15 minutes. Blood pressure was 110/85, and diffuse cardiomegaly was first noted. Serum urea nitrogen was 33 mg./100 ml., and ECG results were unchanged; arm and leg venous pressures were 145 mm. He was readmitted only one month later, his symptoms having progressed, and in addition there was also slight pedal edema, progressive orthopnea and dyspnea on exertion, intermittent abdominal distention, eructation, and many bizarre, apparently functional, complaints often temporarily related to emotional situations. The head and neck flushed a remarkable violaceous hue during Valsalva's maneuver or when the patient was supine, at which time he had grunting respirations and a tense abdomen. The flush disappeared with relaxation. The heart was enlarged almost to the anterior axillary line, a protodiastolic gallop and occasional premature ventricular contractions were noted, and there was a Grade II systolic murmur heard over the ziphoid and lower right sternal border. The liver extended downward five fingerbreadths and was tender. The venous pressure was 225 mm. in the arm and 325 mm. in the leg, dropping to 50 mm. after a 25 pound diuresis, during which time the cardiomegaly decreased. Blood chemistries, including serum urea nitrogen and cholesterol, and urinary 5-hydroxyindole acetic acid (5-HIAA) excretion were normal. An oral glucose tolerance test was normal. The patient did well, with intermittent chlorothiazide diuresis, until one year later, when he developed a "chest cold" with minimal hemoptysis and orthopnea, paroxysmal nocturnal dyspnea, pleuritic left chest pain, and a painful left leg. He was given anticoagulants and was thought to have had a right pulmonary embolus while in the hospital. Because of the plethora of the face and neck while supine, an attempt was made to demonstrate a right atrial thrombus with mediastinal scintiscan, but this was unsuccessful. The patient was again admitted to the hospital in March 1962, with frank congestive heart failure. He again responded and did well on therapy with digitoxin, diuretics, Coumadin anticoagulation, and a low-salt diet.

His last admission was in June 1963, for congestive heart failure. There had also been an increasing frequency in his attacks of facial flushing, these now occurring once a day or more. His physician noted that his weight fluctuated widely, and that when he accumulated edema fluid, the loud systolic murmur at the lower left sternal border was very striking. He also noted that the patient developed extreme neck and face cyanosis after a few seconds in the supine position, which was accompanied by conjunctival suffusion and neck vein distention. He had been very active, in spite of this, until a few days prior to admission. At this admission an arteriogram was interpreted as showing a mass, either a thrombus or a tumor, in the right atrium. Before additional studies could be done, the patient died suddenly.

DISCUSSION OF THE PROBLEM

This patient's illness began with pain in the chest and concluded some 12 years later with abrupt, unheralded death. In the long intervening period, the patient demonstrated the progressive development of in-flow obstruction of the venous circulation. Chest pain, severe venous in-flow block, sudden death—these were the unhappy ingredients of the latter segment of this unfortunate man's life. Let us briefly consider each of these in turn.

Recurrent chest pain such as this patient endured at the introduction of his illness may have a very wide variety of causes, and few complaints try the clinical ingenuity of the physician to a greater extent. In the differential diagnosis of chest pain, x-ray and laboratory procedures may prove helpful, but the pay dirt is generally found in the physical examination and the history—and most especially, in detailed analysis of the latter. In such an analysis the cardinal points are these: The character of the pain, its location and radiation, what causes it to come or increases its intensity, what relieves it, the time relationships, and the phenomena associated with it.

During his lengthy illness, this patient was interviewed by a host of physicians, and his chart is replete with descriptions of the various episodes of chest pain he suffered. One of the more vivid, written by the student who first interviewed him, is as follows:

> Yesterday morning, the patient went to traffic court with his stepson. Upon leaving, he experienced an extremely severe lower substernal pain which is described as dull, nonradiating and nonconstricting, but as if he were hit by a baseball bat. He was not dyspneic. He felt that belching would relieve, but was unable to do so. Shortly thereafter he noted nonradiating pain in both arms from wrists to elbows. The upper arms were free of pain. This arm pain was also quite severe but not as bad as the substernal pain. He went to a local bar where he was given two shots of "peppermint Schnapps," had a bowel movement and felt much better. He became asymptomatic, then proceeded to another bar, where he became totally intoxicated and remembers nothing until 5 A.M. today, when he awoke in his living room. At 6:30 A.M., following intercourse twice, his chest and arm pain returned, more severe this time. He went to the bar, had a few shots and vomited for the first time. He went home and was told "he looked white as a sheet." He was brought to the accident room, where he again experienced pain, but this time it was excruciating and he became nauseated. Following an ECG and administration of 16 mg. of morphine sulfate, he was admitted to the ward.

This description tells us not only about the pain, but also about the man with the pain—aggressive, outgoing, compulsive, perfectionistic—the kind who may have coronary artery disease.

A careful perusal of this description of the patient's chest pain—as well as of the other physicians' reports—brings me to the inevitable conclusion that, whatever else he had, the patient must have had coronary artery insufficiency. The manner in which the pain began, in a setting of emotional and physical stress, its sternal location, its radiation to the neck, shoulders, lower arms, and wrists, its interpretation as dull aching, constriction, or gaseous distension, its short duration, the relief obtained with belching, rest, and nitroglycerine, and the accompanying sweating and great fear of impending death are the classic hallmarks of myocardial ischemia.

But the diagnosis of myocardial ischemia is basically one of exclusion, and there are several matters which we ought to consider before deciding with finality on coronary insufficiency. To become the "devil's advocate" here, he was only in his early 30's when he first had this pain. While all who saw him during his illness took it for granted that he had coronary insufficiency resulting in myocardial infarction, during the acute attacks he had never had fever or leukocytosis, the ECG changes were never classical or specific, and the elevation of transaminase levels was slight.

What about the possibility of some other mechanisms of chest pain? Later in his course, there is very strong evidence that the patient had a pulmonary embolus—or, more likely, several. Could multiple pulmonary emboli have been responsible for these episodes of chest pain from the very beginning? This seems unlikely. While coronary artery insufficiency and pulmonary embolism may present in clinically identical manners and are often mistaken for each other, and, of course, are frequently associated with each other, the type of chest pain which this patient had had repeatedly would be most unusual for pulmonary embolism alone. In this regard, it is interesting to note that later in his illness, when he had what we would regard as the classical presentation of an embolus, he was quick to tell the doctors that this pain was quite distinct from the original pain of his early illness, which had no pleuritic element, and was not consistently associated with any respiratory abnormalities, such as shortness of breath, cough, hemoptysis, rales, or x-ray changes.

Dissecting aneurysm always requires exclusion in these circumstances, but in the first place the patient was not the kind of person who might be expected to have a dissecting aneurysm. He was young and had never had hypertension. There was no history of chest trauma. He had no stigmata of Marfan's disease. Also, there were no alterations in the peripheral pulses during the acute attacks, and no murmurs were heard initially. The pain was never unduly prolonged, nor did it ever radiate to his back. X-rays never showed widening of the aorta. Finally, he fared too well through the years for an individual with repeated, multiple episodes of pain owing to a tearing aorta.

Pericarditis comes to mind, particularly in view of the later development of in-flow venous stasis. But again, the patient's pain was so typical of angina, and the pain of pericarditis does not tend to recur repeatedly for short intervals in a setting of emotional or physical stress, nor does it generally mimic indigestion with bloating or belching, as angina often does and as happened here, nor is radiation to the hands and wrists commonly observed. Finally, no pericardial rubs were ever heard, nor were the ECG changes sometimes accompanying pericarditis noted.

Pulmonary hypertension from any cause may on occasion give rise to a precordial discomfort that is difficult to distinguish from angina. It often has its onset during situations demanding increased cardiac output, as happened here. But it generally does not present with all the flamboyant habiliments of angina which this patient showed, being instead a dull, aching, or distending sensation confined to the precordium. Furthermore, at the time this patient had his initial pains, there was no clinical evidence whatever for the existence of significant pulmonary hypertension.

Striking and dramatic features of the patient's course were the spread of violaceous colors about his face and neck, and the extreme anxiety and agitation he exhibited during acute episodes, sometimes associated with marked sweating and occasionally with deathly pallor. In such a setting, one thinks of some discharge phenomenon, such as a pheochromocytoma. Angina pectoris may, of course, be associated with this, and in addition, a discharging pheochromocytoma may be accompanied by a significant degree of upper abdominal or chest pain, which does not seem to be related to the coronary circulation, and the exact nature of which remains obscure—to me, at least. But this patient's blood pressure was taken repeatedly and was never found to be elevated.

The peculiar discoloration of this patient's head and neck could have been the result of several factors. He had always had a very ruddy coloration and a volatile temper, which was associated with marked flushing. In addition, he had been doing a great amount of drinking, and individuals who do this often acquire vascular dilatation on their faces, necks, and chests. I suspect it was these local vascular peculiarities, plus a marked degree of chronic venous congestion, which accounted for his at times startling violaceous appearance. It seems clear from the record that the appearance of these color changes was directly correlated with venous congestion, a phenomenon which would not make sense, a pheochromocytoma, or a carcinoid, about which we shall have more to say shortly.

Let us now turn to a consideration of the various factors which might have been responsible for the intense in-flow blockage of the venous circulation which this patient evidenced. In general, in-flow obstruction to the venous circulation may result from the following:

1. Obstruction of the vena cava, arising from within or without the vessel. This would include infections, tumors, cysts, aneurysms, forms of arteritis, collagenosis, thrombosis, and so forth.
2. Pericardial disease, wet or dry.
3. Myocardial disease.
4. Endocardial disease.
5. Increased pressure in the peripheral circulation.
6. Increased pressure in the pulmonary circulation.
7. Congenital abnormalities.

A number of these mechanisms we can dispose of readily. The patient had never had systemic hypertension. There were no alterations indicating a congenital abnormality. Vena caval obstruction is unlikely in view of the clear x-ray of the mediastinum and the absence, during the patient's long-drawn-out course, of any evidence of an infectious, neoplastic, or vascular disease likely to be associated with venous thrombosis. Also, there are rampant indications that regardless of the condition of the vena cava, the heart itself was also clearly diseased.

It seems perfectly evident from the record that the patient had at least one, and perhaps several, episodes of pulmonary embolization during the latter part of his illness. Could repeated episodes have led to chronic, severe pulmonary hypertension? This seems unlikely for a number of reasons. First, the P_2 sound was never described as unusually loud. The patient did not develop a marked right axis deviation in the ECG. The lung fields were always described as relatively clear. Repeated x-rays of the chest failed to show any of the telltale changes in the pulmonary vascular patterns sometimes seen in pulmonary embolism. Lung scans were never done, unfortunately. We can conclude with certainty that he did have one or several pulmonary emboli, but the evidence opposes the idea that this could have accounted per se for the in-flow venous obstruction.

So far as wet pericardial disease is concerned, there were never any clinical signs of an appreciable collection of pericardial fluid, and the long-drawn-out clinical course would be incompatible with such a condition, as was the heart scan which was done. Chronic constrictive pericarditis must be given more consideration. But this patient's heart was very large and remained quite active, with distinctly heard sounds. The ECG failed to show appreciable low voltage. X-rays of the chest disclosed congestion of the lung fields, at times, which is unusual in primary pericardial disease. A strong argument against a constricting pericardium was the dramatic response to digitalis and diuretics which the patient repeatedly demonstrated. Once patients with constrictive disease develop a marked degree of in-flow blockage, they do not tend to fare as well as or to respond to treatment in the manner enjoyed by this patient. As already indicated, constrictive disease would not explain well the anginal pain which dominated the early stage of his illness.

The diffusely enlarged heart, the progressive dyspnea, orthopnea, and paroxysmal nocturnal dyspnea, the pulmonary emboli, the development of an arrhythmia and the ECG changes, and the transient systolic murmur are all thoroughly compatible with some kind of primary myocardial disease. There was a family history of heart disease, and one might wonder about a familial myocardiopathy. Rheumatic fever had occurred in the family, and the patient had had frequent sore throats, reminding one of the possibility of rheumatic myocarditis. He had been a heavy drinker, and the setting might have fostered a nutritional myocarditis. However, none of these would be ushered in by the kind of precordial distress which plagued this patient's early illness, and which we have depicted as typical of the distress associated with acute myocardial ischemia, of whatever cause. If this patient *did* have myocardial disease, surely it must have been derived from the myocardial ischemia.

One might well ask at this juncture how such postulated ischemic myocardial disease could account for the progressive in-flow block of the venous circulation which this man developed. There are a number of possible mechanisms:

1. The evolution of diffuse myocardial injury, resulting in right- or left-sided failure, or both. Clinically, this patient gave evidence of both right- and left-sided failure. The lungs were congested, and he had orthopnea and paroxysmal nocturnal dyspnea, as well as marked venous hypertension.

2. The development of a ventricular aneurysm, for which we have no evidence here.

3. Herniation or rupture of the intraventricular septum, for which we have no auscultatory evidence here, and which would be incompatible with both the patient's long course and his good response to therapy.

4. The growth of an intracavitary ball valve thrombus, within either the atria or the ventricles.

The intense cyanosis and other manifestations of congestion that definitely were related to position and posture, plus a filling defect that was described in the angiograms of the right atrium, give real substance to this last possibility. The pulmonary emboli he had could well have originated from such a thrombus in the right heart.

Finally, we come to the endocardium. There were never any clear-cut physical signs of valvular heart disease, and while the marked venous distension and systolic blow to the right of the sternum gave rise to the possibility of tricuspid disease, there were no abnormal pulsations in the neck veins or liver, and the systolic bruit disappeared each time the patient was brought out of congestive heart failure. A primary endocardial disease would not explain the anginal pain of this patient's early illness.

We have already excluded constrictive pericarditis, but what about constrictive endocarditis, better known as endocardial fibroelastosis? In the first place, this is an exceedingly rare condition in the United States. Perhaps the strongest arguments against its presence here are the anginal pains which inaugurated the illness, and the repeated excellent response to therapy, already alluded to. We have seen two patients with mediastinal collagenosis that mimicked endocardial disease, but the angina would not be explained by this disease, either.

For precisely the same reasons that we have mentioned the possibility of an intracavitary ball valve thrombus, we must also review the likelihood of an intracardiac neoplasm, namely, a myxoma. If we can believe the angiograms, such a tumor was perhaps present in the right atrium. The attractive features of this diagnosis are obvious, particularly when it receives support from a shadow on an x-ray plate. However, a recent review of such tumors raises serious doubts in my mind that such a myxoma could have been present. Cramping of the legs, marked weakness, weight loss, dizziness, syncope and convulsions, tachycardia, and arrhythmias are all prominent accompaniments of such tumors in the right heart. None of these were prominent in our patient. Furthermore, precordial pain is most unusual in right-sided myxomas, and typical angina is not reported in any instances of which I am aware. Also, while exertional dyspnea is often present orthopnea and paroxysmal nocturnal dyspnea are uncommon. We have already stressed the fact that left-sided as well as right-sided failure was present here, and in the usual right-sided myxoma, left-sided failure is not prominent.

With myxoma the ECG frequently shows high, peaked P waves and low voltage. None of these changes were noted here. The strongest argument against myxoma is the history of clear-cut anginal pain. It is difficult to understand how a right-sided myxoma could produce such pain. A left-sided tumor may, of course, occlude the coronary vessels with emboli and lead to coronary artery insufficiency, but this patient did not have other features of such a left atrial tumor, such as peripheral emboli, signs of malfunction of the mitral valve, and pronounced left-sided heart failure. The excellent therapeutic response which this patient had would also be contrary to the usual experience with myxomata, as would the very long duration of his pronounced symptoms.

A functioning carcinoid tumor is suggested by a number of features of the patient's course. I have the somewhat unusual distinction of having described in vivid terms one of the earliest cases of carcinoid syndrome seen in this country, although unfortunately I did not recognize what it was at the time. This patient reminds me of the earlier one in that there was marked in-flow stasis, a peculiar systolic murmur, several pulmonary emboli, and a fantastic, lobster-like discoloration of the face and upper trunk. The cardinal manifestations of carcinoid are the flushing phenomenon, diarrhea, episodes of asthma, enlargement of the liver, right heart failure, and auscultatory findings compatible with pulmonic stenosis, tricuspid insufficiency or stenosis, or both. Not all of these features need be present simultaneously. 5-Hydroxyindole acetic acid is present in the urine consistently.

The bizarre play of colors which so impressed those who saw this patient, appearing in a variety of peculiar circumstances, would be thoroughly compatible with carcinoid, as would be his sweating and flushing, although we have already made the point that a dependent position of the head and increased venous pressure seemed the major triggers for these changes, and one might wonder how a carcinoid would be so related to recumbency. Although the patient had no diarrhea, he did become bloated, and this can be considered a part of this symptom complex. His liver was enlarged and the bilirubin level always elevated, and the carcinoid tumor could have been located in the liver. Certainly signs of right-sided failure were predominant. Peculiar behavior such as indulged in by this patient may be a result of carcinoid. On the other hand, he never had diarrhea, abdominal pain, asthma, tachycardia, or weight loss, even though this illness lasted 12 to 15 years. Certainly there were no clear-cut physical signs of pulmonic stenosis or of tricuspid disease, although we must admit that in carcinoid heart disease the physical changes accompanying the alterations of the valves may be minimal, or changing, or not present at all. The murmur which was occasionally heard at the xiphoid could have represented tricuspid disease. But there are two strong points against a functioning carcinoid: (1) the dominance early in the illness of typical anginal pain, and (2) the presence of left-sided heart failure, already alluded to. The valves of the left side are not affected unless there is a patent septum, and no sign of such existed here. Finally, the test for 5-HIAA was negative, and in carcinoid generally is positive.

It seems to me much more logical, therefore, to conclude that this patient had coronary arterial insufficiency at an early age, resulting in angina pectoris and progressive myocardial damage of a diffuse as well as of a focal sort. This basic disorder became complicated by the release of pulmonary emboli, and perhaps also by the growth of a thrombus within the right auricle, all of these elements leading to a marked degree of in-flow venous obstruction.

When death comes with horrible unprepared suddenness "like a thief in the night," it usually is the result of cessation of effective myocardial contractions owing to infarction or ventricular arrhythmia, or to a pulmonary embolus. The stage unfortunately was set just right for any of these events. From a statistical standpoint, it is perhaps most likely that he had an additional myocardial injury.

Why should one so young have coronary disease? There was diabetes in his family, and several of his blood sugars were slightly elevated. He may have had latent diabetes mellitus. Also, he smoked excessively, and his aggressive way of life could have been an additional factor. One always considers congenital anomalies of the coronary circulation in this age group, but the evidence at hand allows us to only make this suggestion. Apparently he did not have syphilis, and there is no reason to anticipate syphilitic aortitis. There was nothing to indicate endocarditis of the aortic valve. Disease of the sinus of Valsalva, either congenital or acquired, would have to be considered, even though there was no indication of actual rupture of a sinus. Sometimes this occurs into the heart muscle at the aortic root, and the course may be more prolonged.

Be that as it may, I believe that coronary artery disease and ischemic myocarditis, with angina pectoris and diffuse as well as focal myocardial damage, were the bases for this patient's trouble. The in-flow obstruction was no doubt the product of these changes, and perhaps also of in-flow blockage induced by formation of a ball valve thrombus in the right atrium. In addition, this may have given rise to pulmonary emboli. His sudden death was probably precipitated by further myocardial injury, or perhaps another pulmonary embolus.

POST MORTEM FINDINGS

Severe coronary artery atherosclerosis. Extensive old myocardial infarction. Long-standing systemic and pulmonary passive congestion.

REFERENCES

Coronary Artery Disease

Andrus, E. C., and Baker, B. M.: Symposium on coronary heart disease, 2nd ed. H. C. Blumgart. (Ed.). American Heart Association, Monograph #2, 1968, p. 44.

Blankenhorn, D. H., et al.: Ischemic heart disease in young adults. Ann. Intern. Med. 69:21, 1968.

Block, W. J., Jr., Crumpacher, E. L., Dry, T. J., et al.: Prognosis of angina pectoris: 6882 cases. JAMA 150:259, 1952.

Friesinger, G. C., Page, E. E., and Ross, R. S.: Diagnostic significance of coronary arteriography. Trans. Ass. Amer. Physicians 83:78, 1970.

Gorlin, R.: Pathophysiology of cardiac pain. Circulation 32:138, 1965.

Graber, J. D., et al.: Ventricular aneurysm. Brit. Heart J. 34:830, 1972.

Harrison, T. R., and Reeves, T. J.: Clinical diagnosis of coronary artery disease. Principles and problems of ischemic heart disease. Chicago, Year Book Medical Publishers, 1968.

PART I / CORONARY ARTERY DISEASE

Herrick, J. B.: Clinical features of sudden obstruction of the coronary arteries. JAMA 59:2015, 1912.
Jenkins, C. D.: Psychologic and social precursors of coronary disease. New Eng. J. Med. 284:244, 1971.
Kannel, W. B., and Feinleib, M.: Natural history of angina pectoris in the Framingham study. Amer. J. Cardiol. 29:154, 1972.
Oberman, A., et al.: Natural history of coronary artery disease. Bull. N.Y. Acad. Sci. 48:1109, 1972.
Richards, D. W., Bland, E. F., and White, P. D.: Twenty-five year follow-up study of 456 patients with angina pectoris. J. Clin. Dis. 4:423, 1956.

Dissecting Aortic Aneurysm

Enselberg, C. D.: The clinical picture of aneurysm of the abdominal aorta. Ann. Intern. Med. 44:1163, 1956.
Hirst, A. E., Jr., Johns, V. J., Jr., and Kime, S. W., Jr.: Dissecting aneurysm of the aorta. A review of 505 cases. Medicine 37:217, 1958.
Lindsay, J., Jr., and Hurst, J. W.: Clinical features and prognosis in dissecting aneurysm of the aorta. Circulation 35:880, 1967.

Pheochromocytoma

Engelman, K.: Principles in the diagnosis of pheochromocytoma. Bull. N.Y. Acad. Med. 45:851, 1969.
Gifford, R. W., Kvale, W. F., Maher, F. T., Roth, G. M., and Priestley, J. T.: Clinical features, diagnosis and treatment of pheochromocytoma. A review of 76 cases. Mayo Clin. Proc. 39:281, 1964.
Moorhead, E. L., Caldwell, J. R., Kelly, A. R., and Morales, A. R.: The diagnosis of pheochromocytoma: Analysis of 26 cases. JAMA 196:1107, 1966.
Page, L. B., et al.: Pheochromocytoma. Disease-A-Month 1:40, January, 1968.
Sjoerdsma, A., Engelman, D., Waldmann, T. A., Cooperman, L. H., and Hammond, W. G.: Pheochromocytoma: current concepts of diagnosis and treatment. Ann. Intern. Med. 65:1302, 1966.

The Carcinoid Syndrome

Grahame-Smith, D. G.: The carcinoid syndrome. Amer. J. Cardiol. 21:376, 1968.
Roberts, W. C., and Sjoerdsma, A.: The cardiac disease associated with the carcinoid syndrome (carcinoid heart disease). Amer. J. Med. 36:5, 1964.

Pericardial Disease

Friedberg, C. K.: Acute Pericarditis. In Diseases of the Heart. 3rd Ed. Philadelphia, W. B. Saunders Company, 1966, pp. 933–965.
McIntosh, H. D.: Pericarditis. Disease-A-Month, 36:1, 1964.
Shabetai, R.: Symposium: pericardial disease. Amer. J. Cardiol. 26:445, 1970.
Wolff, L., and Grunfeld, O.: Pericarditis. New Eng. J. Med. 268:419, 1963.

Endocardial Fibroelastosis

Moller, J. H., et al.: Endocardial fibroelastosis: clinical and anatomic study of 47 patients with emphasis on relationship to mitral insufficiency. Circulation 30:759, 1964.
Sellers, F. J., Keith, J. D., and Manning, J. A.: The diagnosis of primary endocardial fibroelastosis. Circulation 29:49, 1964.

Pulmonary Embolism

Dalen, J. E., and Dexter, L.: Pulmonary embolism. JAMA 207:1505, 1969.
Parker, B. M., and Smith, J. R.: Pulmonary embolism and infarction: a review of the physiological consequences of pulmonary arterial obstruction. Amer. J. Med. 24:402, 1958.
Sokoff, L. A., and Rodman, T.: Acute pulmonary embolism. Amer. Heart J. 74:710, 829; 1967.

Auricular Thrombi and Tumors

Belle, M. S.: Right atrial myxoma. Circulation 19:910, 1959.
Bulray, E. R., and Pomerantz, H. Z.: Mass thrombus of the left auricle. Canad. Med. Ass. J. 84:158, 1961.
Evans, M. E.: Ball thrombus of heart. Brit. Heart J. 10:34, 1948.

Evans, W., and Benson, R.: Mass thrombus of left auricle. Brit. Heart J. *10:*39, 1948.
Goodwin, J. F.: Diagnosis of left atrial myxoma. Lancet *1:*464, 1963.
Hair, T. E., Jr., Orgain, E. S., Sealy, W. C., and McIntosh, H. D.: Myxoma of left atrium: observations on two cases with successful removal and review of diagnostic methods. Amer. J. Med. *32:*560, 1962.
Harvey, W. P.: Clinical aspects of cardiac tumors. Amer. J. Cardiol. *21:*328, 1968.
Surawicz, B., and Ninenberg, M. A.: Association of silent mitral stenosis with massive thrombi in the left atrium. New Eng. J. Med. *263:*423, 1960.
Symposium on cardiac tumors. Amer. J. Cardiol. *21:*307, 1968.

Cardiomyopathy

Friedberg, C. K.: Cardiomyopathy. Symposium. Circulation *44:*935, 1971.
Harvey, W. P., Segal, J. P., and Gurel, T.: The clinical spectrum of primary myocardial disease. Progr. Cardiovasc. Dis., 7:17, 1964.

Aneurysm of Sinus of Valsalva

Kerber, R. E., et al.: Unruptured aneurysm of the sinus of Valsalva producing right ventricular outflow obstruction. Amer. J. Med. *53:*775, 1972.
Wright, J. S.: Ruptured aneurysm of the sinus of Valsalva. Quart. J. Med. *39:*493, 1970.

J A PATIENT WITH ASCITES

THE CLINICAL PROBLEM

A 53 year old black laborer was admitted for the second time on September 2, 1965, with a chief complaint of increasing abdominal girth. A brother of the patient had been in a tuberculosis sanitorium during the year prior to this admission. The patient had worked as a laborer at a steel company for 20 years. He had smoked one and a half packs of cigarettes a day for 30 years and had drunk heavily for many years. The patient's past general health was good and he had had no serious illnesses. In April of 1965, he had been admitted to The Johns Hopkins Hospital for the first time for repair of a torn anterior cruciate ligament in his right knee. At that time, his blood pressure (single determination) was 190/130 mm. Hg. His temperature on admission was 99.2 degrees, and he maintained a low-grade fever throughout his hospital stay. Hematocrit was 42 ml./100 ml.; serum urea nitrogen, 100 mg./100 ml.; serum alkaline phosphatase, 4.7 King-Armstrong units; total serum bilirubin, less than 0.8 mg./100 ml. He was discharged from the hospital five days following repair of his knee injury. The patient was followed closely in the Orthopedic Outpatient Department and showed good recovery of function of his right knee. In mid-July, he noted the onset of anorexia and a sensation of epigastric fullness after eating a small amount of food. This occurred with each meal, and caused him to reduce his food intake. Subsequently, generalized weakness and malaise began. There was no nausea, vomiting, diarrhea, or abdominal pain. In early August, the patient observed gradually increasing abdominal girth, and by mid-August he had noticed shortness of breath on exertion and later two-pillow orthopnea. During this period, he lost 28 pounds. On admission to the hospital, the patient was seen to be depressed and cachectic. Vital signs were normal except for a temperature of 101.4 degrees. The abdomen was protuberant and tense, with shifting dullness and a definite fluid wave. One observer felt the liver edge at the level of the umbilicus, but other observers could not confirm this. The spleen was not palpable, there was no distention of the superficial abdominal veins, and no telangiectases were seen. On admission to the hospital, the patient's hematocrit was 42 ml./100 ml., and the red cells were normal on smear. The white blood cell count was 38,500/cu. mm., with 8 percent juvenile neutrophils, 87 percent polymorphonuclear leukocytes, 2 percent lymphocytes, and 3 percent monocytes. The platelet count was 819,000/cu. mm. Urinalysis was normal except for three to four white blood cells per high power field. The stool was guaiac negative. Results of a first strength purified protein derivative test were negative. X-ray films of the abdomen showed haziness suggestive of ascites. Paracentesis yielded 2000 cc. of clear yellow fluid with a specific gravity of 1.016; the fluid contained 780 white blood cells per cubic millimeter, the majority of which were "polys." Cytologic examination, smears, and cultures for pyogenic organisms and tubercle bacilli were all negative. Serum urea nitrogen was 41 mg./100 ml; sodium, 135 mEq./liter; potassium, 6.7 mEq./liter; chlorides 93 mEq./liter; and CO_2 combining power 21.0 mEq./liter. The serum calcium was 9.0 mg./100 ml., phosphorus was 6.0 mg./100 ml., and fasting blood sugar was 100 mg./100 ml. The serum albumin was 3.4 gm./100 ml. and serum globulin was 3.0 gm./100 ml. The serum glutamic oxaloacetic transaminase (SGOT) level was 67 Karmen units/ml. and the serum glutamic pyruvic transaminase (SGPT) was 37 Karmen units/ml. The serum alkaline and acid phosphatase levels were normal, the total serum bilirubin content was 1.3 mg./100 ml., with 0.6 mg. of direct reacting bilirubin, and the prothrombin time was greater than 80 percent of normal. Sputum smears and cultures were negative for pyogenic organisms and acid fast bacilli. Blood cultures were also negative. An hepatic scintiscan showed slight hepatomegaly without discrete filling defects, but with some generalized decrease in uptake. A barium enema was normal. A GI series revealed a normal "C" loop and duodenal bulb and no evidence of esophageal varices. An ill-defined filling defect at the esophagogastric junction was noted and was thought to result from extrinsic pressure. Intravenous pyelograms revealed bilateral decrease in function, of greater degree on the right side. There was poor visualization of the pelvo-calyceal system and of the renal outline on the left. Gastric washings were negative for tumor cells. Gastroscopy, done on the tenth hospital day, revealed atrophic gastritis and a small ulcer on the lesser curvature of the stomach, with "both benign and malignant features." Esophagoscopy showed no varices or bleeding sites; reflux of gastric contents into the lower esophagus was noted. In the hospital, the patient showed daily afternoon temperature spikes in the range of 100 to 102 degrees. The white blood cell count was persistently elevated between 19,000 and 39,000/cu. mm. The serum urea nitrogen rose to 67 mg./100 ml. A sudden episode of gastrointestinal bleeding occurred, which required the administration of two units of blood and then subsided spontaneously; bright red blood was obtained in the gastric contents at that time. On the twelfth hospital day, a repeat paracentesis was done; the fluid contained 640 white blood cells per cubic millimeter, 95 percent of which were mononuclear cells. The fluid protein was 3.7 gm./100 ml., with an albumin-to-globulin ratio of 1.7:2.0. Therapy was begun with para-aminosalicylic acid (PAS), streptomycin, and isoniazid, but the patient died shortly afterward.

DISCUSSION OF THE PROBLEM

This patient's final illness commenced very insidiously, and in a sense right under the eyes of the orthopedic surgeons, who were following his postoperative course in their clinic. Everything appeared to be going well until mid-August, when suddenly it became evident that he was a very sick man indeed. Thereafter, his health deteriorated rapidly.

The clinical course of his disease was characterized by a profound constitutional reaction, with marked weakness, malaise, fatigability, anorexia, and weight loss, but by a scarcity of focal manifestations, the only ones being epigastric fullness and early filling of the stomach. The most striking physical alteration was ascites, which occurred in the absence of edema of the legs or of other tissues. These changes were associated with a moderate temperature elevation, leukocytosis, and thrombocytosis as well.

In analyzing a clinical problem of this sort, in which one is confronted with the insidious onset of a series of totally nonspecific manifestations, it is helpful to select the most prominent objective alteration, then list all of the various types of clinical disorders in which this feature may be encountered, and finally select from this list the one condition which seems to explain most appropriately all of the facts at hand. This patient's ascites seems to be such an alteration.

The principal causes of ascites may be categorized as follows:
1. Blockage of the venous return to the right heart.
2. Blockage of the inferior vena cava above the hepatic veins.
3. Blockage of the hepatic veins (so-called Chiari syndrome).
4. Diffuse diseases of the liver.
5. Blockage of the portal veins.
6. Peritoneal inflammation.
7. Abnormalities of fluid and electrolyte balance and of serum proteins.
8. Extrusion of blood, urine, and chyle.

Fortunately, several of these etiologies can quickly be eliminated. The facts that the neck veins were flat, the liver was not significantly enlarged, and there was no pedal edema exclude in-flow blockage at the level of the heart. The absence of appreciable hepatic enlargement and edema of the lower extremities likewise eliminates blockage of the vena cava above the hepatic veins. Absence of liver enlargement also militates against the likelihood of

Chiari's syndrome, as does the lack of hepatic pain and tenderness, both common accompaniments of hepatic vein occlusion. The mere fact that the fluid accumulation was confined entirely to the abdominal cavity excludes fluid, electrolyte, or serum protein alterations as major factors in the formation of the ascites, and the fluid obtained was obviously not blood, urine, or chyle.

We are left, then, with three general causative mechanisms: (1) some diffuse disease of the liver, (2) blockage of the portal veins, or (3) peritoneal inflammation. From this point, our analysis of the facts must proceed more cautiously.

It seems to me rather unlikely that this patient had intrinsic liver disease extensive enough to have been solely responsible for the degree of ascites he exhibited, even though his habitual intake of alcohol makes such a possibility theoretically plausible.

In the first place, the patient had none of the customary hallmarks of parenchymal liver disease, such as spider telangiectasia, palmar erythema, and so forth, although, mind you, such classical features are by no means consistently present. Nor were there any indications of the development of a collateral venous circulation, either over the abdominal wall or in the esophagus, but these also are not always present.

Furthermore, the laboratory evidence does not indicate severe parenchymal disease of the liver. However, it should be pointed out that at times ascites secondary to cirrhosis may occur in the face of surprisingly scant laboratory abnormalities in terms of the serum bilirubin, transaminases, alkaline phosphatase, and prothrombin time. Alteration of the serum protein partition and BSP retention may be the only indicants of disordered hepatic function, in such instances. On two occasions in the past year, we have seen elderly females who were admitted with massive ascites. There was little or nothing in the history, physical examination, or laboratory studies to indicate cirrhosis of the liver, yet this condition was discovered at operation.

In this patient, the serum proteins were just a little unusual. A bromsulphalein test was unfortunately not done. Perhaps we should mention the fact that the serum sodium was reduced, and the serum nitrogen was elevated, both of which changes may accompany disease of the liver.

This patient's ascitic fluid might also be challenged as not being the sort usually found in pure intrinsic disease of the liver; you will recall that the specific gravity was 1.016, the fluid protein content 3.7 gm./100 ml., and the cell count several hundreds of cells per cubic millimeter. These findings give the fluid more of the character of an exudate than of a pure transudate, such as would result from uncomplicated hepatic disease.

However, former experiences have made us somewhat leery of relying too much upon minor distinguishing features in ascitic fluid in making the differential diagnosis. The distinctions between transudates and exudates may not be clear-cut, and early in the course of an illness, exudative fluid may resemble a transudate. Also, disorders generally producing transudates may become complicated by other disease processes and result in the accumulation of an exudate, as for example, the not unusual situation of cirrhosis of the liver complicated by tuberculous peritonitis.

Therefore, although we believe that the evidence for parenchymatous liver disease is slim, it may still be worthwhile to explore this possibility a little more thoroughly before dismissing it. Again, although this patient's liver scan was reported as indicative of parenchymal disease, experience has taught us that liver scans can be misleading, just as clinical observation and analysis can be.

For the reasons already outlined, alcoholic cirrhosis appears to be an unlikely explanation for the total course of events. The possibility of a focal or diffuse hepatoma, developing in a background of mild cirrhosis, is less easily dismissed, but the liver was not appreciably enlarged, and there was no abdominal discomfort, significant jaundice, or elevation of the alkaline phosphatase level, which are frequent accompaniments of such tumors. A syphilitic hepar lobatum is unlikely also, in view of the lack of hepatic enlargement and negative serology test results. The patient had undergone an operation in which he was given fluorothane, but the chemical changes noted are not those of acute, fulminant, toxic hepatic necroses. In a Negro male with liver disease, one should always consider the presence of sarcoidosis, but there was no hint of sarcoid in any of its other customary locations. For the same reason, the suggestion of amyloidosis would be no more than a guess. A liver abscess, and in particular an amebic abscess, is suggested by the fever and the marked degree of leukocytosis. However, the scan failed to indicate such a lesion. Leukemia comes to mind in view of the very high WBC count, and also the thrombocytosis, but none of the other changes characteristic of such a process were present. The absence of appreciable jaundice excludes any form of chronic obstructive biliary process.

This patient was noted to have had hypertension in the past, and he clearly had some sort of renal disease, evidenced by nitrogen retention and poor visualization of the kidneys by the intravenous pyelograms. He was noted to have some sort of an ulcerating lesion in his stomach, from which he ultimately bled. He had fever, leukocytosis, and thrombocytosis as well, and had suffered profound weight loss.

Each of these pieces of clinical evidence points to the possibility that he might have had polyarteritis. Only in the last few years have we come to realize that polyarteritis nodosa (PAN) may present with alterations which are principally, or even totally, related to malfunction of the liver. Recently I observed a patient on my rounds, an elderly female with ascites and hepatomegaly, who had all of the hallmarks of nutritional, or perhaps posthepatitic, cirrhosis. If she didn't have either of these, we were certain she would prove to have a malignancy, perhaps a primary cancer, in the liver. However, biopsy of her liver showed PAN!

I can only say that the patient we are considering here could have had PAN, but again I have to fall back upon the impression that the evidence for diffuse, severe, intrinsic liver disease is not outstanding, and that the ascitic fluid may well have been exudative. Also, during the course of the patient's final illness, there were no muscle or joint pains, no neuropathy, no abdominal pain, no strikingly abnormal elements in the urine, and, as a matter of fact, no hypertension, all of which usually accompany a severe, progressive arteritis.

Other types of processes which might have caused diffuse involvement of the liver are metastatic tumor, a lymphoma, or a granulomatous infection, such as tuberculosis or histoplasmosis. However, when metastatic tumor or a lymphoma is confined to the liver, and does not involve the peritoneal surfaces or produce blockage of the portal veins, massive ascites does not generally ensue. In contrast, a granulomatous infection of the liver, such as tuberculosis, may be associated with ascites, a possibility which will be given further consideration shortly.

There is some debate over whether or not blockage of the extrahepatic portal veins can produce ascites in man in the complete absence of some type of disturbance of the liver. Suffice it to say that the most common causes of acquired extrahepatic portal vein blockage are infections and tumors, which often involve the liver concomitantly and to a greater or lesser extent than the portal veins. Also, these same processes not infrequently involve the peritoneal surfaces, and the resultant degree of ascites may be a product of three factors: (1) liver involvement, (2) portal vein obstruction, and (3) peritoneal inflammation. This patient's ascites may well have had such a threefold etiology. Obstruction of the portal veins is often associated with splenomegaly and anemia, neither of which was noted here, and with the production of an ascitic fluid that generally contains less protein than reported here. It seems unlikely, therefore, that the *primary* process here was blockage of the portal veins, although it could have been an associated and secondary phenomenon.

We come finally, then, to the question of whether or not peritoneal inflammation was a major factor in this patient's ascites. This seems entirely likely, in view of the matters already discussed, particularly the fact that the ascitic fluid had exudative qualities. We must re-emphasize the point just made, however, that when peritoneal inflammation is a prime factor in the formation of ascites, there may be concomitant involvement of the liver and portal veins by the same disease process. Such could well have happened here.

The most common causes of peritoneal inflammation resulting in ascites are tumor implants and infection. The tumor usually originates within the gastrointestinal tract, pancreas, or ovaries, but sometimes arises outside the abdominal cavity, as, for example, a seminoma in the male.

Surely this patient's entire clinical course cries out "diffuse malignancy!" Its insidious onset and relentless progression, the prominence of the constitutional reaction, and the dearth of focal manifestations are all very typical of such processes, as are the persistent fever and the thrombocytosis. Sharply elevated WBC counts are, of course, not a rare accompaniment of a variety of neoplasms and, in addition, it was thought that this chronically ill person had a urinary tract infection complicating his basic illness.

If he had a malignancy, where did it arise? Obviously, it could have arisen in a large number of areas, and the information we are given here provides material for speculation, but not solid data for firm conclusions.

The only localizing features of this patient's course are these:
1. The sensation of postprandial fullness, his original complaint.
2. Epigastric tenderness.
3. The visualization of some type of ulcerous-appearing lesion on the lesser curvature of the stomach.
4. The gastrointestinal hemorrhage.

In addition to these is the fact that he drank too much, and, as you well know, hepatomas, pancreatic carcinoma, and gastric carcinoma are more frequent in those who imbibe excessively. Finally, the patient was thought to have atrophic gastritis, and I believe some observers feel that in association with this, there is an increased occurrence of carcinoma.

The features pointing to the possible presence of a gastric tumor, perhaps a carcinoma or lymphosarcoma, should therefore be manifest. The excessively high white blood cell count might point suggestively to a lymphoma as the more likely of the two, although, as already stressed, any tumor can on occasion be associated with leukocytosis. Another possibility to be considered would be perforation of the stomach affected by tumor, with a walled-off abscess accounting for the fever and leukocytosis, but there was no history of such an acute intra-abdominal incident, and the abdominal signs never keenly suggested this possibility.

Because this patient's serum urea nitrogen rose progressively as his ascites increased, one would have to consider the possibility of retroperitoneal fibrosis occurring concomitantly with gastric carcinoma, as sometimes happens. But the intravenous pyelograms failed to show obstructive uropathy, which makes this event a poor bet.

Militating against carcinoma of the stomach is the x-ray appearance of the stomach which, but for the lesions on the lesser curvature, appears to be normal. Furthermore, reliable observers considered the lesions on the lesser curvature as more likely to be extrinsic than intrinsic.

The facts that this patient's gastric ulcers were located high on the lesser curvature of the stomach near the esophagus, and were thought by radiologists to result from some process extrinsic to the stomach, should immediately direct one's attention to carcinoma of the tail of the pancreas, for it is at the very area of the stomach affected that the two organs are very contiguous. And there are *many* features of the patient's course pointing to carcinoma of the tail of the pancreas:
1. His alcoholic abuse, already alluded to.
2. The very insidious, silent, stealthy onset and progression of his disease. Truly, in this disorder, death comes "like a thief in the night."
3. The sensation of epigastric fullness, associated with mild tenderness.
4. The profound anorexia, and the wasting of the soft tissues.
5. The nature of the ascites, with high protein content, indicative of peritoneal seeding. In addition, of course, it is not rare for pancreatic car-

cinoma to obstruct the portal vein, and also to spread to the liver, resulting in the trivalent type of ascites already described.

6. Finally, this patient may well have succumbed as a result of pulmonary embolus, and while pulmonary emboli are not infrequently the coup de grâce in many forms of malignant new growths, they occur particularly commonly in tumors of the pancreas.

The only finding at all out of the ordinary is the WBC count, but it was associated with a thrombocytosis and hence may have been the leukemoid reaction of malignant tumor, a not uncommon accompaniment of pancreatic carcinoma. Also, in a patient so debilitated, there may have been other causes of leukocytosis, such as basilar pneumonia or a urinary infection, and this patient's WBC count and fever did decrease when he was placed on antibiotics. Bacteria were present in his urine.

However, there is another affliction of the pancreas which deserves comment, in view of the brisk leukocytosis, and that is an acute pancreatitis. Not too commonly, the inflammatory process associated with severe pancreatitis may result in portal vein thrombosis and ascites, and, as you know, bacterial suppuration sometimes follows pancreatitis. Therefore, could this entire course of events have followed an acute pancreatitic episode in a chronic alcoholic? This is an intriguing possibility, and would neatly explain the marked leukocytosis and fever, as well as the extrinsic gastric lesion. But, on the other hand, there was never a history of an acute episode, and the abdominal findings were not those of an intra-abdominal abscess. As already stressed, the dominant feature of the onset of this patient's illness was slow, quiet stealth, quite the opposite of the beginnings of an acute pancreatitis.

For the same reason, we can exclude other localized suppurative processes within the abdominal cavity, such as might have resulted from a ruptured appendix, peptic ulcer, or diverticulum.

While the quiet insidiousness of the earliest manifestations of this patient's disease makes localized suppuration unlikely, these same clinical features are often the hallmark of another type of bacterial infection, which should top everyone's list of likelihoods in these circumstances because it is readily curable—to wit, tuberculosis.

Several pieces of clinical evidence point to tuberculosis in these particular circumstances:

1. His brother was said to have tuberculosis.

2. The patient was drinking too much, and he may have had hepatic cirrhosis. It is a well-known fact that in this era, tuberculous peritonitis occurs more frequently in association with cirrhosis of the liver than in any other situation. For this reason, tuberculous peritonitis requires consideration in any patient with cirrhosis who develops ascites.

3. The patient was wasted and febrile.

4. He had a very high WBC count and, of course, a leukemoid reaction may be a part of disseminated tuberculosis, which may be true of thrombocytosis as well.

5. The ascitic fluid contained considerable protein and many cells.

6. The serum sodium and chloride levels were depressed, the serum urea nitrogen was elevated, and his blood pressure, formerly noted to be considerably elevated, was depressed.

7. The liver scan suggested diffuse parenchymal changes, and these could have been the result of tuberculosis.

8. While the changes in the intravenous pyelograms were obviously far from typical, it is conceivable that the renal alterations also may have resulted from tuberculosis.

Clearly, disseminated tuberculosis with adrenal insufficiency and peritonitis could have been present here, although clinical evidence of some weight can be marshalled against such an explanation. The patient was not reported as having night sweats, a common feature of disseminated tuberculosis. There was no history of abdominal pain or tenderness, often a prominent feature in tuberculous peritonitis. The abdomen was not doughy, and no masses were ever felt within it, as sometimes occurs when the omentum and gut become involved in the plastic inflammatory process. Diarrhea or tympanites are sometimes a part of such a process, but these were not noted here. On the abdominal films, the barium loops do not appear to be gathered in adherent clusters, as frequently is the case in the gluey peritonitis of tuberculosis. As far as the liver is concerned, the serum alkaline phosphatase level was normal, although in tuberculous hepatitis, it is frequently elevated. Also, the patient's chest film was clear, although he had been sick for several months. If tuberculosis were present, one might have expected the occurrence of miliary pulmonary lesions, although recent experiences have taught us that disseminated tuberculosis can indeed occur in the complete absence of visible x-ray changes in the lungs. More weight should be given to the negative tuberculin test, but this demands cautious interpretation, as it may be negative despite a widespread infection, and also because the test was carried out only to the first strength. Finally, it seems to me that the ulcerative lesion on the patient's lesser gastric curvature would perhaps be unusual in tuberculous peritonitis, although I suppose it could have been a granuloma, a so-called "stress" ulcer, or a nest of tuberculous lymph nodes.

In conclusion, it seems to me that the two most likely explanations for the course of events described here are carcinoma of the tail of the pancreas, and tuberculous peritonitis with disseminated infection involving liver and adrenal glands. Of the two, I favor carcinoma of the pancreas, for the reasons I have attempted to outline, but it is so difficult to distinguish these two conditions on unassailable clinical grounds that I am confident I would have treated this patient for tuberculosis strenuously, while attempting to get objective evidence that he actually had a carcinoma. In addition, I believe he had a mild degree of hepatic cirrhosis, and also some type of chronic nephritis, perhaps pyelonephritis. I believe that he probably ultimately died of a pulmonary embolism.

POST MORTEM FINDINGS

Tuberculous peritonitis. Fatty liver with early cirrhosis.

REFERENCES

General

Berner, C., Fred, H. L., Riggs, S., and Davis, J. S.: Diagnostic probabilities in patients with conspicuous ascites. Arch. Intern. Med. *113*:687, 1964.
Hyman, S., Villa, F., and Steigmann, F.: Mimetic aspects of ascites. JAMA *183*:651, 1963.
Lesser, G. T., et al.: Chylous ascites—newer insights. Arch. Intern. Med. *125*:1073, 1970.

Liver Disease

Alpert, E., et al.: A fetoprotein in human hepatoma. Gastroenterology *61*:137, 1971.
Atkinson, M., and Losowsky, M. S.: The mechanism of ascites formation in chronic liver disease. Quart. J. Med. *30*:153, 1961.
Benner, E. J., and Labby, D. H.: Hepatoma: clinical experience with a frequently bizarre tumor. Ann. Intern. Med. *54*:620, 1961.
Fenster, L. F., and Klatskin, G.: Manifestations of metastatic tumor of the liver. A study of 81 patients subjected to needle biopsy. Amer. J. Med. *31*:238, 1961.
Guckian, J. C., and Perry, J. E.: Granulomatous hepatitis. An analysis of sixty-three cases and review of the literature. Ann. Intern. Med. *65*:1081, 1966.
Jeske, R. H., and Laurence, B. H.: Familial cirrhosis with autoimmune features and raised immunoglobulin levels. Gastroenterology *59*:546, 1970.
Levine, R. A.: Amyloid disease of the liver: correlation of clinical, functional and morphologic features in 47 patients. Amer. J. Med. *33*:349, 1962.
MacDonald, R. A.: Primary carcinoma of liver: a clinicopathologic study of one hundred eight cases. Arch. Intern. Med. *99*:266, 1957.
MacDonald, R. A., and Mallory, G. K.: The natural history of postnecrotic cirrhosis: a study of 221 autopsy cases. Amer. J. Med. *24*:334, 1958.
Maddrey W., Johns, C. J., and Iber, F.: Sarcoidosis and chronic hepatic disease. Medicine *49*:375, 1970.
Mistilis, S. P., and Blackburn, C. R. B.: Active chronic hepatitis. Amer. J. Med. *48*:484, 1970.
Ratnoff, O. D., and Patek, A. J., Jr.: The natural history of Laennec's cirrhosis of the liver: analysis of 386 cases. Medicine *21*:207, 1942.
Ross, R. S., Iber, F. L., and Harvey, A. M.: Serum alkaline phosphatase in chronic infiltrative disease of the liver. Amer. J. Med. *21*:850, 1956.
Sherlock, S., and Shaldon, S.: Etiology and management of ascites in patients with hepatic cirrhosis. Gut *4*:95, 1963.
Witte, M. H., et al.: Physiological factors in cirrhotic ascites. Gastroenterology *61*:742, 1971.

Tuberculosis

Burock, W. R., and Hollister, R. M.: Tuberculous peritonitis. A study of 47 proved cases encountered by a general medical unit in 25 years. Amer. J. Med. *28*:510, 1960.
Gonnella, J. S., and Hudson, E. K.: Clinical patterns of tuberculous peritonitis. Arch. Intern. Med. *117*:164, 1966.
Korn, R. J., Kellow, W. F., Heller, P., Chomet, B., and Zimmerman, H. J.: Hepatic involvement in extrapulmonary tuberculosis. Amer. J. Med. *27*:60, 1959.
Rich, A. R.: The pathogenesis of tuberculosis. 2nd ed. Springfield, Ill., Charles C Thomas, 1951.
Sing, M. M., Bhargara, A. M., and Jain, K. P.: Tuberculous peritonitis: pathogenesis, diagnosis and therapy. New Eng. J. Med. *281*:1091, 1969.
Stead, W. W.: The pathogenesis of tuberculosis among older persons. Ann. Rev. Resp. Dis. *91*:811, 1965.
Terry, R. B., and Gunnar, R. M.: Primary miliary tuberculosis of liver. JAMA *164*:150, 1957.

Pancreatic Carcinoma

Arlen, M., and Brockunier, A., Jr.: Clinical manifestations of carcinoma of the tail of the pancreas. Cancer 20:1920, 1967.
Cliffon, E. E.: Carcinoma of pancreas. Amer. J. Med. 21:760, 1956.
Dreiling, D. A., Janowitz, H. D., and Perrier, C. V.: Pancreatic inflammatory disease. New York, Harper & Row, 1964.
Duff, G. L.: The clinical and pathological features of carcinoma of the body and tail of the pancreas. Bull. Johns Hopkins Hosp. 65:69, 1939.
Gullick, H. D.: Carcinoma of the pancreas, a review and critical analysis of 100 cases. Medicine 38:47, 1959.
Serebro, H. A.: A diagnostic sign of carcinoma of the body of the pancreas. Lancet 1:85, 1965.

Obstruction of Hepatic and Portal Veins

Clain, D., Freston, J., Kreel, L., and Sherlock, S.: Clinical diagnosis of the Budd-Chiari syndrome. Amer. J. Med. 43:544, 1967.
Hepatic vein occlusion. Brit. Med. J. 3:550, 1971.
Maddrey, W. C., Sen Gupta, K. P., Basu Mallik, K. C., Iber, F. L., and Basu, A. K.: Extrahepatic obstruction of the portal venous system Surg. Gynec. Obstet. 127:989, 1968.
Ormond, J. K.: Idiopathic retroperitoneal fibrosis: an established clinical entity. JAMA 174:1561, 1960.
Parker, R. G. F.: Occlusion of the hepatic veins in man. Medicine 38:369, 1959.

Whipple's Disease

Isenberg, J. I., et al.: Ascites with peritoneal involvement in Whipple's disease. Gastroenterology 60:305, 1971.

K A PATIENT WITH CRYPTOCOCCAL MENINGITIS

THE CLINICAL PROBLEM

This 65 year old Negro male janitor was admitted for evaluation of headache and progressive confusion of one month's duration. He had been a heavy drinker. One month prior to admission, he began to have severe frontal and facial headaches with an associated gradually progressive anorexia, confusion, and lethargy. His daughter noted clear drainage from the left ear. Three weeks prior to admission, his vision became blurred, and two weeks prior to admission, his right arm and hand began to shake. He developed urinary incontinence and became essentially uncommunicative. He was seen to be an acutely ill, wasted, somnolent elderly male who responded to shouted direct commands. Blood pressure, 185/112; pulse, 92; respirations, 25; temperature, 100 degrees. Bilateral arcus senilis with irregular pupils that reacted sluggishly to light, bilateral 4+ papilledema with narrowed arterioles, vascularization about the right macula, one flame hemorrhage, and multiple exudates; absent left tympanic membrane, with foul, purulent drainage; dental caries. Neck: marked rigidity. Heart: No cardiomegaly, but soft basilar systolic murmur was present. Lungs: clear to percussion and auscultation. Abdomen: no palpable masses; hypoactive bowel sounds. Rectum and genitalia: within normal limits. Neurological findings: The patient spoke rarely but without dysarthria; bilateral Kernig signs were present; there was slight flattening of the right nasolabial fold with equivocal right Babinski's sign; reflexes symmetrical and without clonus. Blood: hematocrit, 47 ml./100 ml.; WBC count, 5900/cu. mm., with 14 percent juvenile neutrophils, 70 percent polymorphonuclear leukocytes, 4 percent lymphocytes, and 10 percent monocytes; platelets adequate; 2 percent atypical lymphocytes; occasional target cells. Urine: specific gravity, 1.018; pH 5.0; protein, 4+; sugar, negative; acetone, negative; erythrocytes and 5 to 7 leukocytes per high power field. Spinal fluid: pressure, 280 mm. water; slightly cloudy; Pandy's test, 3+; 2 to 3 RBC's; 504 WBC's (92 percent polymorphonuclears and 8 percent monocytes); rare gram-positive diplococci stated to be present within polymorphonuclear cells, but no organisms grown on culture. Gram stain of ear drainage showed mixed flora; no cultures recorded. Chemical tests: serum urea nitrogen, 41 mg./100 ml., rising progressively to 79 mg./100 ml.; blood sugar, 108 mg./100 ml.; sodium, 145 mEq./liter, falling to 126 mEq./liter; potassium, 5.8 mEq./liter, falling to 4.6 mEq./liter; chloride, 110 mEq./liter, falling to 85 mEq./liter; carbon dioxide content, 23.8 mEq./liter, falling to 16.2 mEq./liter; calcium, 9.4 mEq./liter, falling to 8.3 mEq./liter; phosphate, 3.3 mg./100 ml., rising to 7.4 mg./100 ml.; total serum protein, 6.7 g./100 ml., falling to 4.7 g./100 ml., with albumin-to-globulin ratio of 2.6:4.1, falling to 1.1:3.6; uric acid, 19.0 mg./100 ml. Standard test for syphilis, negative. Purified protein derivative test not performed. X-rays: chest films showed marked cardiomegaly, predominantly left ventricular, with calcified nodes in the right hilar area and a small granuloma in the left upper mediastinum; skull films normal except for a suspicion of chronic mastoiditis on the left; cerebral arteriograms showed stenosis of the origin of the external carotid artery in the neck, rather marked cerebral arteriosclerosis, no filling of the anterior cerebral vessels, and questionable ventricular dilatation. Electrocardiogram: left axis deviation, delayed precordial transition, and ST–T wave changes suggestive of ischemia. Shortly after admission, therapy was begun with Keflin and chloromycetin, and cerebral arteriograms were carried out. During the arteriogram procedure, the patient developed focal seizures of the right face and arm. Anticonvulsant therapy was started, and he was taken to the operating room, where burr holes were made and a left ventricular tap, a left simple mastoidectomy, and a left frontal sinus trephine were performed. Postoperative diagnoses were: acute meningitis, acute and chronic mastoiditis, no epidural abscess. Penicillin (20,000,000 units) and 100 mg. of Colistin per day were added to his antibiotic regime, but the patient continued to be febrile. Shortly thereafter, grand mal seizures commenced and continued until the time of death.

DISCUSSION OF THE PROBLEM

Three features of this unfortunate patient's illness seem self-evident:
1. He had meningeal irritation.
2. There was increased intracranial pressure of an appreciable degree.

3. There was diffuse brain injury.

The presence of meningeal irritation was manifested by the marked, persistent stiffness of the patient's neck and the positive Kernig signs, associated with increased white blood cells and protein in the spinal fluid. The increased pressure of the spinal fluid was evident from the papilledema, the confusion, the obtundity, and the headaches, as well as by the single measurement of spinal pressure of 290 mm. water. That the brain injury was diffuse was indicated by the presence of the changing, bilateral neurological alterations, the profound unresponsiveness, and the focal as well as generalized seizures.

With the firm conviction that these three cardinal features were indeed present, the next step is to ask, "What types of disease processes are most likely to produce the triad of meningeal irritation, increased intracranial pressure, and diffuse brain injury in these particular clinical circumstances?"

Unfortunately, we do not have several pieces of information that are almost vital for definitive diagnosis in this type of problem. Among these are culture and chemistry of the spinal fluid, serology of the spinal fluid, and the results of blood cultures, if any were obtained, and of skin tests for tuberculosis. It should be noted that all of these tests, while affording essential and perhaps even life-saving information, are quick, easy and very inexpensive to accomplish.

We would list these types of disease processes as follows (these are not necessarily listed in the order of their statistical likelihood):

1. Some type of vascular disease.
2. Some new growth (lymphoma/myeloma).
3. Leukemia.
4. Granulomatous process (sarcoid).
5. Amyloidosis.
6. An infection.
7. A collagen-vascular disorder.
8. Unusual process, such as thrombotic thrombocytic purpura.

Happily, we can readily dispose of several of these possibilities.

The patient's peripheral blood smear was normal, he was not anemic, there was no obvious depression of the platelet count, and he showed no bleeding tendency or enlargement of the lymph nodes, liver, or spleen that would suggest a leukemic process.

While sarcoid is capable of producing the three features we are centering on, it is generally a much more slowly evolving and benign course than the fulminant process described here.

The type of peculiar renal change noted here, with proteinuria and little else, would be quite compatible with amyloidosis, even in the face of hypertension, and amyloidosis could also explain the episode of heart failure. However, I am not aware that amyloidosis by itself has ever induced the degree of meningeal irritation indicated here. Furthermore, amyloidosis tends to affect the peripheral and autonomic nervous structures more often than the brain. Also, there was no evidence of bleeding into the skin or of deposition of amyloid in the soft tissues.

We come now to categories less easily excluded. The rapid and diffuse nature of the changes in the central nervous system, together with fever and uremia, makes one consider thrombotic thrombocytopenic purpura. (TTP). Also, the patient's blood smear was said to show some burr cells. On the other hand, the platelet count was not observed to be decreased, there was no anemia, and the spleen was not felt. It should be mentioned, however, that TTP has been described in the absence of anemia, platelet depression, and splenomegaly. Stronger points against the presence of TTP are the marked degree of meningeal irritation in the absence of red blood cells in the urine. Finally, this is an unusual disorder, especially in elderly males.

There is nothing about this 65 year old male patient's history to suggest a chronic, recurrent, episodic, multiorgan disease such as systemic lupus erythematosus (SLE), although the interesting renal changes recorded here are often seen in this disease, and the serum globulin level was elevated. Also, an LE test was negative. Therefore, if the patient had a collagen-vascular disorder, some form of an acute arteritis would have been much more likely than SLE. His age, his sex, the diffuseness of the brain injury, the fever, the antecedent severe diastolic hypertension, and the episode of heart failure obviously all point to the possibility of an arteritis. Giving additional strength to this suggestion is the description of marked muscle wasting, often a prominent accompaniment of polyarteritis nodosa (PAN).

This patient is said to have had severe headaches and also marked facial pain, and the latter, in particular, should lead to the suspicion of temporal arteritis. In this disorder, which is, of course, a manifestation of giant cell arteritis, diffuse brain damage may occur. However, there are two features of this patient's course which act against the diagnosis of an arteritis: (1) the degree of meningeal irritation, in the absence of RBC's in the spinal fluid, and (2) the nature of this patient's renal status. While meningitis has been described as occurring in uncomplicated arteritis, it must be unusual in the absence of some degree of subarachnoid bleeding. To have a patient die in uremia, with hypertension from an aggressive arteritis, and yet to have only albumin in the urine must be unusual. I can imagine only one circumstance in which this might happen, and that would be if there were renal vein thrombosis in association with the arteritis. Such can occur. We have actually observed such an occurrence in two patients with active SLE. But still, this is an unusual happening, particularly in the absence of hematuria and pain in the region of the kidneys, although these are by no means constantly present. We can only conclude that while an acute arteritis is a challenging explanation for almost all of the facts here, there are a few which don't quite fit without forcing.

Let us now turn to other forms of vascular disorders. A subdural hematoma, likely in an alcoholic patient with headaches, confusion, obtundity, and a shifting neurological pattern, seems excluded by the presence of outspoken meningeal signs, as well as by the nature of the spinal fluid changes, and the negative arteriograms and air studies.

A diffuse, severe degree of degenerative occlusive vascular disease, with thrombosis and perhaps small hemorrhages and even embolism of arteriosclerotic plaques, warrants more serious consideration. There seems no doubt this patient had diffuse vascular disease. His blood pressure was significantly elevated; there were marked changes in his eye grounds, with small aneurysms; his heart was enlarged, and the ECG showed ischemic changes; the cholesterol level was elevated. Finally, there were sclerotic changes noted in the arteriograms, to which, it will be recalled, he reacted very poorly, a characteristic occurrence in patients with diffuse cerebrovascular disease. Also, the burr cells noted in his blood smear may be seen in association with damaged blood vessels. Perhaps this entire chain of events, including the episode of heart failure, was the result of a progressive, malignant form of degenerative vasculitis.

Inviting as this formulation is superficially, there are two factors that militate against it, namely:

1. The marked signs of meningeal irritation in the absence of RBC's in the spinal fluid.

2. Most important, the renal changes described are not those of severe, diffuse or focal renovascular disease, in which one would certainly expect at least a few RBC's.

Hence, while the patient obviously had a severe degree of vascular degeneration, there must have been other factors causing his ultimate demise.

Metastatic tumors may, of course, invade the meninges and also produce diffuse neurological changes. A wide variety of tumors may do this, but we think immediately of carcinoma of the lung, the thyroid gland, the breast, melanoma, and lymphomata. It should be emphasized that in such circumstances, the primary tumor, whatever its site, may be silent. This is particularly true of carcinoma of the lung, in which even the chest film may be clear despite extensive meningeal and brain involvement.

This patient's age, the profound wasting of his muscles, his weight loss of 35 pounds, his fever, the failure to culture any organisms from the spinal fluid, the elevation of his serum uric acid, and the diffuseness of the neurological alterations, despite negative x-ray studies, are all features pointing to widespread involvement of his brain and meninges by a malignant tumor.

However, there are sound reasons to conclude this did not occur. First, there were no obvious evidences of a parent tumor elsewhere, for whatever this is worth. Second, the neurological alterations shifted very rapidly, which is perhaps unlikely in tumor. Third, x-ray studies failed to give any hint of a large mass lesion in the brain. Fourth, the intensity of the meningeal signs noted here was perhaps more than is generally attributed to tumor metastases. Fifth, one would be hard put to explain the unusual renal picture described here, unless the patient had had a renal vein thrombosis in association with a tumor. Such could have occurred, and we cannot exclude it, but it is an unusual happening, especially in the absence of RBC's in the urine and of pain in the kidney region, as already emphasized.

We come, then, to the conclusion that this patient must have had some sort of infection. In elderly persons, bacterial endocarditis is being seen with

PART K / A PATIENT WITH CRYPTOCOCCAL MENINGITIS

increasing frequency, and the mortality in such persons is excessively high, chiefly because the diagnosis is not correctly made or is arrived at too late. In the elderly, bacterial endocarditis can present in such a fashion the physician is convinced the patient has some sort of degenerative or neoplastic process. Such confusing presentations infrequently involve the central nervous system.

This patient represents an excellent example of this diagnostic dilemma. He was elderly, he had bad teeth, he had been plagued by boils, he suffered from fever and wasting, he had had an episode of heart failure, and he died in uremia. It is true that there was no clubbing, splenomegaly, petechiae, or significant anemia, but these alterations may not be seen in 30 to 40 percent of patients with bacterial endocarditis.

A strong argument against the presence of endocarditis, however, is the nature of the renal changes, for uremia with a clear urine but for albuminuria must be unusual, indeed, in bacterial endocarditis.

Syphilis, tuberculosis, and cryptococcus are common infections to be excluded in this type of setting of alcoholism, and the possibility that this wasted patient may have had some underlying disorder producing chronic disability and perhaps altered immune reactivity would particularly favor tuberculosis or cryptococcus.

It is true that this patient's serology was negative, but unfortunately no studies were reported on the spinal fluid, and of course, negative serology doesn't exclude meningovascular syphilis. However, the predominance of polymorphonuclear cells in the spinal fluid would be unlikely at this stage in meningovascular syphilis, in which disorder the meningeal signs also are often not as prominent as they were here.

The fact that no organisms were immediately seen or cultured would favor a tuberculous or cryptococcal infection, and it is impossible to exclude either, but, again, at this stage of these two infections, the spinal fluid generally is not filled predominantly with polymorphonuclear cells. Neither tuberculosis, cryptococcal infection, or syphilis would offer a very satisfactory answer to the renal changes seen here. While syphilis may induce a nephrotic picture, this usually occurs during the secondary stage of the infection.

A viral meningoencephalitis, which can indeed run a fulminant course such as occurred here, is also suggested by the failure to report the presence of bacteria in the spinal fluid, but once again the nature of the cellular response in the spinal fluid—not the renal alterations—fails to give this suggestion credence.

In recent years, meningococcal meningitis has not been a stranger among us, but this patient's course seems too "indolent" and long-drawn-out to be well explained on such a basis. Without specific treatment, one might have expected the patient to have long since succumbed.

Finally, none of these infections take into consideration the facts that this patient was known to have a chronically draining left ear, that x-rays indicated a chronic mastoiditis, and that at operation both acute and chronic mastoiditis, as well as meningitis, were reported to have been found.

It seems inescapable to me that this focus of infection in the ear was the parent site of the infection, which later involved the meninges and brain substance widely—probably by way of the meninges, the venous sinuses, and the brain substance itself—with a cerebritis, resulting in multiple small areas of infection, infarction, and small abscesses.

Whether one or several organisms were involved seems a moot point. While such chronic ear infections often result from staphylococcus, streptococcus, pneumococcus, *Haemophilus influenzae*, or *H. pyocyaneus*, they may also be mixed infections. Not infrequently, in such circumstances, it may be highly difficult to demonstrate the responsible organism in smears. Also, fungi may secondarily take up an abode in such a chronically infected area, particularly if the patient is chronically debilitated, as this one was.

But how could one relate such an infection to the particular changes noted in this patient's urine? It seems to me entirely likely that he had a multiple myeloma, a condition that would readily explain the course of events in the kidneys. It would also explain the wasting and weight loss, as well as the elevated serum uric acid level and the episode of gout, although the latter feature is somewhat confused by the presence of uremia and the administration of thiazide drugs. However, it will be recalled that the episode of pain in the patient's great toe took place at a time when he was not clearly uremic.

The association between multiple myeloma and infection is well known, and I believe we are being confronted by still another example of it. Its association with pneumococcal infections is particularly common, and pneumococcus may well have been the responsible organism, although other types of infection, including those from cryptococcus and other fungi, may also complicate the course of myeloma, leading ultimately to the death of the patient. A degree of amyloidosis of the kidneys, may, of course, have been an accompaniment of the myelomatous process.

In conclusion, we believe this patient had multiple myeloma, with myeloma kidney. He had, in addition, diffuse vascular degeneration. We conclude that his death was the result of an infection, perhaps pneumococcal in origin, or perhaps a result of a mixed group of organisms, which began in the left ear, and after remaining localized for a time, disseminated itself via the meninges, the venous sinuses, and the brain substance itself, with resultant cerebritis.

POST MORTEM FINDINGS

Cryptococcal meningitis.

REFERENCES

Thrombotic Thrombocytopenic Purpura

Amorosi, E. L., and Ultmann, J. E.: Thrombotic thrombocytopenic purpura: Report of 16 cases and review of the literature. Medicine 45:139, 1966.

PART K / A PATIENT WITH CRYPTOCOCCAL MENINGITIS 285

Laszlo, M. H., Alvarez, A., and Feldman, F.: The association of thrombotic thrombocytopenic purpura and disseminated lupus erythematosus. Ann. Intern. Med. 42:1308, 1955.

Lukes, R. J., Rath, C. E., Stuessy, C. H., and Mailliard, J.: Thrombotic thrombocytopenic purpura—clinical and pathological findings in 49 cases. Blood 17:366, 1961.

Polyarteritis

Rose, G. A.: Natural history of polyarteritis. Clinical and pathologic findings in 111 proved cases. Brit. Med. J. 2:1148, 1957.

Giant Cell Arteritis

Hamilton, C. R., Shelley, W., and Tumulty, P. A.: Giant cell arteritis: including temporal arteritis and polymyalgia rheumatica. Medicine 50:1, 1971.

Forms of Meningoencephalitis

Beeson, P. B., and Hankey, D. D.: Leptospiral meningitis. Arch. Intern. Med. 89:575, 1952.

Bindschadler, D. D., and Bennett, J. E.: Serology of human cryptococcosis. Ann. Intern. Med. 69:45, 1968.

Butler, W. T., Alling, D. W., Spickard, H., and Utz, J. P.: Diagnostic and prognostic value of clinical and laboratory findings in cryptococcal meningitis. New Eng. J. Med. 270:59, 1964.

Carpenter, R. R., and Petersdorf, R. G.: Clinical spectrum of bacterial meningitis. Amer. J. Med. 33:262, 1962.

Clark, E. G., and Danbolt, N.: Oslo study of the natural course of untreated syphilis. Med. Clin. N. Amer. 48:613, 1964.

Farmer, T. W., and Janeway, C. A.: Infections with the virus of lymphocytic choriomeningitis. Medicine 21:1, 1942.

Gray, M. L., and Killinger, A. H.: *Listeria monocytogenes* and *Listeria* infections. Bact. Rev. 30:309, 1966.

Hoeprich, A. D.: Infection due to *Listeria monocytogenes*. Medicine 37:143, 1958.

Holden, E. M., Eagles, A. Y., and Stevens, J. E., Jr.: Mumps involvement of the central nervous system. JAMA, 131:382, 1946.

Johnson, R. T., and Johnson, K. P.: Slow and chronic virus infections of the CNS. In Recent Advances in Neurology. Fred Plum (Ed.). Philadelphia, F. A. Davis, 1969.

Johnson, R. T., and Mims, C. A.: Medical progress. Pathogenesis of viral infections of the nervous system. New Eng. J. Med. 278:23, 84; 1968.

Leider, W., Magoffin, R. L., Lennette, E. H., and Leonards, L. W. R.: Herpes simplex virus encephalitis: Its possible association with reactivated latent infection. New Eng. J. Med. 273:341, 1965.

Lennette, E. H., Magoffin, R. L., and Knouf, E.: Viral central nervous system disease. JAMA 179:687, 1962.

Miller, S. K., Hesser, F., and Tompkins, V. N.: Herpes simplex encephalitis. Report of 20 cases. Ann. Intern. Med. 64:92, 1966.

Mosbery, W. H., Jr., and Arnold, J. G., Jr.: Torulosis of the CNS—review. Ann. Intern. Med. 32:1153, 1950.

Munt, P. W.: Miliary tuberculosis in the chemotherapy era. Medicine 51:139, 1972.

Quade, F., and Kristensen, K. P.: Purulent meningitis: Review of 685 cases. Acta Med. Scand. 171:544, 1962.

Swartz, M. N., and Dodge, P. B.: Bacterial meningitis—a review of selected aspects. New Eng. J. Med. 272:725, 779, 842, 898, 954, 1003; 1965.

Welshimer, H. J., and Winglewish, H. G.: Listeriosis—summary of 7 cases of *Listeria* meningitis. JAMA 171:1319, 1959.

Wolf, R. E., and Birbara, C. A.: Meningococcal infections at any Army training center. Amer. J. Med. 44:243, 1968.

New Growths in the CNS

Brain, L.: The neurological complications of neoplasms. Lancet 1:179, 1963.

Dinsdale, H. B., and Taghavy, A.: Carcinomatosis of meninges. Canad. Med. Ass. J. 90:505, 1964.

Fischer-Williams, M., Bosanquet, F. D., and Daniel, P. M.: Carcinomatosis of meninges. Brain 78:42, 1955.

Griffin, J. W., et al.: Lymphomatous leptomeningitis. Amer. J. Med. 51:200, 1971.

Maloney, J. V., Jr., et al.: Carcinoma of the lung. Ann. Intern. Med. 64:165, 1966.

Skoog, W. A., and Adams, W. S.: Multiple myeloma. Calif. Med. 99:106, 1963.

Sparling, H. J., Jr., Adams, R. D., and Parker, F., Jr.: Involvement of nervous system by malignant lymphoma. Medicine 26:285, 1947.

Bacterial Endocarditis and Central Nervous System

Traut, E. F., Carter, J. B., Gumbiner, S. H., and Hench, R. N.: Bacterial endocarditis in the elderly: report of 94 autopsied cases. Geriatrics 4:205, 1949.

Tumulty, P. A.: Management of bacterial endocarditis. Geriatrics 22:122, 1967.

L A PATIENT WITH THE HAMMAN-RICH SYNDROME

THE CLINICAL PROBLEM

This 45 year old white nun was admitted to the hospital on June 15, 1968, with a two week history of dyspnea on exertion. There was no prior history of cardiopulmonary disease except for a murmur noted five years earlier, which was thought to be the result of a ventricular septal defect. There was no history of chest pain, cough, recent respiratory infection, or occupational exposure. Past history and systems review were negative except for questionable presence of Raynaud's phenomenon. On admission, the patient was thought to have acute pulmonary edema. Blood pressure was 90/50; pulse, 124; respirations, 28; temperature, 97 degrees. She had distended neck veins and moist rales throughout both lung fields. Chest x-ray revealed pulmonary congestion and accentuated vascular markings, with mild cardiomegaly. The electrocardiogram revealed sinus tachycardia. Complete blood count revealed the following: hematocrit, 47 ml./100 ml.; hemoglobin, 16.4 g./100 ml.; WBC 24,500/with 89 segmented neutrophils and 3 band cells. Urinalysis was normal except for trace amounts of acetone. LE cells were not found. The patient was digitalized and underwent diuresis on admission. After an episode of hemoptysis on June 16, she was heparinized and treatment with Keflin and streptomycin was instituted. Systolic pressure remained between 80 and 100, with adequate urine output. Cultures revealed Group A beta hemolytic streptococci in the sputum, 10,000 colonies of *E. coli* in the urine, and no bacterial growths in blood cultures. Her chest x-ray was unchanged. She developed a phlebitis of the right arm near the site of catheterization. Sinus tachycardia persisted. The patient was started on a Decadron regimen. Chest x-rays again revealed bilateral infiltrates and cardiomegaly. Tachycardia continued. Assisted respirations were begun via endotracheal intubation. Pink, frothy sputum was suctioned out, culture showed no growth. Blood gases: pH 7.40; pCO_2, 40 mm. Hg; oxygen saturation, 94 percent of capacity. There was gradual improvement, with mild clearing on x-ray. Then, the temperature spiked to 103 degrees with recurrence of clinical pulmonary edema. Kanamycin was added to the treatment regimen, and the endotracheal tube was removed. The chest later showed clinical improvement and the patient's condition became more stable. Klebsiella was cultured from the sputum. On

July 4, there was recurrence of anxiety and of tachycardia and tachypnea. Fine, diffuse rales were heard throughout her lungs. Chest x-ray showed diffuse, extensive patchy nodular infiltrates. Steroid therapy was pushed. However, persistent tachycardia and tachypnea continued. Skin and muscle biopsy (forearm) showed "acute capillaritis." Chest x-ray revealed increased infiltrates and almost complete consolidation. The patient became semi-conscious. On July 16, she complained of sudden, severe left upper quadrant pain and of jaundice. The abdomen was noted to be distended and somewhat rigid, with depressed bowel sounds; diastase, 800 units. Coma, shock, and death occurred within hours. Acid fast bacilli cultures were subsequently negative in two tests.

DISCUSSION OF THE PROBLEM

The significant features of this patient's illness appear to be these:
1. She was only 45, and had enjoyed good health, although she was suspected of having had a ventricular septal defect and Raynaud's phenomenon.
2. Her illness began abruptly, with exertional dyspnea, and within a few days her respirations had to be assisted and she required constant oxygen, despite which her respiratory distress worsened.
3. In addition to respiratory insufficiency, she had cardiac failure, and this appeared very early in her illness.
4. After intensive therapy with anticoagulants, digitalis, diuretics, antibiotics and steroids, there was a short-lived period of betterment in her condition, which led to cessation of treatment, following which she became more ill.
5. She succumbed just six weeks after the onset of her symptoms, in a setting of an acute abdominal incident with jaundice and shock.

Determination of the specific cause of this patient's fulminant illness is excessively difficult, because a very wide variety of different disease processes can produce the changes noted here, and the data we are given do not allow us to select one from others with a strong degree of assurance, for many of the facts are non-specific in nature.

The various kinds of disease processes which may produce a clinical course such as this may be categorized as follows:
1. An infectious process.
2. An abnormality of the heart or of the pulmonary vessels.
3. A so-called "collagen-vascular" disease.
4. A granuloma, such as sarcoid.
5. A neoplasm.
6. A peculiar disorder of unknown etiology such as the Hamman-Rich disease (so-called interstitial pneumonitis), or histiocytosis X, or TTP (thrombotic thrombocytopenic purpura).

Let us briefly explore the likelihood of each of these in turn.

When you come right down to it, not too many disease processes will bring death to a previously well person through cardiac and respiratory failure in only six weeks. An infection is surely one of these. What might its nature have been?

A viral pneumonitis associated with a viral myocarditis comes immdiately to mind. While such infections are generally mild, they can become fulminant, and secondary bacterial invasion is always a possibility. We recently saw a young woman overwhelmed in but 10 days by Hong Kong influenza with pneumonitis and myocarditis. However, this patient's history relates none of the usual constitutional accompaniments of such a viral infection, including coryza, cough, substernal soreness, musculoskeletal aching, feverishness, or chills. Also, when admitted two weeks after the onset of her first symptoms, the clinical changes were chiefly those of pulmonary edema, not of a pneumonitis. In the cases of fulminant viral infection of the lungs I have encountered, evidences of bronchial and bronchiolar obstruction with asthmatic wheezes were prominent. None were described here.

Both psittacosis and Q fever may rapidly and seriously affect the lungs and heart, early death sometimes ensuing. In both of these a WBC count of 24,000/cu. mm. would not be unusual. But, again, the onset of severe dyspnea without fever or other evidences of an infection would be odd. It would also be peculiar for the initial chest film to be clear except for some congestion owing to heart failure. For similar reasons, such infections as tuberculosis or histoplasmosis seem unlikely.

It appears that the only infection which these circumstances support is bacterial endocarditis. Indeed, there are a number of features firmly buttressing this diagnosis. For example, the patient was suspected of having a ventricular septal defect, an excellent nidus for such an infection. In septal endocarditis, the vegetations usually form first on the right or pulmonary side of the shunt, and hence, the earliest manifestations are often respiratory in nature, including dyspnea, cough, asthma, pneumonia, pleurisy, lung abscess, pulmonary infarction, and so forth. In addition, a mitral systolic murmur was described for the first time. Not infrequently, after a shunt has become infected, secondary infection of one of the valves of the left heart ensues. Such could have happened to this patient's mitral valve.

The episodes of pulmonary edema could have resulted from pulmonary embolization or from an acute myocarditis, which is a not uncommon accompaniment of bacterial endocarditis, caused either by microinfarcts from small coronary emboli, or by a diffuse myocarditis secondary to hypersensitization to bacterial proteins.

Furthermore, the patient transiently improved when antibiotics were given and grew worse when they were halted. Finally, the terminal episode, marked by sudden abdominal pain and shock, is the sort which not infrequently complicates and terminates bacterial endocarditis, when, as a result of either embolism or acute arteritis, there is an acute pancreatitis, splenic rupture, or a mesenteric artery catastrophe.

Indeed, the evidence favoring endocarditis is strongly impelling, but there are features which make it less than conclusive. For example, by far the most commonly occurring clinical manifestations of bacterial endocarditis are those resulting from infection, and yet, at the time of her admission, this patient was afebrile, and none of the usual constitutional accompaniments of an infection were described. Also, this patient's course was so acute that if she did have bacterial endocarditis, the infecting agent must have been a highly invasive and destructive organism. Statistically, *Staphylococcus* would be most probable, and this organism is usually easily cultured. It is true that *Klebsiella* was cultured repeatedly from the sputum, but endocarditis from gram-negative organisms is unusual. On the other hand, 15 to 20 percent of patients with infective endocarditis have negative blood cultures, and this percentage is even higher in instances of right-sided endocarditis.

A much stronger point against the presence of an acute endocarditis resulting from an invasive, destructive organism is the fact that the pulmonary lesions that developed never suppurated or broke down into small abscesses, which would have been anticipated.

Finally, the spleen was not felt, nor were there renal alterations. While it has been found that these changes may not be present in up to 40 percent of patients with endocarditis, they generally do occur when there is an invasive, destructive infection.

The lymphatic spread of a tumor throughout her lungs seems to be excluded by the sudden onset and brief course of this illness in the face of previous good health. Also, as previously stressed, the initial x-ray showed chiefly vascular congestion of the lungs, and this would be hard to explain on the basis of tumor unless the patient was producing pulmonary emboli consisting of masses of tumor. Such can indeed happen, as you know. The tumors most often responsible for this unusual presentation are carcinoma of the liver, the kidney, the pancreas, and the breast. None of the information indicates the presence of any of these malignant neoplasms in this woman, unless the terminal episode could have been associated with pancreatic carcinoma.

In the absence of constitutional signs of tumor or infection, sarcoidosis of the lungs and of the heart comes to mind. Sometimes sarcoid may set in acutely and terminate rapidly. However, no hilar adenopathy was described, nor was there enlargement of the peripheral lymph nodes, spleen, or liver. No lesions were described in the eyes, skin, joints, or muscles. The serum calcium level was normal, as was that of the serum proteins. The WBC count was briskly elevated. Certainly there was nothing to indicate cor pulmonale, which would be expected to accompany a more long-standing pulmonary fibrotic process.

When confronted with a young female having a likely history of Raynaud's phenomenon, whose illness is dominated by changes stemming from both pulmonary and cardiac failure, the possibility of a "collagen-vascular" disorder looms very large indeed. The fact that improvement seemingly came with administration of large dosages of Decadron, and rapid death followed its abrupt cessation, further strengthens this suspicion, for abrupt stoppage of steroids is well known to precipitate a so-called crisis in collagen disorders, and is always to be avoided. In addition to systemic lupus erythematosus (SLE), we must examine the likelihood of other members of this spectrum of diseases being present, including polyarteritis nodosa (PAN), scleroderma, and Wegener's granulomatosis.

In each of these conditions, both the pulmonary parenchyma and the pulmonary vasculature may be affected, singly or together, producing the sort of alterations noted in this patient's lungs. In all of these disorders, myocarditis may ensue. In each, intra-abdominal vessels may undergo acute changes, concluding with rupture or thrombosis, and leading to the kind of acute abdominal incident which terminated this patient's illness. Each disorder may, at times, begin very acutely, out of the blue, and rage to a rapid end. Clearly, this group of disorders must be reviewed with great circumspection.

Involvement of the lungs in SLE is very common. The typical change is an atelectasizing pneumonitis, most prominent in the lower lung fields and producing areas of plate-like atelectasis. However, diffuse alterations such as noted here are encountered, though infrequently. We are now beginning to recognize that involvement of the pulmonary vessels in SLE may produce edema or hypertension and, eventually, cor pulmonale. Secondary bacterial infection is very frequent, and we recall the repeated culturing of *Klebsiella* from the patient's sputum. But, once again, there are reasonable diagnostic doubts that challenge eager acceptance of the diagnosis of SLE. These include (1) the very abrupt onset, not associated with any constitutional elements, and the absence of fever when admitted; (2) the lack in her past history of episodes of illness indicating the presence of a chronic, episodic, polyorgan system disorder, such as lupus; (3) the absence of renal or pleural involvement; and (4) the normal serum globulin level and the WBC count of 24,000/cu. mm.

The WBC count of 24,000/cu. mm. is more suggestive of PAN, but several of the characteristic features of this disorder were absent, including fever at the outset, myalgias, arthralgias, neuropathy, renal changes, elevation of the blood pressure, and eosinophilia. The last, while often absent in PAN, is common when the lungs are widely affected by this disorder.

Recently, instances of Wegener's granulomatosis have been described in the absence of involvement of the kidneys or upper respiratory passages. However, the x-ray changes noted here are not those of Wegener's granulomatosis, in which the presence of confluent patches of pneumonitis, often leading to cavitation, is usual.

The history of Raynaud's phenomenon, the absence of constitutional reactions, such as fever, and so forth, and the initial presentation with pulmonary edema and heart failure but with relatively clear lung fields, are all features characteristic of scleroderma of the lungs and heart. We now know that visceral scleroderma may occur in the absence of scleroderma of the integument. There may be marked alterations in the pulmonary vasculature, and little or none in the parenchyma of the lungs, or the changes in the latter may appear belatedly. Myocarditis and pericarditis leading to congestive failure are common. How reminiscent of this patient's illness are these remarks! But here again we strike shoal waters. Unless this patient was sick longer than has been recorded, her course was too precipitous for the usual instance of scleroderma. Despite the history of Raynaud's phenomenon, no sclerosis was described in her fingers. She had no telangiectasia, and there was no history of dysphagia, nor was there evidence of renal scleroderma or hypertension. A WBC count of 24,000/cu. mm. is not seen in scleroderma unless there is secondary infection.

The patient's unremitting course and the diffuse pulmonary changes, which were only transiently responsive to treatment, suggest some unusual process, such as the acute interstitial pneumonitis of Hamman-Rich or histiocytosis X. These disorders sometimes seem to start very abruptly, and may exactly mimic an infectious process, a high WBC count sometimes being present, as well as a fluctuating fever. There may be a rapid downhill course, despite the strongest supportive measures. Persistent tachycardia and tachypnea, despite assisted respirations and oxygen administration, are characteristic. However, in most instances, the course of these disorders is measured in months and not weeks, as happened here. For example, most patients with acute interstitial pneumonitis live six months or longer. When heart failure develops, it is generally cor pulmonale, for which we have no evidence here. Both of these processes lead to marked structural alterations in the lungs, due to fibrosis. None were observed here. There was no evidence of histiocytosis elsewhere.

Thrombotic thrombocytopenic purpura may produce the kind of alterations described here through the occlusion of many small vessels, eventuating in respiratory and myocardial failure, and in acute abdominal conditions of a wide variety, such as hemorrhagic pancreatitis. However, several of the cardinal features of this disorder were absent, including a hemolytic anemia, peculiar RBC forms (such as helmet cells and schizocytes), thrombocytopenia, central nervous system alterations, and renal failure. It is hard to select this diagnosis in the face of these absences.

This patient had been informed she might have a ventricular septal defect. Could such a shunt have led to pulmonary hypertension and the events noted here? This possibility seems excluded by the dearth of any indication of right heart failure, as already stressed. If, in fact, she had a septal defect, it must have been a small one of no dynamic consequence.

Sometimes cardiac murmurs are misinterpreted by all of us. Perhaps she had some acquired endocardial lesion. In a female of this age, the most likely acquired lesion would be a rheumatic mitral valve disease.

A possibility never to be overlooked, because of present-day therapeutic possibilities, is silent mitral stenosis. As emphasized years ago by the brilliant physician Soma Weiss, the customary clinical presentations of mitral stenosis are sometimes replaced by those indicative of primary pulmonary disease, including dyspnea, cough, hemoptyses, episodes of pneumonitis, and other respiratory abnormalities, which result from marked changes in the pulmonary vascular bed secondary to the mitral lesion. And, of course, patients with rheumatic mitral valvulitis often throw emboli, which could have accounted for the acute abdominal incident. Against this tempting thesis, however, is the abrupt onset of her severe respiratory distress, and the often stated absence of evidence of right heart failure.

It is a wise clinical rule to consider the possibility of a myxoma of the left auricle whenever there is reason to question the likelihood of rheumatic mitral stenosis, for the two conditions can exactly imitate each other. Both are encountered in females in this age group. A myxoma may become symptomatic rather abruptly, and the sudden coming and going of pulmonary edema, such as noted here, is typical, as is failure to respond to treatment for a protracted period. Embolization is another characteristic of myxoma, which could have accounted for the abdominal incident. The patient had a murmur on admission that had not been noted previously. On the other hand, there were no indications of intermittent out-flow obstruction, such as syncope, which is very common with myxoma, or of a relationship between pulmonary edema or murmurs and alterations in body position. Also, the patient's downhill course was too rapid.

We come, then, to the final type of disease mechanism which might have caused her demise, namely, multiple pulmonary emboli, originating from a site unknown. There are a number of factors pointing to such a mechanism:

1. The precipitous, unheralded onset of exertional dyspnea.

2. The persistent, excessive tachycardia and tachypnea despite respiratory assistance and oxygen.

3. Failure to discover on physical examination or in the initial chest film a satisfactory explanation for her intense respiratory distress.

4. The dearth of constitutional accompaniments, such as fever and indications of toxicity.

5. The rapid and early appearance of pulmonary edema, with the parenchymal alterations lagging behind.

6. To some extent, the patient's respiratory distress and pulmonary edema occurred in episodes. She was described as being anxious and restless, so often accompaniments of embolism. On two occasions, her sputum contained blood.

7. Her lactic dehydrogenase content rose to a high level, in the absence of evidence pointing to either significant liver or muscle injury or acute myocardial infarction.

8. She failed to respond to strenuous therapy.

9. The systolic murmur heard at the time of admission could have been produced by blockage of pulmonary arteries.

The only strong objections to this explanation are the very brisk leukocytosis and the lack of signs of acute pulmonary hypertension. It is, of course, possible that secondary infection may have complicated pulmonary embolism. In this regard, *Klebsiella* were repeatedly grown from her sputum, and the frequency with which gram-negative rod infections are associated with the use of contaminated equipment in respiratory assistance is now being recognized. As for indications of pulmonary hypertension, these often do not accompany pulmonary embolism, and many times one is disconcerted by the report of left ventricular hypertrophy.

The description of the patient's terminal event and the elevated diastase are more indicative of an acute hemorrhagic pancreatitis than of anything else. Other considerations are the rupture of a stress ulcer, or a mesenteric vascular accident. It is hard to relate these directly to multiple pulmonary emboli.

One might think of a paradoxical embolus traveling through the suspected ventricular septal defect and lodging in one of the mesenteric vessels, but in the absence of marked pulmonary hypertension, which was not seen here, this could not happen. This patient was receiving Decadron, and an increased incidence of acute pancreatitis has been ascribed to the administration of steroid hormones.

Also, although we are not informed of the fact, it is conceivable that she was receiving "the pill" for some menstrual problem, and the questioned relationship between oral contraceptives and venous thrombosis and pulmonary embolism is well known to you all. "The pill" may also be associated with the occurrence of acute pancreatitis. Finally, it is likewise conceivable that the acute abdominal incident was consequent to a pancreatic carcinoma, and the relationship between such carcinomas and venous thrombosis and embolism is equally well known.

In summary, it is evident that many considerations enter into the differential diagnosis of this nun's tragic illness. It is exceedingly difficult to cull these out, and to select the single most likely explanation for all that took place. A key point, it seems to me, is the fact that the patient was thought to be in congestive heart failure before extensive parenchymal alterations were noted in the lungs. Therefore, the process must have originated within either the heart or the pulmonary vessels, or both, the parenchymal alterations being secondary phenomena. Also, the process, whatever its nature, was of fulminant character, which could not be checked by strenuous measures, and it caused the death of the patient in a span of but six weeks.

Of the various disease processes discussed, the following three most reasonably explain these basic features:

1. Multiple pulmonary emboli from unknown site.
2. Acute bacterial endocarditis originating on the right side of a ventricular shunt.
3. An acute vasculitis—PAN, to be specific.

It is possible that oxygen intoxication and *Klebsiella* contamination played secondary roles.

Both acute bacterial endocarditis and an acute arteritis afford an excellent unifying explanation for all that happened here, particularly the brisk leukocytosis and the final acute abdominal incident. However, the initial absence of any significant constitutional accompaniments or of evidence of the involvement of other organ systems, in particular, the kidneys, makes me reluctant to adopt either of these explanations. Multiple pulmonary emboli, of obscure origin, seems more probable. I believe the terminal event was acute hemorrhagic pancreatitis, either resulting from the Decadron therapy, or perhaps associated with a carcinoma of the pancreas, which would have set the stage for venous thrombosis and the repeated episodes of embolization. We have already referred to the role the taking of "the pill" might possibly have played in venous thrombosis and embolism, and even of the suspected pancreatitis.

POST MORTEM FINDINGS

Acute interstitial pneumonitis of Hamman-Rich. Acute perforated duodenal ulcer, with widespread peritonitis. Marantic endocarditis of mitral valve. Focal infarction of right kidney.

REFERENCES

Diffuse Lung Disease

Buechner, H. A.: The differential diagnosis of miliary disease of the lung. Med. Clin. N. Amer. 43:89–110, 1959.
Buechner, H. A.: Diffuse pulmonary lesions: the problems of differential diagnosis of probable cases by examination of sputum. Amer. J. Clin. Path. 33:48, 1960.
Gould, D. M., and Dalrymple, G. V.: Radiological analysis of disseminated lung disease. Amer. J. Med. Sci. 238:621, 1959.
James, D. G., and Carstairs, L. S.; Miliary disease of the lungs. In Disease-A-Month. Chicago, Year Book Medical Publishers, July, 1962.
Klassen, K. P., and Andrews, N. C.: Biopsy of diffuse pulmonary lesions: a 17-year experience. Ann. Thoracic Surg. 4:117, 1967.

Hamman-Rich Syndrome

Hamman, L., and Rich, A. R.: Acute diffuse interstitial fibrosis of lungs. Bull. Johns Hopkins Hosp. 74:177, 1944.
Livingstone, J. L., Lewis, J. G., Reid, L., and Jefferson, K. E.: Diffuse interstitial pulmonary fibrosis. Quart. J. Med. 33:71, 1964.
Rubin, E. H., and Lubliner, R.: Hamman-Rich fibrosis of lungs. Medicine 36:110, 1957.
Scadding, J. G., and Hinson, R.: Diffuse fibrosing alveolitis (diffuse interstitial fibrosis of the lungs). Thorax 22:291, 1967.
Wagley, P. F.: A new look at the Hamman-Rich syndrome. Johns Hopkins Med. J. 131:412, 1972.

Pulmonary Embolism

Bain, R. C., Edwards, J. E., Scheifly, C., and Geraci, E.: Right-sided bacterial endocarditis and endarteritis: clinical and pathological study. Amer. J. Med. 24:98, 1958.
Harvey, W. P.: Clinical aspects of cardiac tumors, Amer. J. Cardiol. 21:328, 1968.
McDonald, J. G., et al.: Major pulmonary embolism, a correlation of clinical findings, haemodynamics, pulmonary angiography and pathological physiology. Brit. Heart J. 34:356, 1972.
Owen, W. R., et al.: Unrecognized emboli to the lungs with subsequent cor pulmonale. New Eng. J. Med. 249:919, 1953.
Story, P. B., and Goldstein, W.: Pulmonary embolization from primary hepatic carcinoma. Arch. Intern. Med. 110:262, 1962.

Symbas, P. N., et al.: Atrial myxomas—especial emphasis on unusual manifestations. Chest 59:504, 1971.
Winterbauer, R., et al.: The incidence and clinical significance of tumor embolization to the lungs. Amer. J. Med. 45:271, 1968.

Pulmonary Infections

Aslam, P. H.: Aspergillosis of the lung—18-year experience. Chest 59:28, 1971.
Chanock, R. M.: Mycoplasma infections in man. New Eng. J. Med. 273:1199, 1257; 1965.
Finland, M., and Dingle, J. H.: Medical progress; virus pneumonias; pneumonias associated with known nonbacterial agents; influenza, psittacosis and "Q" fever. New Eng. J. Med. 227:342, 1942.
Mogabgab, W. J.: *Mycoplasma pneumoniae* and adenovirus respiratory illnesses in military and university personnel, 1959–1966. Amer. Rev. Resp. Dis. 97:345, 1968.
Murray, J. F., Haegelin, H. F., and Hewitt, W. C.: Opportunistic pulmonary infections. Ann. Intern. Med. 65:566, 1966.

Sarcoidosis

Boushy, S. F., Kurtzman, R. S., and Anarten, N. D.: The course of pulmonary function in sarcoidosis. Ann. Intern. Med. 62:939, 1965.
Longcope, W. T., and Freiman, D. G.: A study of sarcoidosis. Medicine 31:1, 1952.
Mayock, R. L., et al.: Manifestations of sarcoidosis. Amer. J. Med. 35:67, 1963.
Reisner, D.: Observations on the course and prognosis of sarcoidosis. Ann. Rev. Resp. Dis. 96:361, 1967.
Siltzbach, L. E.: Sarcoidosis: Clinical features and management. Med. Clin. N. Amer. 51:483, 1966.

Mitral Stenosis

Gordon, S. C., et al.: Pathology of the lungs in mitral stenosis in relation to respiratory function and pulmonary hemodynamics. Brit. Heart J. 28:101, 1966.
Mooltin, S. E.: Pulmonary fibrosis in rheumatic heart disease. Amer. J. Med. 33:421, 1962.

Scleroderma

D'Angelo, W. A., Fries, J. F., Masi, A. T., and Shulman, L. E.: Pathologic observations in systemic sclerosis (scleroderma). Amer. J. Med. 46:428, 1969.
Sackner, M. A.: Scleroderma. New York, Grune & Stratton, 1967.
Tumulty, P. A.: Clinical synopsis of scleroderma, simulator of other diseases. Johns Hopkins Med. J. 122:236, 1968.

Systemic Lupus Erythematosus

Gold, W. M., and Jennings, D. B.: Pulmonary function in patients with SLE. Amer. Rev. Resp. Dis. 93:556, 1966.
Harvey, A. M., Shulman, L. E., Tumulty, P. A., Conley, C. L., and Schoenrich, E. H.: Systemic lupus erythematosus: review of the literature and clinical analysis of 138 cases. Medicine 33:291, 1954.

Lymphoma

Garrison, C., Dines, D. E., Harrison, E. G., et al.: The alveolar pattern of pulmonary lymphoma. Mayo Clin. Proc. 44:260, 1969.

Histiocytosis X

Avioli, L. V., et al.: Histiocytosis X, a clinicopathological survey. Medicine 42:119, 1963.
Gracey, D. R., et al.: Primary pulmonary histiocytosis X—electron microscopic study. Chest 59:5, 1971.

Polyarteritis

Rose, G. A., and Spencer, H.: Polyarteritis nodosa. Quart. J. Med. 26:43, 1957.

Wegener's Disease

Cassan, S. M., Coles, D. E., and Harrison, E. G., Jr.: Limited forms of Wegener's granulomatosis. Am. J. Med. 49:366, 1970.
Israel, H. L., and Patchefsky, A. S.: Wegener's granulomatosis of the lung. Ann. Intern. Med. 74:881, 1971.

Walton, E. W.: Giant-cell granuloma of the respiratory tract (Wegener's granulomatosis). Brit. Med. J. 2:265, 1958.

Wegener's granulomatosis. Clinicopathologic Conference, Washington University. Amer. J. Med. 35:384, 1963.

Thrombotic Thrombocytopenic Purpura

Amorosi, E. L., and Ultman, J. E.: Thrombotic thrombocytopenic purpura—Report of 16 cases and review of literature. Medicine 45:139, 1966.

M   A PATIENT WITH CONGESTIVE HEART FAILURE AND AORTIC INSUFFICIENCY

THE CLINICAL PROBLEM

This 62 year old black female cook was admitted to the hospital three weeks before her death with dyspnea, right-sided chest pain, cough, and general malaise. In 1966, a son was treated for tuberculosis. She was known to have the abnormal hemoglobin of the sickle cell trait (Hgb-SA). She was in good health until 1945 when, following pregnancy, she developed asthma, pedal edema, and orthopnea for six weeks. She recovered on outpatient treatment. About the same time, her "nose fell off." A diagnosis of syphilis was made, and she was treated by a course of "needles." In 1960, the patient was seen at The Johns Hopkins Hospital for the first time. She was hypertensive, blood pressure being in the range of 210/110, with grade III fundi. A systolic ejection murmur was described, but no diastolic murmur. She received antihypertensive therapy intermittently. In 1966, the patient was admitted with congestive failure and pulmonary edema, which resolved with diuretics. Phonocardiography was consistent with aortic insufficiency. The electrocardiogram showed left ventricular hypertrophy and sinus tachycardia. Acid fast bacillus culture of sputum was negative. Intermediate tuberculin (PPD) test was negative, as was STS. Left optic atrophy was present. A course of penicillin was given for suspected syphilis. The second admission was in 1968, again with congestive failure. In March 1969, the patient was once more admitted with congestive heart failure and fever. She was treated with diuretics and with ampicillin for pneumonia. Both cough and purulent sputum cleared. No etiologic agent was established. The patient became afebrile, refused cardiac catheterization, and was discharged. In October 1969, the patient was readmitted with congestive failure and was released three weeks prior to the final admission. Two days prior to the last admission, the patient noted ankle edema, increasing dyspnea, and a cough productive of green sputum. The next day right lower pleuritic chest pain developed, with nausea and malaise. On examination, she was described as a well-developed, elderly female in moderate distress, with shortness of breath and chest pain. Blood pressure, 175/90; pulse, 115; respirations, 32; temperature, 100.6 degrees. Nose flat, with loss of nasal cartilage. Pupils unequal and irregular, with right larger than left; right reacted to light and accommodation. Fundi: Marked arteriolar narrowing, arteriovenous nicking. Neck: No significant enlargement of lymph nodes. Neck veins were distended. Thyroid: Not palpable. Trachea in midline. Chest: Poor expansion, but symmetrical. Dullness at right base. Bilateral basilar coarse rhonchi, with scattered expiratory rales; otherwise clear. Heart was grossly enlarged, with a diffuse point of maximal impulse— from left anterior to mid-axillary line. Grade 3/6 blowing diastolic murmur, with 2/6 high-pitched, musical decrescendo murmur along left sternal border. Grade 2/6 harsh systolic murmur conducted to the axilla. There was no opening snap. Pretibial edema, 2+. Pulses 3+ and symmetrical. Abdomen: Liver 6 to 8 cm. below costal margin. Neurological examination: Within physiological limits. Laboratory findings: Hematocrit, 34 ml./100 ml.; WBCs, 8000/cu. mm., with 13 percent juvenile neutrophils, 47 percent polymorphonuclear leukocytes, 24 percent lymphocytes, and 15 percent monocytes; platelets adequate. Serum urea nitrogen, 21 mg./100 ml.; sugar, 125 mg./100 ml.; total protein, 6.7 g./100 ml.; albumin, 2.1 g./100 ml.; alkaline phosphatase, 147 milliunits/ml. (I.U.); serum glutamic oxaloacetic transaminase, 44 Karmen units/ml.; serum glutamic pyruvic transaminase, 13 Karmen units/ml.; bilirubin, 1.5 mg./100 ml.; lactic dehydrogenase, 230 units/ml.; STS, negative; T_4 (thyroxine iodine), 1.9 mcg./100 ml.; PPD, negative. Stool, guaiac negative. Urine: Specific gravity, 1.019; pH 5.5; protein, 1 to 2+. Negative sugar and acetone. No RBCs, and few WBCs. Sputum: Polymorphonuclear leukocytes and gram-positive diplococci, some being intracellular. Electrocardiogram: Left axis deviation, left ventricular hypertrophy, unchanged from previous ECG except for sinus tachycardia. Chest film: Huge heart, tortuous aorta, right lower lobe infiltrate and effusion. The right lobe effusion was tapped, and 700 cc. of fluid was obtained. Specific gravity, 1.022; 25,000 cells/cc., 75 to 80 percent being polymorphonuclear leukocytes; sugar, 122 mcg./100 ml.; protein, 2.7 g. Subsequent taps showed 700 cells/ cc., mainly mononuclear.

With diagnosis of congestive heart failure and pneumococcal pneumonia, treatment was begun with diuretics and penicillin. The patient's temperature fell slowly over six days. Thoracentesis was performed four times during hospitalization. No positive cultures were obtained. The patient suffered two episodes of shortness of breath, tachycardia, and diaphoresis on the fifth day. She recovered with diuresis. The pleural effusion cleared over seven days. From the eighth day onward, the patient had a fluctuating fever of 99 to 101 degrees. Hematocrit reading fell to 26 ml./100 ml. Reticulocytes were 3.7 percent of erythrocytes. Cultures of blood and pleural fluid were sterile. Penicillin was discontinued on the nineteenth day. No change was noted in heart murmur. No peripheral petechiae were seen. On the twenty-third hospital day, the patient became uncooperative and somewhat confused. A lumbar puncture showed approximately 100 WBC/cu. mm., all mononuclear leukocytes. Brain scan was normal. No bacteria seen on gram stain. Serology was negative. Negative routine bacteriological cultures. No localizing neurologic signs were demonstrated. Penicillin and chloramphenicol were given intravenously. Her mental status declined. Tachycardia and tachypnea developed, and she expired on the twenty-fifth hospital day.

DISCUSSION OF THE PROBLEM

The dominant feature of this patient's long-drawn-out illness was congestive heart failure. For fully 25 years, she was in and out of hospitals, accident rooms, and clinics suffering from varying degrees of heart failure, her condition worsening relentlessly.

Many of the physicians who saw her took it for granted that her heart failure was the result of syphilitic cardiovascular disease. Such taking of things for granted by clinicians is one of the built-in dangers of having a chronic illness, and forming the habit of challenging all features of a patient's illness is a clinical must.

Frequently, *several* factors may be playing a role in the genesis of congestive heart failure, although only one may be predominant. Some of these factors may be remediable, and others irreversible. It is, therefore, a serious error to think only in terms of *the* cause of heart failure, for to do so may mean therapeutic opportunities are overlooked.

The best way to screen out such causative factors is to apply the approach Dr. Louis Hamman taught us.

He categorized the general factors in production of congestive heart failure as follows:
1. Pericardial disease.
2. Myocardial disease.
3. Endocardial disease.
4. Increased pressure in the pulmonary circulation.
5. Increased pressure in the systemic circulation.
6. Congenital abnormalities.

To this listing we have added two additional factors:
7. Trauma.
8. Conditions arising primarily outside the heart, but exactly imitating intrinsic cardiac disease, such as mediastinal fibrosis.

One should become compulsive and obsessive about this list, and repeatedly scan it analytically, even though the etiology of a patient's heart failure seems too tiresomely obvious.

Let us briefly apply this approach here.

1. There was never any clinical evidence of a pericardial effusion, and the great enlargement of the heart and the intensive diastolic murmurs noted here would not accompany constrictive pericardial disease.

2. The very great enlargement of the cardiac chambers, the ECG abnormalities, the progressively falling blood pressure, the decreasing response to specific therapy, and the sudden death all point to myocardial disease. Several elements, no doubt, were important in its genesis: (a) The patient had a valvular abnormality which mechanically greatly increased the work of the

PART M / HEART FAILURE AND AORTIC INSUFFICIENCY

heart muscle. (b) The mechanical abnormality—namely, aortic insufficiency—was of a type which could interfere with coronary artery perfusion. (c) The patient was known to have had hypertension for years, with degenerative changes having taken place in her eye grounds. Several expert observers concluded that hypertension contributed more to her failure than did the aortic insufficiency. (d) There was a strong evidence that she had syphilis. As you well know, for years there has been disagreement regarding the relationship between syphilis and myocarditis. Nevertheless, I recall the instances in which Dr. Arnold Rich made a diagnosis of syphilitic myocarditis when confronted with a patient who had both syphilis and myocarditis, and no other apparent reason for myocardial injury, despite the absence of any specific histologic alterations in the myocardium. (e) This patient was reaching an age at which degenerative vascular changes begin to appear, and, as already emphasized, she did have hypertension and eye ground changes.

Therefore, while we do not believe that myocardial disease was the *only* factor in this patient's heart failure, her myocardium was certainly abnormal, as a result of an interplay of the several factors we have just reviewed.

3. That endocardial, and specifically valvular, factors were important here seems indisputable, and was the item upon which all of those who saw the patient dwelt. What was its nature?

While a variety of murmurs were depicted, the one which attracted the most comment was a decrescendo ("diamond-shaped") diastolic murmur originating at the base of the heart. Because of its character, many listeners came to an instant conclusion of "aortic insufficiency." Let me give a warning here of the diagnostic booby-trap of blithely and uncritically relating a diastolic murmur heard in the aortic area to aortic insufficiency. A host of other conditions may generate just such a diastolic murmur, including the following:

1. Pulmonic insufficiency.
2. Dissecting aneurysm.
3. Ruptured sinus of Valsalva.
4. Vascular tumors.
5. Coronary artery fistula.
6. Pulmonary arteriovenous fistula.
7. Patent ductus arteriosus.
8. Mediastinal fibrosis.

It is a sound rule to question the diagnosis of aortic insufficiency in congestive heart failure, unless, in addition to the diastolic murmur, some peripheral manifestations of aortic insufficiency are also present.

I was somewhat disconcerted in reading this patient's chart to note the long and vivid descriptions of the heart sounds, with little or no attention being paid to other manifestations of abnormal flow dynamics.

Nevertheless, I believe that the patient's widened pulse pressure is sufficient evidence to indicate that she did have, dynamically speaking, a significant degree of insufficiency of the aortic valve.

The next question is—what caused it? It was concluded in comments on the chart that syphilis was the causative factor, because of the history of syphilis, the disappearance of the soft tissues of the nose, the pupillary changes, and the questionable optic atrophy. Before agreeing with this diagnosis, however, I think we should, once again, briefly challenge it. The patient had her first episode of swelling, dyspnea, and so-called asthma when she was only 38 and, interestingly, this took place shortly after delivery. Also, and as already emphasized, the characteristic features of her clinical course were its chronicity and episodicity, its ups and downs. These features are typical of rheumatic heart disease.

As a matter of fact, up until the 1950's or so, episodicity of heart failure was used as an important differential point between syphilitic disease and rheumatic disease of the heart: it was thought that a patient with syphilitic aortic insufficiency, once heart failure set in, underwent progressive and inexorable deterioration, without showing episodic periods of stability such as occur in rheumatic heart patients. However, this clinical assumption was subsequently restudied, and, as so often happens when one takes a second look, was found to be invalid. Patients with syphilitic aortic disease may indeed pursue a chronic, intermittent course exactly similar to that of the rheumatic patient.

More significantly, in this particular case, no one ever thought that this patient's mitral valve was affected, or that there was a significant degree of aortic stenosis, and it would be most unusual for a female to have pure aortic insufficiency as the sole manifestation of rheumatic valvular disease.

Again, in Boston a few years ago, I overlooked the diagnosis of healed bacterial endocarditis in circumstances exactly similar to these. In this day and age, when almost anyone with a fever, for whatever cause, is given a course of antibiotics, it is inescapable that we will see patients who present with valvular disease resulting from healed bacterial endocarditis, whose initial episode was camouflaged by antibiotics. We can only say that for this patient we have no historical grounds for such a suspicion.

Finally, she did not have rheumatoid disease or evidences of systemic lupus, there was no history of traumatic injury to her chest, and she had not taken Sansert for migraine headaches.

We conclude, therefore, that this patient's aortic insufficiency was, in fact, the result of syphilis.

So now let us quickly conclude Dr. Hamman's outlined approach: We have already alluded to the potential role of systemic hypertension in her failure. In checking her blood pressure values, when she was resting in the hospital and was not in heart failure, her hypertension was only moderate. Dr. Hamman emphasized repeatedly the need to be critical in evaluating the role of hypertension in patients while they are in congestive heart failure, for the hypertension may actually be only a manifestation of the congestion, not the cause of it. The description of the patient's eye grounds, however, indicates that she did have a significant degree of hypertension.

Her renal function remained good, and her urinary sediment was never remarkable. There was no history of urinary tract infections. Why did she have hypertension?

In reviewing the chart, I was impressed by the number of times she was described as becoming suddenly short of breath, and of sweating a great deal, and hence, I wondered about a pheochromocytoma, although at such times dramatic changes in the blood pressure were not noted. Statistically, however, it is more likely that she had essential hypertension with secondary degenerative vascular alterations in the kidneys.

Could she have had hypertension in the pulmonary circulation? Surely this patient's course clamors "Watch for recurrent pulmonary embolism!" For example, her first episode of dyspnea and so-called "asthma" began shortly after delivery, and thereafter, for 25 years, she had recurrent episodes of dyspnea and sweating. In the 10 months prior to her death, she had had two episodes of so-called "pneumonia," with bilateral effusions, although, peculiarly, no significant organisms were ever cultured from the sputum, blood, or chest fluid. In so very many cases in this setting, lower lobe "pneumonia" proves to be pulmonary embolism at post mortem. Also, let us not forget that this patient died abruptly.

We can quickly dispose of the remaining factors on Dr. Hamman's list, for, as already mentioned, there was no history of trauma, mediastinal fibrosis much more often mimics mitral than aortic disease, and I don't know any congenital disorder which would follow this patient's pattern.

In summary, then, our analysis to this point makes us conclude that the patient did, in fact, have aortic insufficiency. Syphilis seems its most likely cause. Other factors contributing to her unfortunate predicament appear to be systemic hypertension, recurrent pulmonary embolism, and myocardial injury, the latter being the result of several processes, including the aortic valve leakage, syphilis, hypertension, and degenerative vascular changes.

Lastly, what brought her long illness to its climax?

When you are caring for a patient with chronic, congestive heart failure, such as this patient, and her health begins to fade and dwindle, there are a number of causative factors you should review, in a systematized fashion, lest you overlook something remediable:

1. Poor patient cooperation with diet and medications.
2. An inadequate therapeutic program.
3. Iatrogenic factors—overusage of digitalis and diuretics, leading to conduction abnormalities, hypokalemia, and hyponatremia.
4. The onset of an arrhythmia.
5. The occurrence of pulmonary embolism.
6. Progression of the natural course of the basic disease process.
7. The development of myocardiopathy.
8. The onset of a hypermetabolic state, including fever and hyperthyroidism.
9. The development of anemia, anoxia, obesity, pregnancy and other factors requiring increased cardiac output.

10. The onset of a serious depressive-anxiety state.

11. The inception of some complicating disorder, and in particular, a neoplasm or some infectious process.

A perusal of this list reveals a number which clearly have no pertinency here.

For example, the patient was reasonably cooperative and was being treated very intensively, at times too much so, for she developed electrolyte imbalance, but this was rapidly recognized and corrected. There was no arrhythmia, and no indications of renewed or acute myocardial injury clinically or electrocardiographically. Her metabolic state had been carefully studied and was judged to be normal. Although she became anemic, her health had begun to dwindle before this became a significant factor. Anxiety and depression were not a problem, nor was an increased work load imposed, other than through mild fever and anemia.

On the other hand, certain of these categories have very real pertinency here. For example, we have already referred to the likelihood that this patient was having recurrent pulmonary emboli. In addition, during the last months of her life, she lost some 30 pounds, and her final weeks were accompanied by unexplained fever, pleural effusions, mental confusion, and presence of increased cells in the spinal fluid, indicating that some new disease process had come into being. What was its nature? Could she have acquired infective endocarditis, perhaps during the course of her pneumonic episode? Did cerebral emboli or cerebritis account for her confusion and spinal fluid alterations? Although none of the so-called classical features of infective endocarditis were present, such as clubbing, petechiae, hematuria, and so forth, in a significant portion of patients with endocarditis, some or all of these features may be absent. However, their complete absence reduces somewhat the statistical likelihood of this infection. Also, blood cultures were sterile, reducing the likelihood even further, although certainly not eliminating it.

Likewise, the possibility of neoplasm—particularly, in view of the chest findings, bronchiogenic carcinoma with metastases to the brain—deserves consideration. However, the brain scan was normal. In this setting, with rapid deterioration and sudden death as well, an infectious process is more to be favored.

Before turning to other types of infection she might have had, let us not forget that this patient was known to have an SA hemoglobinopathy. While this abnormality usually behaves benignly, in certain circumstances it may greatly exacerbate, producing vascular thrombosis in the lungs, brain, and elsewhere. Two of the circumstances in which this may occur were present in the terminal weeks of this patient's illness—namely, fever and anorexia. We will recall that during this period her hematocrit values fell from 35 to 25 ml./100 ml., and she had a reticulocytosis. However, this is an exceedingly rare occurrence, seen only in situations of dire stress, and is not generally accompanied by presence of mononuclear cells in the spinal fluid.

Those who managed this patient's terminal illness thought that she had pneumococcal pneumonia with empyema, and in this setting one should also wonder about a complicating lung abscess, pneumococcal endocarditis, or a brain abscess. But the cultures of her blood, sputum, and the chest fluid were sterile, her WBC count was not elevated, the brain scan was normal, and there was no mention of headaches. Finally, her temperature failed to respond to very brisk antibiotic therapy.

Therefore, a granulomatous infection due to tuberculosis or a fungal agent would seem much more likely. The long-drawn-out, debilitating illness which this patient endured would be fertile soil for such an infection. Dissemination into the central nervous system is indicated by the terminal cerebral alterations and the nature of the changes in the spinal fluid.

We conclude, therefore, that the most reasonable explanation for the course of this patient's long illness is:

1. She had aortic insufficiency resulting from syphilis, with syphilitic aortitis as well.

2. In addition, she had hypertension, probably essential in nature.

3. Several processes had affected her myocardium, including the dynamic effects of her leaking valve, the hypertension, degenerative vascular disease, and syphilis, as well.

4. Her course became complicated by repetitive pulmonary emboli.

5. Lastly, she developed a disseminated granulomatous infection, most likely tuberculosis.

We have, then, yet another example of sickness and death resulting from concomitance of a complex of common diseases.

POST MORTEM FINDINGS

Generalized tuberculosis of lymph nodes, liver, spleen, kidney, lungs, and pleura. Subacute tuberculous meningitis of the brain and spinal cord. Biventricular hypertrophy and dilatation of the heart. Chronic congestion of lungs and liver. Syphilitic aortitis, with aneurysmal dilatation of thoracic aorta.

REFERENCES

General

Hamman, L. A.: Diagnosis of the causes of heart failure. New Eng. J. Med. *219:*289, 1938.
Levine, S. A., and Harvey, W. P.: Clinical Auscultation of the Heart. 2nd ed. Philadelphia, W. B. Saunders Company, 1959.
Runco, V., and Booth, R. W.: Basal diastolic murmurs. Amer. Heart J. *65:*697, 1963.
Runco, V., Molnar, W., Meckstroth, C. V., and Ryan, J. M.: The Graham Steell murmur versus aortic regurgitation. Amer. J. Med. *31:*71, 1961.

Aortic Valve Lesions

Bland, E. F., and Wheeler, E. O.: Severe aortic regurgitation in young people. New Eng. J. Med. 256:667, 1957.
Bleich, A., and Lewis, J.: Aortic regurgitation in the elderly. Amer. Heart J. 71:627, 1966.
Frank, M. J., Casanegra, T., and Levinson, G. E.: Evaluation of aortic insufficiency. Circulation 28:723, 1963.
Hamman, L.: Diagnostic implications of aortic insufficiency. Cincinnati J. Med. 25:95, 1944.
London, S. B., and London, R. E.: Production of aortic insufficiency by imperforated aneurysm of sinus of Valsalva. Circulation 24:1403, 1961.
Reppert, E. H.: Aortic valve lesions. Amer. Heart J. 76:136, 1968.
Roberts, W. C.: Anatomically isolated aortic valvular disease. The case against its being of rheumatic etiology. Amer. J. Med. 49:151, 1970.
Segal, J. P., Harvey, W. P., and Hufnagel, C. A.: A clinical study of 100 cases of severe aortic regurgitation. Amer. J. Med. 21:200, 1956.
Spagnuolo, M., et al.: Natural history of rheumatic aortic regurgitation. Circulation 44:368, 1971.

Syphilitic Aortic Regurgitation

Hamman, L. A., and Rich, A. R.: Clinical pathological conference; case of syphilitic myocarditis. Internat. Clin. 4:221, 1934.
Heggtveit, A. A.: Syphilitic aortitis—a clinicopathologic autopsy of 100 cases, 1950 to 1960. Circulation 29:345, 1964.
MacFarlane, W. V., Swan, W. G., and Irvine, R. E.: Cardiovascular disease in syphilis. A review of 1330 patients. Brit. Med. J. 1:827, 1956.
McCann, J. S., and Porter, D. C.: Calcification of the aorta as an aid to the diagnosis of syphilis. Brit. Med. J. 1:826, 1956.
Webster, B., et al.: The natural history of syphilitic aortic insufficiency. Amer. Heart J. 46:117, 1953.

Bacterial Endocarditis

Cohen, L. and Freedman, L. R.: Damage to aortic valve as cause of death in bacterial endocarditis. Ann. Intern. Med. 55:562, 1961.
Hamman, L.: Healed bacterial endocarditis. Ann. Intern. Med. 11:175, 1937.
Hughes, P., and Gould, W. R.: Bacterial endocarditis, changing disease. Quart. J. Med. 35:511, 1966.
Robinson, M. J., and Reudy, J.: Sequelae of bacterial endocarditis. Amer. J. Med. 32:910, 1962.

Lupus of the Heart

Hejtmancik, M. R., et al.: The cardiovascular manifestations of systemic lupus erythematosus. Amer. Heart J. 68:301–8, 1963.

Sickle Cell Anemia

Charache, S., and Page, D. L.: Infarction of bone marrow in the sickle cell disorders. Ann. Intern. Med. 67:1195, 1967.
Diggs, L. W.: Sickle cell crisis. Amer. J. Clin. Path. 44:1, 1965.
Smith, E. W., and Conley, C. L.: Sicklemia and infarction of the spleen during aerial flight. Bull. Johns Hopkins Hosp. 96:35, 1955.

Pulmonary Embolism

Freiman, D. G., Suyemoto, J., and Wessler, S.: Frequency of pulmonary thromboembolism in man. New Eng. J. Med. 272:1278, 1965.
Parmley, L. F.: Clinically deceptive massive pulmonary embolism. Chest 58:15, 1970.

Granulomatous Infections

Munt, P. W.: Miliary tuberculosis in the chemotherapy era. Medicine 51:139, 1972.
Utz, J. P.: The spectrum of opportunistic fungus infections. Lab. Invest. 2:1018, 1962.

N A PATIENT WITH COMPLICATED, CHRONIC, EPISODIC, POLYORGAN SYSTEM DISEASE

THE CLINICAL PROBLEM

This was the sixth admission for this 57 year old unemployed landscape gardener and coal yard worker, who complained of increasing weakness and shortness of breath over the week prior to admission. From 1941 until 1944 he had worked in a chromate factory, and had developed a nasal septal perforation. He drank heavily prior to gastric surgery in 1955.

His first hospital admission, in January 1951, was with a three week history of a chest cold which progressed to pleurisy and shortness of breath. He also developed a swollen, lacrimating left eye. He had a fever of 101 degrees and a blood pressure of 188/110. He had periorbital edema, chemosis, conjunctivitis, a nasal septum perforation, erythematous pharynx, and generalized shotty lymphadenopathy. Lungs were unremarkable except for slight dullness and bronchovesicular breath sounds in the right subclavicular area. There was slight cardiomegaly and, along the left sternal border, a systolic blowing murmur, mild pretibial edema, and three finger hepatomegaly. The liver was firm, smooth, and nontender. Chest films revealed a pneumonitic process in the right upper lobe, with strandlike densities extending to the hilum and probably partial right middle lobe atelectasis. The possibility that this could represent tuberculosis was raised by the radiologist. Hematocrit, 34 ml./100 ml.; WBC count, 10,200; differential count, normal; urine revealed slight proteinuria and microscopic hematuria; stool, guaiac negative. Routine blood, sputum, urine, and nasopharyngeal cultures were unremarkable. Five 24 hour sputum cultures for acid fast bacilli were negative. The STS was positive. The tuberculin test (O.T.) was positive at 1:1000, negative at 1:10,000. The patient was given 600,000 units of penicillin a day for 18 days, with partial resolution of the pneumonitis. He was lost to follow-up, but apparently did well until 1954, when he was again treated for pneumonia. He developed abdominal pain and had an upper gastrointestinal hemorrhage, for which he underwent subtotal gastric resection at another hospital in 1955. Cholecystectomy was performed at the same time. Digitalis was discontinued at this time, and he developed intermittent dyspnea, anginal pain, and paroxysmal nocturnal dyspnea. He was again hospitalized elsewhere in 1958 because of anemia, nausea, vomiting, and abdominal pain. He was transfused and started on iron therapy, and was again treated for syphilis as a result of a positive STS. He developed painful swelling of his major joints and great toe and had a serum uric acid content of 12 mg./100 ml. He was admitted to this hospital for the second time in June 1958 for evaluation of his anemia. Physical findings were essentially unchanged except that the lungs were clear and the liver was down only 2 cm. There were multiple joint deformities and a mild hemiparesis. Electrocardiogram was unchanged, and the lung fields were clear on X-ray. The cause of his anemia was not found. He was given three transfusions. In August 1959 he began to lose weight, and in October, when he was admitted for the third time, his hematocrit dropped from 37 to 32 ml./100 ml. Blood pressure was 205/120, physical findings unchanged except for Grade II hypertensive retinopathy, bilateral parotid gland enlargement, a normal thyroid gland, and a small prostate. He had persistent guaiac-positive stools, but sigmoidoscopy, proctoscopy, gastroscopy, and X-ray studies failed to demonstrate a source. It was felt that the patient had panhypopituitarism, and he was started on thyroid extract, 64 mg. per day, but this did not alter his hematocrit readings or reticulocyte count. Again, in the outpatient department, he continued to be weak, had chronic arthritis with acute gouty attacks, redeveloped hypertension, and was admitted in May 1961 to confirm the diagnosis of panhypopituitarism. Blood pressure was 200/120, physical findings unchanged. Hematocrit, 26 ml./100 ml., WBC count and differential count normal; stools only intermittently positive for occult blood; platelet count, 298,000/cu. mm.; RTCF reactive; old tuberculin, 1:10,000 positive. Phenolsulphonphthalein excretion was 37 percent total; urea clearance, 27–29%. Sialogram revealed diffuse parotid enlargement only. There was some improvement after he was started on 20 mg. of hydrocortisone per day. He was again seen sporadically in the clinic, having had syncopal episodes in August, with carpal spasm, and recurrent gout. He was continued on colchicine, digitalis, Benemid, ferrous sulfate, thyroid extract, and replacement prednisone, but had episodes of weakness, syncope, anorexia, nausea, and diarrhea, the last a persistent problem. By January 1963, he had two pillow orthopnea and nightly paroxysmal nocturnal dyspnea, increasing exertional dyspnea, and dependent edema. He was examined by members of the Connective Tissue Clinic, who felt there was little evidence for sarcoidosis, but a Kveim test biopsy revealed "possible sarcoidal reaction, compatible with suspicious Kveim test." His fifth hospital admission was in February 1963 for further evaluation. Physical findings were unchanged. Hematocrit, 28 ml./ 100 ml.; WBC count, 4400/cu. mm., with moderate shift to the left. Parotid biopsy was normal; liver biopsy revealed a few round aggregates of epithelioid cells, thought probably to represent "healing granulomas." Venous pressure was normal, thyroid studies again were compatible with hypothyroidism. The patient had a persistent fever of 99 to 101.6 degrees, and a throat culture was positive for beta hemolytic streptococci. His fever did not respond to penicillin therapy.

After discharge, the patient remained extremely weak and essentially bedridden, but he took fluids and medications religiously. He noticed increasing dyspnea at rest and, three days prior to final admission, developed fever, night sweats, and multiple shaking chills. At the time of the last admission, his blood pressure was 180/100, pulse 80 and regular.

The patient was a chronically ill, dyspneic black male. Unimpressive shotty lymphadenopathy was noted. Eyes revealed only marked arcus senilis and arteriolar narrowing, with increased light reflex and arteriovenous nicking. There was a large nasal septal defect and bilateral enlargement of the parotids, with patent Stensen's ducts. The glands were firm and nontender. Lungs were filled with rales to the scapular angles bilaterally. Other findings: heart, moderately enlarged; aortic second sound, accentuated and tambouric; no murmurs or rubs; neck veins flat; peripheral arteries tortuous; pulses good; no cyanosis or clubbing; abdomen not tender; liver down five fingerbreadths and very tender; and a splenic tip easily palpable. There were no masses, and the bowel sounds were hypoactive. Genitalia normal, with soft, normal-sized testes. Extremities showed osteoarthritic changes. The prostate was very small. Neurological findings were within physiological limits.

Hematocrit, 33 ml./100 ml., with normochromia, normocytosis, target cells, and a few stippled RBC's. WBC count, 6000/cu. mm., with 38 percent juvenile neutrophils, 38 percent segmented neutrophils, 20 percent lymphocytes, 4 percent monocytes, 900,000 platelets. Urinalysis normal except for 3 + proteinuria. Stool guaiac negative. O.T., 1:10,000 negative. Serum urea nitrogen, 59 mg./100 ml.; carbon dioxide content, 12.8 mEq./liter; chloride, 120 mEq./liter; sodium, 139 mEq./liter; potassium, 6.4 mEq./liter; phosphorus, 2.4 mg./100 ml.; alkaline phosphatase, 4.1 King-Armstrong units; amylase, 85 Somogyi units/hr.; bilirubin, 0.8 mg./100 ml.; total serum proteins, 5.2 g./100 ml., albumen/globulin ratio, 1.5:3.7; cerebrospinal fluid normal. Throat, stool, urine, and CSF cultures negative; sputum clutures showed pure, heavy growth of Klebsiella. Chest and abdominal x-rays normal.

The patient was felt to have septicemia or miliary tuberculosis and appropriate therapy was begun. A hepatic scintiscan showed hepatomegaly only. Lupus erythematosus preparation was negative. Two 24 hour sputum samples and gastric washing for acid-fast bacilli were negative. However, he did not respond to therapy and died shortly.

DISCUSSION OF THE PROBLEM

A superficial perusal of the history of this patient's illness creates the illusion of being lost in an impenetrable forest of data from history and physical examination, and an overwhelming number of laboratory tests. Whenever he begins to feel lost, the wise clinical explorer comes to a dead stop, and looks about to see if he can find some landmarks which will point the way to a clearing.

Perhaps we can secure our first landmark by searching through this mass of data and discovering what the general characteristics of the course of this illness were. My analysis would list them as follows:
  1. It was a chronic illness, covering a span of not less than 12 years.
  2. The illness evolved in an episodic fashion.
  3. There were periods of exacerbation mingled with periods of remission.
  4. There was progressive, relentless deterioration of the patient's health.

5. A large number of different organ systems were affected by illness, singly and in confusing combination.

Now we are beginning to get our bearings, so to speak. So let us look for additional landmarks.

Certain general manifestations of disease dominated the course of his illness. These included marked weight loss, weakness, easy fatigability, anorexia, nausea, abdominal pain, diarrhea, recurrent fever, and night sweats.

In addition to these manifestations which formed the backdrop of his clinical course, there was altered function of an amazing number of specific organ systems, as follows:

1. The heart was enlarged, and the patient ultimately had congestive heart failure. He had angina pectoris. His blood pressure was persistently elevated, although its height fluctuated considerably.

2. The kidneys became insufficient, and he developed hypochloremic acidosis.

3. There were several attacks of pneumonitis.

4. The central nervous system became implicated through the development of a transient hemiparesis, and a symmetrical polyneuropathy, which was principally sensory in type.

5. There was chronic bilateral parotid gland enlargement.

6. Shotty lymph gland enlargement was noted.

7. He had chronic, recurrent polyarthritis.

8. There was marked wasting and atrophy of the neck and shoulder girdle muscles.

9. The liver was enlarged and found to contain small granulomata.

10. There was enlargement of the spleen.

11. Gastrointestinal dysfunction was manifested by abdominal pain, which resulted in removal of both the gallbladder and a portion of the stomach but without relief, and by recurrent diarrhea, with blood in the stools.

12. He was considered to have hypothyroidism, and perhaps even hypopituitarism, although there was great disagreement about the latter.

13. He had a severe, very long-standing anemia, which at times had some of the characteristics of an iron deficiency anemia, but at others seemed to result from bone marrow suppression. On one occasion he had a distinct thrombocytosis.

Now, at this stage of our exploration, we have obtained some definite landmarks. Let us next consider up what paths they might lead us. This is best done by asking ourselves the following question: What different kinds of disease processes are characterized by the involvement of many organ systems chronically and episodically over a long span of time, in association with fever, weight loss, and general debility?

It seems to me that there are 10, as follows:

1. Sarcoidosis.

2. Amyloidosis.

3. Collagen-vascular disease such as polyarteritis nodosa or systemic lupus erythematosus.

4. Disseminated infection of a chronic granulomatous type, such as tuberculosis, histoplasmosis, or syphilis.

5. A widely disseminated tumor, either a carcinoma, lymphoma, or myeloma.

6. A blood dyscrasia, such as leukemia, primary anemia, or myeloid metaplasia.

7. Some poison, drug or toxin.

8. An endocrine disturbance.

9. Degenerative vascular disease.

10. Macroglobulinemia of Waldenström or other primary dysproteinemia.

The landmarks we have chosen have led us to a variety of possible paths out of this forest of facts.

Some of them we can readily reject. For example, there was no history of exposure to toxic substances, other than chromate, which per se would not produce these changes. Degenerative vascular disease could only explain the cardiorenal alterations, which were only one segment of the patient's illness. His peripheral blood and bone marrow, though studied through the years, failed to show any changes ascribable to leukemia. Myeloid metaplasia would neatly explain the anemia, elevated uric acid level, and enlarged liver and spleen, but the bone marrow and peripheral blood studies excluded such a process. There was, indeed, some indication of hypothyroidism, and perhaps even of hypopituitarism, but these would have to be regarded as secondary and not primary phenomena, since a large number of the changes observed in this patient do not occur in these endocrine conditions when they are primary.

A duration of 10 to 15 years would make a malignant neoplasm unlikely, although we realize more and more that the life story of malignant tumors may be much longer than we had previously imagined. Also, the very wide variety of clinical alterations which tumors may produce by virtue of their endocrine and metabolic effects, and their association with the appearance of peculiar protein materials, are only now being appreciated. The fact that the patient had been exposed to chromate obviously makes one think of carcinoma of the lung. Also, we have learned in recent years to consider the presence of new growths in obscure problems in which there is hyperuricemia, such as occurred here, since occasionally this chemical change is the single clue to the presence of a hidden malignancy. But not once through all these years did any neoplasm suggest its presence focally, and the elevated blood pressure and renal insufficiency would be difficult to explain on such a basis, to name but one obvious objection.

The patient's serum was never shown to contain peculiar proteins, and the bleeding tendency, Raynaud's phenomenon, eye ground changes, and other evidences of sludged blood so typical of Waldenström's disorder were never present.

It appears from the serological studies which were done that the patient probably had syphilis, but this alone could not cause all the changes seen in this patient. Disseminated tuberculosis and histoplasmosis cannot be discarded quite as readily. As already emphasized, this was a wasting illness, with fever and sweats. It began with a pulmonary lesion at the right apex, and terminated with a large liver containing granulomata. How like tuberculosis is this sequence! But again, there were so many features of this patient's illness which would be foreign to tuberculosis, such as the hypertension, heart failure, renal insufficiency, parotid enlargement, and arthritis. Also, 10 to 15 years is an excessive duration for disseminated tuberculosis, and during this long span of time some dissemination to the lungs should have been anticipated, but this never occurred. The differential white count never showed a monocytosis. The patient's tuberculin sensitivity remained only mild throughout. Repeated attempts to culture tubercle bacilli were unrevealing. Again, disseminated histoplasmosis in a Negro tends to be rapidly fatal.

Amyloidosis would explain some but not all of these happenings. Peripheral neuropathy, enlargement of the liver and spleen, renal insufficiency, hypothyroidism and even hypopituitarism, anemia, and joint pains may all be part of amyloidosis. But hypertension is, of course, unusual, the renal alterations in amyloidosis are more nephrotic in type, and the pneumonia, bilateral parotid enlargement, and recurrent abdominal pain with diarrhea would not be well answered by such a diagnosis. Nor did the patient have any bleeding into the skin, common in amyloidosis, nor were deposits of amyloid noted in any of the soft tissues. Results of chemical tests of the liver were not those usually associated with amyloidosis, elevated alkaline phosphatase being the typical alteration in this disorder. No amyloid was seen in the liver biopsy.

Sarcoidosis has to be given thorough consideration. The very duration of the disease, with relative benignity for years, makes one think of sarcoid. The initial pulmonary infiltrate, while far from typical, could have been sarcoid, as could the general glandular enlargement. The red, swollen eye described on the patient's first admission, is found in sarcoid, the diagnosis sometimes being facilitated by conjunctival biopsy. Parotid enlargement is a well known hallmark of sarcoid, as is arthritis, and muscular wasting (of a striking degree in this patient) is sometimes so extensive in sarcoid as to mimic some primary muscle disease. Hypothyroidism may be due to sarcoid, and of course, sarcoid occasionally implicates the pituitary gland, as might have happened in this instance. This patient had diarrhea and a low serum carotene, and as you know sarcoid is one of the more common causes of secondary sprue. The hepatic and splenic enlargement would fit sarcoid perfectly, and we must recall that tiny granulomata were seen in the liver biopsy. He even had a questionably positive Kveim test.

But again, there are some features which do not fit the diagnosis of sarcoid as neatly as they should, and make it a diagnostic path down which we do not choose to walk, even cautiously. In the first place, if we think of the four tissues which are most often affected by sarcoid, namely, skin, lymph glands, lungs, and liver, we have very little evidence of significant involvement by sarcoid. It is true that there were granulomata in the liver, but not very impressive ones, and the liver chemistries did not show the high elevation of alkaline phosphatase generally present with sarcoidosis. Marked hypertension has not been a striking feature of the patients I have seen with sarcoid. A transient hemiparesis must be quite unusual in sarcoid, as is recurrent severe abdominal pain associated with bloody diarrhea. A pronounced chronic anemia is not a common feature of sarcoid. Also, the patient was sensitive to tuberculin, and no increase was seen in the serum globulin or calcium levels although repeatedly sought.

This brings us to the only path which is still left open, the possibility of some type of collagen vascular disease, in particular polyarteritis nodosa. We say "in particular" because systemic lupus erythematosus is the only other likely member of this group of disorders, and the degree of hypertension, the presence of a peripheral neuritis, the abdominal complaints, and the absence of increased gamma globulin and of LE cells make SLE considerably less likely than PAN, though one should not overstress these features. It can be impossible to distinguish an acute arteritis from SLE, and they of course can be concurrent.

There is really nothing in this patient's long-drawn-out, complicated course which is not quite typical of polyarteritis nodosa. If we reconsider the episode of pneumonia which first brought him to Hopkins in 1951 we see in it features quite characteristic of PAN. The peculiar reddening and swelling of the left eye, with periorbital edema, is just the sort of event which occurs in PAN. We had just recently discharged from the hospital a patient with PAN who had exactly the same sort of atelectasizing pneumonitis described in this protocol and also a red eye. The pneumonic episode was even then associated with marked hypertension, early congestive heart failure, and an unexplained anemia, as well as abnormal urine.

This patient was made miserable by repeated episodes of abdominal pain and diarrhea, sometimes containing blood. It seems no adequate explanation for this was ever discovered. He was initially said to have gastric ulcers, but it is interesting that when the surgeons removed part of his stomach for the supposed ulcers, they also took out the gallbladder, creating in my mind a reasonable doubt that the real cause of his trouble was ever actually found. Subsequently, his entire GI tract was restudied on two occasions, with great care, and no abnormality was revealed to account for the pain and diarrhea. This kind of frustrating history is so typical of polyarteritis, in which the patient has recurrent episodes of acute abdominal pain or diarrhea, suggesting this or that diagnosis, but no confirmation is obtained when specific studies or even exploratory laparotomy are performed. A variety of ulcerative lesions in the GI tract are of course not uncommon in PAN.

Hypertension and progressive renal insufficiency, often associated with cardiac failure such as occurred here, are, of course, the trademarks of advancing PAN. It is of interest that fluctuating blood pressure, sometimes to the extent that a pheochromocytoma is suspected, may be seen, and this patient's pressure did vary considerably. Angina may accompany these changes, as it did here.

Involvement of the central nervous system occurs with great frequency in PAN, a whole host of alterations being seen, depending upon the region of the CNS implicated by the arteritis. This patient had a transient hemiparesis, and also peripheral neuritis. A symmetrical peripheral neuropathy, in which the predominant complaint relates to sensory alterations, just as happened here, is a common abnormality.

Cotton wool spots were described by one observer in this patient's fundi. Cytoid bodies are not uncommon in PAN, and are well worth searching for in obscure or complicated illnesses.

The sort of chronic anemia which this patient had—perhaps best characterized as a bone marrow suppressive anemia, although iron deficiency may also have played a role—is often a part of PAN. An increased platelet count has been observed many times during the course of PAN, and it is of great interest that this patient's platelet count was 900,000.

If this patient had PAN, one might ask: Why didn't he have leukocytosis or eosinophilia? Actually, more patients with PAN do not have eosinophilia than do, and whereas a WBC count of 20,000 to 40,000 cu. mm. is not uncommon, the WBC count is not always elevated.

Bilateral parotid gland enlargement, as well as the whole panoply of changes of Sjögren's syndrome, has been described in PAN, which makes some observers conclude that this is another member of the spectrum of autoimmune disorders.

What about the question of hypopituitarism and hypothyroidism? I am not an erudite enough endocrinologist to be sure whether or not this patient had either of these abnormalities. The studies which were done certainly seem to have excluded the possibility of panhypopituitarism, but the pituitary may, of course, be affected in such a way as to lose some, but not all, of its functions. There seems to be stronger evidence for hypothyroidism, but again, this was a very chronically ill individual, with much wasting, and in these circumstances one may be misled into thinking a patient has organic hypothyroidism, when actually nature has simply turned down the metabolic thermostat during the stressful period. I wouldn't be surprised if this had happened here. It is of interest, however, that in one place in the chart the patient recorded that he had had a goiter at one time, and so had his uncle, and since we have postulated a Sjögren's-like enlargement of the parotids, perhaps he may have also had auto-immune disease of the thyroid, or Hashimoto's struma. While I have never personally come across impairment of the pituitary in PAN, certainly vascular thrombosis or hemorrhage is a common cause of pituitary injury, and I don't see why this could not take place in PAN. Finally, amyloidosis, which may be associated with PAN, could produce either thyroid or pituitary dysfunction, or both.

This patient had a great deal of muscular wasting, and this is exceedingly common in PAN, sometimes mimicking primary muscular atrophy. Also, he had recurrent polyarthritis. This could have been the result of gout, since his uric acid level was persistently elevated, but it does seem to me that he never got the relief from antigout measures which might have been expected if gout alone was present, and I wonder if PAN might not also be playing a role in the joint changes, which sometimes are mistaken for gout or even rheumatoid arthritis.

Splenic enlargement, seen in this patient, is present in about one third of the patients with PAN. But what about the liver enlargement, and the histological diagnosis of granulomata?

One of the things we have learned about PAN in recent years is the frequency with which the liver is affected by PAN. As a matter of fact, PAN is the most common cause of infarction of the liver. Granulomata, as described in this patient, are not infrequent. The alterations in the liver may conclude with a picture which can be mistaken for hepatitis or cirrhosis. Hemorrhages may occur in the capsule of the liver and present as mass right upper quadrant lesions which can be erroneously regarded as huge cysts, tumors, or inflammatory masses. Hence, the changes noted in this patient's liver actually favor the diagnosis of PAN.

The general characteristics of this patient's course, which we established as our first landmark, are exactly like those of PAN. Chronicity, episodicity, exacerbations and remissions, progressive deterioration, confusing polyorgan system involvement—this is the typical course of PAN, as this peculiar inflammation of blood vessels flares and subsides, now in this part, now in that, over a span sometimes covering many, many years. The general manifestations which formed the background for the polyorgan changes this man endured, and which constituted our second landmark, were also very typical of PAN—relentless weight loss, weakness, fatigue, recurrent fever, sweats and chills, anorexia and nausea.

It seems to me that having found our bearings and having followed our landmarks, we are now out of the forest, and that it is clearly evident that this patient must have had PAN. However, we should point out that a characteristic feature of all patients with collagen vascular disease is this: their course is frequently complicated by the development of a secondary infection, which they do not handle well, and which often overwhelms them. Among these are miliary tuberculosis, generalized fungus infections, and septicemias of all sorts. Over and over again such complicating infections are found only at post mortem, the unfortunate mistake being made of assuming during life that their manifestations were all part of the parent disease. Such may have happened here.

POST MORTEM FINDINGS

Miliary tuberculosis of lungs, liver, spleen, kidney, bone marrow, lymph nodes, papillary muscle of left heart, thyroid, adrenal. Marked pulmonary edema. Severe arterio- and arteriolosclerotic nephritis. Cardiac hypertrophy. Partial obstruction of pancreatic duct. Severe pancreatic fibrosis.

REFERENCES

Polyarteritis

Baker, A. L., et al.: Polyarteritis with Australian antigen-positive hepatitis. Gastroenterology 62:105, 1972.
Bleehan, S. S., et al.: Mononeuritis multiplex in polyarteritis nodosa. Quart. J. Med. 32:193, 1963.
Dahl, E. V., Baggenstoss, A. H., and Deweerd, J. H.: Testicular lesions of periarteritis nodosa with special reference to diagnosis. Amer. J. Med. 28:222, 1960.
Frohnert, P. P., and Sheps, S. G.: Long term follow-up study of periarteritis nodosa. Amer. J. Med. 43:8, 1967.
Gocke, D. J., et al.: Association between polyarteritis and Australian antigen. Lancet 2:1149, 1970.
Rose, G. A.: The natural history of polyarteritis. Brit. Med. J. 2:1148, 1957.
Rose, G. A., and Spencer, H.: Polyarteritis nodosa. Quart. J. Med. 26:43, 1957.

Waldenström's Macroglobulinemia

Cohen, R. J., Bohannon, R. A., and Wallerstein, R. O.: Waldenström's macroglobulinemia. Amer. J. Med. 41:274, 1966.
MacKenzie, M. R.: Macroglobulinemia. Calif. Med. 108:136, 1968.
McCallister, B. D., et al: Primary macroglobulinemia: review. Amer. J. Med. 43:394, 1967.

Amyloidosis

Brandt, K., Cathcart, E. S., and Cohen, A. S.: Clinical analysis of 42 patients with amyloidosis. Amer. J. Med. 44:955, 1968.
Cohen, A. S.: Medical progress. Amyloidosis. 277:524, 574, 628; 1967.

Sarcoidosis

Israel, H. L.: The diagnosis of sarcoidosis. Ann. Intern. Med. 68:1323, 1968.
Lordon, R. E., et al.: Sarcoidosis: Clinical evaluation of the alterations in delayed hypersensitivity. Ann. Rev. Resp. Dis. 97:1009, 1968.
Mandel, W., et al.: Bibliography of sarcoidosis: 1878–1963. U.S. Public Health Service, Publication No. 1215.
Siltzback, L. E.: Clinical features of sarcoidosis. Med. Clin. N. Amer. 51:483, 1967.

Granulomatous Infections

Parsons, R. J., and Zarafonetis, C. J. D.: Histoplasmosis in man: report of 7 cases and review of 72 cases. Arch. Intern. Med. 75:1, 1945.
Pfuetze, I. C. H., and Radner, D. B.: Clinical Tuberculosis—Essentials of Diagnosis and Treatment. Springfield, Ill., Charles C Thomas, 1966.
Rich, A. R.: The Pathogenesis of Tuberculosis. 2nd ed. Springfield, Ill., Charles C Thomas, 1951.
Stead, W. W.: The pathogenesis of pulmonary tuberculosis among older persons. Amer. Rev. Resp. Dis. 91:811, 1965.

O A PATIENT WITH AMYLOIDOSIS

THE CLINICAL PROBLEM

This 32 year old white housewife was admitted in May 1953 complaining of intermittent vomiting of 18 months' duration. She knew nothing of her family's medical history. Her general health had been excellent, although for the year prior to the present illness she had had episodes of peculiar darting pains in her legs, and had noticed blood in her urine. She had always been dark skinned.

In the summer of 1951, she developed fatigue, malaise, anorexia, weakness, and nausea and vomiting, which soon became associated with weight loss. Later, diarrhea began. X-ray studies were unrevealing. Her weight loss became marked. Systolic blood pressure was 69 to 80. A diagnosis of gastric neurosis was made. The patient's vision then became impaired. When in the erect position, she fainted several times. Blood pressure was 116/86 lying, 70/58 sitting, and unobtainable standing. A right nephropexy was done because of unexplained hematuria, but this continued, as did weight loss, profound weakness, and postural hypotension.

Physical examination: Temperature 97.8 degrees; pulse, 84; respirations, 16; blood pressure, 105/80; supine, 80/60 sitting, unobtainable standing. Thin, listless, chronically ill emaciated white female, looking older than her stated age, who became dizzy on standing. Skin dark, dry, and loose, with periocular dark rings, pigmented moles on arms, and numerous bruises on legs and back. No enlargement of lymph nodes or thyroid. Lungs clear to percussion and auscultation. Heart not enlarged. Pulses present, but weak. Abdomen flat. Spleen palpable. Unpigmented nephropexy scar. Neurological examination showed large pupils, irregular right pupil, no reaction to light by either pupil, minimal pupillary contraction on accommodation, good vision, full fields, no cranial nerve abnormality, generalized muscular weakness and wasting, no definite ataxia, sluggish tendon reflexes, absent ankle jerks, normal plantar reflexes, no loss of vibratory or position sense in feet, decreased and delayed awareness of pin pricks in legs, and no pain on squeezing of Achilles tendons. Laboratory findings: Hematocrit, 34.8 ml./100 ml.; hemoglobin, 11.5 g./100 ml.; RBCs, 4.2 million/cu. mm.; reticulocytes, 0.7 percent; erythrocyte sedimentation rate, 35; WBCs, 6800/cu. mm., with 1 percent juvenile neutrophils, 50 percent polymorphonuclear leukocytes, 1 percent eosinophils, 1 percent basophils, 40 percent lymphocytes, and 7 percent monocytes. Urine: yellow; specific gravity, 1.015; negative sugar and albumin; 3 to 7 WBC and occasional epithelial cells. Stool: Brown and guaiac negative (twice). Nonprotein nitrogen, 28 mg./100 ml.; sugar, 76 mg./100 ml.; carbon dioxide content, 29.2 mEq./liter; chloride, 100.4 mEq./liter; sodium, 140 mEq./liter; potassium, 4.0 mEq./liter; calcium, 10.7 mg./100 ml.; phosphorus, 4.1 mg./100 ml.; albumin-to-globulin ratio, 4.0:2.6; cholesterol, 210 mg./100 ml.;

cephalin cholesterol flocculation, 2+; thymol turbidity, 5.9 units; alkaline phosphatase, 2.9 King-Armstrong units; bilirubin, less than 0.8 mg./100 ml.; STS, negative. Lumbar puncture: Opening pressure, 80 mm. water; 7 RBCs/cu. mm. and no WBCs; Pandy test, 4+; protein, 388 mg./100 ml.; colloidal mastic test results (8 tubes): 2-3-3-2-2-1-1-0; sugar, 56 mg./100 ml. (blood sugar, 92 mg./100 ml.); chloride, 119 mEq./liter. Electrocardiogram: Left axis deviation and abnormal precordial transition. Chest x-rays and skull x-rays were normal. Course: On the fourteenth hospital day, an exploratory operation was done. Her subsequent course was downhill.

DISCUSSION OF THE PROBLEM

As usual, we begin consideration of this patient's problem by winnowing out those features of her illness which seem to be most pertinent.

1. She was a white female of 32 years.
2. Her illness began so insidiously that we are not even certain of the date of its inception. Did it begin two years before her admission, or actually 4 to 5 years prior to this, when she began to have peculiar knife-like, darting pains in her legs and feet?
3. The illness was long-drawn-out, lasting for at least two years, and possibly six years or even longer.
4. It became associated with profound weight loss and debility, but without fever or sweats.
5. A striking feature was three sorts of neuromuscular disorders, which may be categorized as follows: (a) symmetrical, bilateral peripheral neuritis, (b) pupillary abnormalities and failing vision, (c) muscle wasting and weakness. The profound degree of postural hypotension she developed may indicate the presence of a fourth sort of neurological disorder, which we might characterize as a do-it-yourself sympathectomy. While postural hypotension is not at all uncommon in any sort of wasting disorder, or in any disorder affecting the tone or activity of the peripheral musculature, the degree of hypotension manifested by this patient strikes me as being considerably more than one generally sees in these circumstances, and raises the possibility of some process actually affecting the sympathetic nerves and ganglia per se.
6. These neurological alterations were associated with interesting spinal fluid changes. There was considerable protein in the fluid, but no cells, and pressure was normal.
7. From a symptomatic standpoint, these features of her course stand out: (a) She had episodes of intractable vomiting lasting several days, in the absence of abdominal pain, toxicity, headache, or indications of intestinal obstruction, (b) She was beset by profound weakness and fatigue, (c) She had disabling hypotension, already described.

Now, from the standpoint of clinical analysis, it will perhaps be most rewarding if we ask what disease mechanisms are most likely to produce the type of neuromuscular alterations we have just described, in association with an extreme degree of wasting and weakness, and then see how the more minor elements of her illness fall into place as we go along.

I would categorize the mechanisms of disease which might produce these neuromuscular changes as follows:
1. A nutritional disorder.
2. A metabolic-endocrine dysfunction.
3. An infection.
4. A neoplasm.
5. A collagen-vascular disorder.
6. A granulomatous process.
7. A disorder of the reticuloendothelial tissues, in particular the plasma cell-lymphocyte axis, leading to the production of peculiar protein materials or amyloid.

Let us briefly review these categories, and see if we can ferret out those most meaningful in terms of this particular patient's illness.

When this patient was first admitted, she was considered to have a peculiar personality, and she gave a life history of "nerves." It was initially postulated that her vomiting might be psychogenic, and her neuromuscular changes secondary to malnutrition. But a number of factors militated against the likelihood of this, including the eye changes, the spinal fluid alterations, and the palpable spleen. In addition, there were none of the usual hallmarks of malnutrition, including dermatitis, keilosis, sore tongue, liver dysfunction, and so forth.

Diabetes mellitus would offer an elegant explanation for the neurological findings noted here, for of course diabetic neuropathy can exactly mimic syphilitic tabes dorsalis, but this patient did not have diabetes.

Apathetic hyperthyroidism is suggested by the description of prominent eyes, increased skin pigmentation, profound weakness, and wasting of subcutaneous fat and muscles, and also by the enlarged spleen, but the type of neurological disorder observed here is not seen in hyperthyroidism, so far as I am aware.

Adrenal insufficiency was seriously considered by those who saw her on the ward, and a number of tests were done to exclude it. However, she had the wrong sort of pigmentation, and it seems unlikely that she would have survived so long if she had had adrenal insufficiency severe enough to account for all the changes she showed. In this regard, it is perhaps significant that she had no trouble during the nephropexy operation, which might well have proved fatal had she actually had significant adrenal inadequacy. Also, the normal serum urea nitrogen and other chemical data conflict with a diagnosis of Addison's disease, and the type of neurological changes seen here do not occur in this disorder.

Porphyria is a possibility, and the pigmentation of her skin, the passage of dark urine which became darker in the sun, as well as the debility, wasting, and peripheral neuropathy, spurred a quest for porphyrins in the urine, which were not found. One might have suspected that such would be the case, what with the pupillary changes and the excessive protein in the spinal fluid, not to mention the enlarged spleen and the total absence of abdominal distress in association with the protracted vomiting.

The profound weakness and wasting which characterized this patient should early awaken one to the likelihood of some disseminated infection, such as tuberculosis or a fungus such as histoplasmosis. Such infections may be associated with postural hypotension, or with a peripheral neuropathy. However, she never had persistent fever or sweats, and the erythrocyte sedimentation rate was normal. Her chest film was reported to be clear. Finally, the abnormal pupillary responses, and the finding of protein but no cells in the spinal fluid, would be odd for any disseminated infection.

Syphilis would of course adequately explain the neurological peculiarities, but tests for syphilis in the spinal fluid and serum were all negative. Furthermore, she had never had any girdling pains in association with the spells of vomiting, and syphilis affecting the central nervous system would not offer a very good explanation for her profound constitutional reaction.

For some of the very same reasons that an infection is unlikely, malignant tumor becomes likely—namely, the presence of excessive weakness and wasting in the absence of sweats and fever. It might be argued that the patient's course was too long-drawn-out for a malignant growth, but I am convinced that tumors often have a much longer life span than is recognized by some observers. In recent years, we have become aware that tumors are not infrequently associated with myopathy, as well as with peripheral neuropathy and a variety of other neurological alterations only now beginning to be understood. The history of headaches and numbness of the left side of the body when lying on the right side suggests an intracranial mass lesion of some type or a vascular abnormality. Profound nausea and vomiting may occur in these circumstances.

Against the existence of a malignancy, however, are a number of points. First, the type of pupillary changes described here are not, to my knowledge, a part of the neuropathy of tumors. Second, a tumor invading the meninges should be associated with an increased number of cells in the spinal fluid, or decreased sugar content, or both. Neither was present here. Third, intracerebral metastases are unlikely because there were no evidences of increased pressure, or of clouding of the sensorium, or of any focal alterations whatever. The patient remained alert and bright, although there was some question of the acuteness of her memory. Finally, the history and physical examination offered no likely site of origin of a new growth. One would think of a bronchogenic carcinoma in this setting, but the lungs were clear, and she was too young for this to be a probable occurrence. Her vomiting led to suspicion of GI tract disease, but all x-rays were negative. She was too young for the usual pancreatic cancer. She had had hematuria, but the intravenous pyelograms were unremarkable. There were no significant findings in the pelvis.

She also was too young for myeloma, and there were no bone changes, no alterations in the serum proteins, or no protein in the urine. But she was in the correct age group for a lymphoma, and her spleen was enlarged. Lymphomata may implicate the spinal cord or infiltrate the meninges or, less often, appear as intracerebral mass lesions, but as we have already indicated, the kind of changes noted clinically and in the spinal fluid would not fit this particular bill.

We come now to the collagen diseases. Polyarteritis is suggested by the marked weakness and wasting, and certainly myositis and polyneuritis are common stigmata of this disorder. The enlarged spleen, the spells of hematuria, the vague pains in the legs, and the anemia are also compatible. But again, she was a relatively young female. Fever was not prominent, and it usually—but not always—is present in polyarteritis. There were no episodes of sweating, and no signs of toxicity, although she was extremely debilitated. The sedimentation rate was normal. She had no myalgias or arthralgias, nor were there any skin eruptions or nodules. There was no abdominal pain despite all the vomiting. The blood pressure was normal, and the urine was clear. The spinal fluid protein was too high for a simple, commonplace polyneuritis stemming from polyarteritis, and there were no cells to indicate an active vasculitis. There were no indications of any focal brain damage. Also, the pupillary changes would be difficult to explain on the basis of polyarteritis.

Similar and other arguments make systemic lupus erythematosus unlikely. There was no antecedent history suggesting an episodic, recurrent polysystem disorder. There was too much wasting and debility, and not enough constitutional reaction in terms of toxicity, sweats, fever, increased sedimentation rate, and so forth. There were no skin eruptions, painful joints, serositis, renal abnormalities, or serum protein peculiarities. Furthermore, peripheral neuritis is very uncommon in lupus in our experience. Focal vascular lesions in the central nervous system are seen, but when they do occur they are not usually associated with the spinal fluid alterations noted here. Lastly, the eye signs this patient manifested are not ones we have ever observed in SLE.

Sarcoidosis is a possibility not to be discarded too quickly. As already mentioned, this patient was very chronically ill, with marked weight loss, weakness, and general debility, and yet had had little or no fever or sweats or other evidences of a constitutional reaction. It is this sort of paradoxical situation which should always make one think of sarcoid. Muscle wasting was a prominent feature of this patient's illness, and of course we have learned in recent years that weakness and wasting of muscles may be the predominant changes in sarcoidosis. On the other hand, the tissues most commonly affected by sarcoid were—at the least—not obviously implicated in this patient. These include the skin, lymph glands, lungs, and liver. I am especially interested in the fact that there was no good indication of sarcoid in the liver, for many of the patients I have seen with sarcoid, who showed the severe degree of wasting and debility manifested by this patient, did have involvement of the liver.

Although I could accept the kind of spinal fluid changes noted here as perhaps being the product of a granuloma, such as sarcoid, I have never seen this disorder produce a symmetrical polyneuritis such as this patient was considered to have, nor the type of pupillary changes noted. Sarcoid usually affects the central nervous system by spreading itself about the base of the brain, involving one cranial nerve after another. Less often granulomata may coalesce in the brain substance, resulting in the effects of a mass lesion.

We come, therefore, to the final category of disease mechanisms which might produce the changes we have singled out for explanation—namely, the production of some peculiar protein material, such as macroglobulin or amyloid. As we all know, the production of such substances is thought by some to be the result of an aberration on the part of certain mononuclear cells, in particular the plasma cells. At times this disorder appears to be a secondary response to a wide variety of different agencies, most of which we have already considered in our differential diagnosis. At still other times, however, the disordered functioning of these cells has no obvious cause, and we call it "primary." There is some indication that in at least some such instances, genetic factors may be at work, since the disorder may have a familial transmission.

Failing vision, weight loss, great debility, muscle weakness, and wasting are all common features of macroglobulinemia. Peripheral neuropathy and various abnormalities of the CNS are seen. The spleen is often enlarged. Anemia is common. Bleeding into the skin, prominent in this patient, is commonplace. However, bleeding from the mucous membranes of the nose and mouth is most frequent, and this patient had no such bleeding. There were a number of other hallmarks of macroglobulinemia that were not shown by this patient. She never had joint pains or Raynaud's phenomenon. Her eye grounds did not show the telltale tortuosity and dilation of the vessels, with hemorrhages and exudates typical of the "sludged blood" of macroglobulinemia. Her blood did not form rouleaux when it was withdrawn, nor was there an increased serum globulin level. One would be hard put to explain the kind of spinal fluid changes noted here on the basis of macroglobulinemia, in which the central nervous system alterations are secondary to a vasculitis. Also, how could one explain the intractable vomiting and the extremely low blood pressure?

We come, therefore, to the inevitable conclusion that the abnormalities occurring in this young woman must have been due to very widespread distribution of amyloid.

Since amyloid may be deposited in any of the tissues of the body, an exceedingly complex variety of symptoms and signs may be associated with the disorder, and there is no typical picture. This patient's course, however, illustrates in a terrible but vivid manner many of the alterations which are frequently part of its natural history. Profound weakness, weight loss, and debility without fever or evidences of an active inflammatory reaction are common general manifestations. Purpura and bleeding into the skin and elsewhere occurs with great frequency, just as it did here. Bleeding from the urinary tract, as evidenced by this patient early in the course, is seen. Involvement of the muscles may be widespread, resulting in atrophy and weakness.

The vitreous body of the eye may be a focus of amyloid deposits, resulting in impairment of vision, as happened here. Vomiting and diarrhea may result from infiltration of the walls of the gut by amyloid, or from involvement of autonomic fibers.

Most indicative of amyloidosis in this patient were the neurological abnormalities. As we initially postulated, whatever was wrong had resulted in involvement of muscles, peripheral nerves, perhaps brain and meninges, and possibly also the sympathetic nervous system, in view of the marked degree of postural hypotension that she had. Furthermore, this had been accompanied by increased protein, but no cells, in the spinal fluid. Infiltration of amyloid into these affected tissues is one of the few ways we can imagine such a sequence of events could have been brought about. Finally, the pupillary changes stressed repeatedly in this discussion are typical of amyloidosis.

We started our discussion by wondering when this patient's illness actually began. Looking back, it probably commenced many years prior to admission, when she began to have darting, burning pains in her legs and feet. These symptoms are typical of a chronic polyneuritis, such as is produced by amyloidosis.

Having concluded that she had amyloidosis, the final matters for disposal are whether it was primary or secondary, and if primary, was it of the familial sort?

As you are well aware, in the past attempts have been made to separate out different types of amyloidosis based upon such distinctions as whether this, that, or the other organ system was or was not implicated. As knowledge of this disorder has increased, many of these distinctions have proved to be invalid and worthless. For example, in the earlier literature involvement of the pupils and the central nervous system is said to be unusual in secondary amyloidosis, but common in the familial, primary type.

We can only conclude that this patient had severe, generalized amyloidosis. Since there was no obvious associated disease at the time she was under observation, we shall call this primary amyloidosis. While there is no family history available, she was swarthy in appearance, and familial amyloidosis has most frequently been reported in those of Portuguese extraction. The changes she showed fit the descriptions of familial amyloidosis very exactly.

POST MORTEM FINDINGS

Primary amyloidosis.

REFERENCES

General

Thomas, J. E., and Schirger, A.: Orthostatic hypotension: Etiologic considerations, diagnosis and treatment. Med. Clin. N. Amer. 52:809, 1968.
Wagner, H. N., Jr.: Orthostatic hypotension. Johns Hopkins Med. J. 105:322, 1959.

Diabetes

Martin, M. M.: Diabetic neuropathy. Brain 76:594, 1953.
Rundles, R. W.: Diabetic neuropathy. Medicine 24:111, 1945.
Warren, S., and LeCompte, P. M.: The Pathology of Diabetes Mellitus. Philadelphia, Lea & Febiger, 1952.

Syphilis

Spingarn, C. L., and Hitzig, M. W.: Orthostatic circulatory insufficiency: its occurrence in tabes dorsalis and Addison's disease. Arch. Intern. Med. 69:23, 1942.
Wooften, A. C., and Diebert, A. V.: Postural hypotension in tabes dorsalis. Amer. J. Syph. 27:616, 1943.

Addison's Disease

Blizzard, R. M., Chee, D., and Davis, W.: The incidence of adrenal and other antibodies in the sera of patients with idiopathic adrenal insufficiency Clin. Exper. Immunol. 2:19, 1967.
Guttman, P. H.: Addison's disease: statistical analysis of 566 cases and study of pathology. Arch. Path. 10:742, 895; 1930.
Irvine, W. J., et al.: A clinical and immunological study of adrenocortical insufficiency (Addison's disease). Clin. Exper. Immunol. 2:31, 1967.
Tarkington, R. W., and Lebovitz, H. E.: Extra-adrenal endocrine deficiencies in Addison's disease. Amer. J. Med. 43:499, 1967.

Porphyria

Mahood, W. H., and Killough, J. H.: Acute intermittent porphyria. Ann. Intern. Med. 64:259, 1966.
Riehards, F. F., and Brinton, D.: Peripheral neuropathy and porphyria. Brain 85:657, 1962.

Sarcoidosis

Camp, W. A., and Frierson, J. G.: Sarcoidosis of central nervous system. Arch. Neurol. 7:432, 1962.
Hook, O.: Sarcoidosis with involvement of the CNS. Arch. Neurol. Psychiat. 71:554, 1954.

New Growths and the CNS

Brain, Lord R., and Norris, F. H.: The remote effects of cancer on the nervous system. Cont. Neuro. Symp. I. New York, Grune & Stratton, 1965.
Brain, R.: Neurological complications of neoplasms. Lancet 1:179, 1963.
Brain, R., and Hanson, R. A.: Neurological syndromes associated with carcinoma; the carcinomatous neuromyopathies. Lancet 2:971, 1958.
Croft, P. B., and Wilkenson, M.: Carcinomatous neuromyopathy. Lancet 1:184, 1963.
Dinsdale, H. B., and Taghary, A.: Carcinomatosis of the meninges. Canad. Med. Ass. J. 90:505, 1964.
Fischer-Williams, M., et al.: Carcinomatosis of the meninges. Brain 78:42, 1955.
Gain, G. O., and Karr, J. P.: Diffuse leptomeningeal carcinomatosis. Neurology 5:706, 1955.
Hughes, I. E., Adams, J. H., and Ibert, R. C.: Invasion of the leptomeninges by tumors; the differential diagnosis from TBC. J. Neurol. Neurosurg. Psych. 26:83, 1963.
Newman, M. K., and Gujmo, R. J.: Neuropathies, myopathies, and occult malignancies. JAMA 190:575, 1964.
Sparling, H. J., Jr., et al.: Involvement of the CNS by malignant lymphoma. Medicine 26:285, 1947.
Williams, H. M., et al.: The pathogenesis of neurological complications in patients with lymphomas and leukemia. Cancer 11:76, 1958.

Polyarteritis

Moskowitz, R. W., Baggenstoss, A. H., and Slocumb, C. H.: Histopathologic classification of periarteritis nodosa: Study of 56 cases confirmed at autopsy. Mayo Clin. Proc. 38:345, 1963.
Rose, G. A.: The natural history of polyarteritis. Brit. Med. J., 2:1148, 1957.
Rose, G. A., and Spencer, H.: Polyarteritis nodosa. Quart. J. Med. 26:43, 1957.

Systemic Lupus

Glaser, G. H.: Neurologic manifestations in collagen diseases. Neurology 5:751, 1955.

Johnson, R. T., and Richardson, E. P.: Neurological complications of systemic lupus. Medicine 47:337, 1968.

Waldenström's Macroglobulinemia

Cohen, R. J., Bohannon, R. A., and Wallerstein, R. O.: Waldenström's macroglobulinemia. Amer. J. Med. 41:271, 1966.
Darnley, J. D.: Polyneuropathy in Waldenström's macroglobulinemia. Neurology 12:617, 1962.
Dutcher, T. F., and Fahey, J. L.: Histopathology of macroglobulinemia of Waldenström. J. Nat. Cancer Inst. 22:887–917, 1959.
Forget, B. G., Squires, J. W., and Sheldon, H.: Waldenström's macroglobulinemia with generalized amyloidosis. Arch. Intern. Med. 118:363, 1966.
Waldenstrom, J.: Macroglobulinemia in immunological diseases. M. Samter (Ed.). Boston, Little, Brown & Co., 1965.

Amyloidosis

Alruzzo, J. L.: Amyloidosis—A study of its pathogenesis. Arthritis Rheum. 14:457, 1971.
Andrade, C., et al.: Hereditary amyloidosis. Arthritis Rheum. 13:902, 1970.
Barth, W. F., et al.: Primary amyloidosis—15 patients. Amer. J. Med. 47:259, 1969.
Brandt, K., Cathcart, E. S., and Cohen, A. S.: Clinical analysis of course and prognosis of 42 patients with amyloidosis. Amer. J. Med. 44:955, 1968.
Calkins, E., and Cohen, A. S.: Diagnosis of amyloidosis. Bull. Rheum. Dis. 10:215, 1960.
Chambers, R. A., et al.: Primary amyloidosis with reference to CNS. Quart. J. Med. 27:207, 1958.
Klyle, R. A., and Bayrd, E. D.: "Primary" systemic amyloidosis and myeloma. Arch. Intern. Med. 107:344, 1961.
Mahloudji, M., et al.: The genetic amyloidoses; with particular reference to hereditary neuropathic amyloidosis. Medicine 48:1, 1969.
Rukavina, J. G., et al.: Primary systemic amyloidosis, a review of 28 cases with emphasis on familial form. Medicine 35:239, 1956.
Sullivan, J. F., et al.: Amyloid polyneuropathy. Neurology 5:847, 1955.
Wiernik, P. H.: Amyloid joint disease. Medicine 51:465, 1972.

Hyperthyroidism

Chapman, E. M., and Maloof, F.: Bizarre clinical presentations of hyperthyroidism. New Eng. J. Med. 254:1, 1956.
Hidden hyperthyroidism. Lancet 4:386, 1970.
Millikan, C. H., and Haines, S. F.: Thyroid gland in relation to neuromuscular disease. Arch. Intern. Med. 92:5, 1953.
Solomon, D. H., and Chopka, I. J.: Graves' disease, 1972. Mayo Clin. Proc. 47:801, 1972.
Solomon, D. H., et al.: Hyperthyroidism. Ann. Intern. Med. 69:1015, 1968.
Symposium on Graves' disease. Mayo Clin. Proc. 47:801, 1972.

P   A PATIENT WITH CHRONIC UREMIA

THE CLINICAL PROBLEM

This 47 year old white male research chemist with a history of known chronic renal disease was admitted to the chronic hemodialysis program. At age 18, the patient had had a "strep throat," which was followed by the appearance of very dark urine. At age 21, he experienced an episode of grossly bloodly urine and was told he had red cell casts. A second such episode occurred later that year. Over the next 20 years (1943 to 1963), examinations revealed intermittent red cells and red cell casts, but the blood pressure remained normal and there was no known increase in serum urea nitrogen, no edema, and no depression of serum albumin. In 1963, the patient began to have headaches, and epistaxis and one syncopal episode occurred. He consulted his physician, who told him his blood pressure was 250/140. Over the succeeding five years, he was given a variety of antihypertensive medications, with steadily decreasing results. He also had a recurrent mild pedal edema, for which he had been given Esidrix and Aldactone on different occasions. As late as early 1968, the serum urea nitrogen was between 25 and 30 mg./100 ml. During the five weeks prior to admission, he had intermittent and progressive vomiting, frequently bilious, but not blood-tinged. He also had intermittent episodes of loose but not watery diarrhea, without melena. On admission, the patient was seen to be a well developed, well nourished white male in no distress. Pulse, 80; respirations, 16; no fever; blood pressure, 165/95. Skin: Uremic frost reported by one observer. Fundi showed moderate arteriolar narrowing, no hemorrhages or exudates; discs were flat. The pharynx showed no inflammation. The neck was supple. There was dullness at lung bases; few rales at left base. The point of maximal impulse was almost in anterior axillary line. Loud to-and-fro pericardial rub was heard. The liver was down 3 cm. below the costal margin and tender. The spleen was not felt. There was no edema, and pulses were good. No cyanosis or clubbing was present. Normal results on neurological examination. On admission, these findings were recorded: hematocrit, 26.5 ml./100 ml.; WBCs, 13,300, with 6 percent juvenile neutrophils, 88 percent segmented neutrophils, 1 percent eosinophils, 5 percent lymphocytes; serum urea nitrogen, 282 mg./100 ml.; sugar, 147 mg./100 ml.; carbon dioxide content, 20.7 mEq./liter; chloride, 83 mEq./liter; sodium, 143 mEq./liter; potassium, 5.5 mEq./liter; calcium, 8.6 mg./100 ml.; alkaline phosphatase, 10.4 King-Armstrong units; total protein, 6.5 g./100 ml.; albumin, 3.1 g./100 ml.; serum glutamic oxaloacetic transaminase, 87 Karmen units/ml.; phosphate, 20.2 mg./100 ml.; uric acid, 23.4 mg./100 ml.; creatinine, 15.5 mg./100 ml.; amylase, 215 Somogyi units/100 ml. Urinalysis not recorded, apparently because the urine output was extremely low. Hemodialysis was carried out, with the following pre- and postdialysis values recorded: serum urea nitrogen, 339 mg./100 ml.; falling to 107 mg./100 ml.; potassium, 5.8 mEq./liter, falling to 3.8 mEq./liter; carbon dioxide content, 14.5 mEq./liter, rising to 16.3 mEq./liter; creatinine, falling from 15.5 to 11.3 mg./100 ml.; hematocrit, 25.5 ml./100 ml., rising to 31 ml./100 ml. Weight loss: 2.8 kg. Blood pressure: 190/85, rising to 190/90. During dialysis, the patient developed an irregular cardiac rhythm, which proved to be a multifocal atrial tachycardia on ECG. The following day, a second dialysis was performed, during the course of which he sat up, vomited, became hypotensive (90/60 to 90/40), and had a grand mal seizure. He was thereafter placed on phenobarbital and Dilantin, and the seizures did not recur. Blood pressure recovered spontaneously and was recorded as 180/70 at the end of dialysis. Following the third dialysis, the patient complained of some slight anterior chest pain differing from that he had experienced before. Blood pressure was maintained at the same level. The neck veins were flat. The heart sounds were distant. No pericardial rub was heard. Shortly afterward, the patient became unresponsive and died.

DISCUSSION OF THE PROBLEM

Whatever else may have been wrong with this patient's health, it seems incontrovertible that he was uremic when admitted. It is exceedingly important to develop a well organized clinical approach to the patient with uremia, now that measures are available which can, in certain circumstances, completely reverse uremia, or at least bring it under control for prolonged periods.

In general, the following categories of disease may be causative in inducing the uremic state:

1. Extrarenal factors, including: dehydration, anoxia, hypotension and shock, anemia of a severe degree, acute hemorrhage, electrolyte imbalances.
2. Obstruction to the out-flow of urine.
3. Obstruction of blood flow to or from the kidney, occurring extrarenally.
4. The use of some drug or toxin, and one might include here hemolytic processes.
5. Intrarenal factors, and these are further subdivided into diffuse or focal parenchymal alterations.

Let us analyze the course of this patient's illness in terms of these categories, and see what develops. In making such an analysis, we must give particular attention to those factors affording therapeutic opportunities.

First, extrarenal factors: these very commonly exaggerate the effects of some pre-existing renal abnormality, causing a well compensated renal disease to decompensate. Often they are so readily correctible that it is a shame that they are overlooked. In this day, when a variety of highly potent diuretics are being employed lavishly, but frequently unwisely, water and electrolyte imbalances are among the very first items to be carefully checked. However, in this patient's illness, a review of the data we are given does not support the role of any such extrarenal factors.

The next category is obstruction to urine out-flow. This is another category to be given special attention, because such obstruction not infrequently is present in settings in which it is least anticipated. I recall a black female patient who died in uremia, we thought because of chronic pyelonephritis. Now, pyelonephritis is often too ready an explanation for renal insufficiency in females. In this instance, we failed to heed the historical item that several years before her death, she had been given pelvic radiation for some gynecological condition. At post mortem examination, her uremia was discovered to be due to ureteral obstruction secondary to radiation fibrosis. There was no pyelonephritis. It is important to emphasize the fact that this unfortunate lady had no symptoms whatever indicative of obstruction, and that she continued to the very end to have an appreciable output of urine. Failure to realize that obstructive uremia can exist in the face of a sizeable urinary output, and in the absence of any of the classical accompaniments of a renal blockage, were features which misled us, and which will continue to mislead others.

While the history of the patient we are now considering indicates some type of very long-standing parenchymal renal disease, we must not forget that patients with hitherto well handled parenchymal renal disease may subsequently develop some obstructive process, such as renal calculi or prostatism, which may tip the balance. Sometimes, in dealing with such problems, it is wise to catheterize the ureters, even though the evidence at hand weighs against obstruction. For often one can't be certain.

I believe this was just such a situation, for the striking feature of this patient's long-drawn-out illness is the fact that he somewhat abruptly developed profound uremia, although he was known to have had some sort of renal disease for many years. It is possible that two elements were producing his end-stage uremia: (1) some chronic intrarenal disorder, and (2) an obstructive process which might have been remediable. The information we have simply does not positively exclude such a sequence.

So far as renotoxic agents are concerned, there was no history of their ingestion. In this regard, however, one has to take a meticulous history, for today drugs are prescribed with such abandon. Also, the patient may be taking a drug for some condition so unrelated to his kidneys, in his judgment, that he doesn't bother to mention it. Two common examples of this not rare phenomenon are ergosterol poisoning, the ergosterol being taken for arthritis, and the milk-alkali syndrome in the chronic dyspeptic patient.

Extrarenal obstruction to the flow of blood to or from the kidneys is another category demanding most thoughtful analysis because specific therapeutic measures are available—an operation or anticoagulants, whichever the case may be.

It is essential to appreciate the fact that extrarenal obstruction to blood flow to and from the kidneys can suddenly complicate the course in patients who have a variety of long-standing parenchymal disorders of the kidney. Thus, Dr. Carlos Hamilton and I described the development of renal vein thrombosis in a patient with chronic renal lupus. I will never forget a delightful physician-friend who had chronic glomerulonephritis, well compensated. Abruptly, his compensation broke, he developed marked hypertension, and he subsequently died with uremia. The final clinical diagnosis was end-stage glomerular disease. However, post mortem examination disclosed how important it is always to challenge the most obvious diagnosis. My friend was found to have unilateral renal artery obstruction, of recent origin, in addition to chronic glomerulonephritis. Surgical correction might have been feasible.

Obviously, a similar event is suggested here, for after 20 years of well handled renal disease without hypertension or nitrogen retention, this patient developed a marked degree of hypertension, and then, at a later date, abruptly developed uremia.

As far as the diagnosis of renal vein thrombosis is concerned, I have found it impossible to secure for myself diagnostic criteria which are consistently helpful, for this lesion is being described as present in instances in which it actually does not exist. For example, I once saw a youngster with the nephrotic syndrome. Special x-ray studies were interpreted as showing unequivocal renal vein thrombosis, although at post mortem none was found. It's comforting, though disconcerting, to realize that radiologists aren't infallible, either.

All one can say is that the classical features of renal vein thrombosis were not present here, but I'm sure that they often are not, despite the presence of this abnormality. However, one should not dismiss this possibility altogether, since this patient may have died suddenly as the result of pulmonary embolus, as we shall shortly discuss, and pulmonary embolization is not infrequently the first presentation of renal vein thrombosis.

However, from the facts we are given, if this patient had an extrarenal vascular obstruction, it seems more likely to me that it was in the arterial rather than the venous component of the circulation. In considering renal arterial obstruction, one must include such agencies as renal emboli associated with bacterial endocarditis, mural thrombi, myxoma, marantic endocarditis, pieces of arteriosclerotic plaques, and so forth, but there is no evidence for any of these.

Before leaving this category of vascular blockage, we should include an uncommon cause of such blockage which may take place in either the arterial or the venous circulation, although more often venous—namely, renal carcinoma. Such tumors are well known to invade and grow through the renal arteries and veins, even sometimes spreading across the vena cava to implicate the vessels of the opposite kidney. Pulmonary embolization is a not rare accompaniment of such events. Certainly, this patient with 20 years of chronic renal disease could have died as a result of unexpected development of renal carcinoma. I don't see how we can reasonably say more than that this is one additional mechanism of renovascular obstruction, favored diagnostically by those clinicians who like to reach for a fast curve ball.

In analyzing renal parenchymal factors, I like to follow the diagnostic legacy of Dr. Louis Hamman, and divide such factors into (1) those which affect the kidneys focally, and (2) those which affect the kidneys diffusely.

It should be said at the outset that this clinical differentiation is of only limited value because not infrequently, diffuse and focal processes may present in exactly similar clinical guises, and, furthermore, a process which starts focally may terminate diffusely. Pyelonephritis would be a typical example. We are all well aware that even the pathologists, with all the advantages and "security" their microscopes provide, not too rarely can only tell us that a kidney is "end-stage," the origin of the nonspecific alterations remaining obscure, and if the pathologists sometimes have trouble in making such diagnoses, we clinicians should feel fortunate indeed that we are ever correct.

The typical clinical setting of focal renal disease is one in which the patient, despite varying degrees of renal insufficiency, is able to get along well for at times surprisingly long periods of time, voiding a urine which while not normal, is not particularly abnormal in terms of casts, and so forth. The classical example of such a focal disease would be cystic disease of the kidneys. The kidneys of patients with this condition cannot maintain normal function, but they may function well enough to sustain the patients for a very long period, and the urine they produce is the product of relatively normal glomeruli.

In contrast, the patient with diffuse disease, once renal insufficiency has developed, tends to become progressively worse, and his urine is "sick" because it is the product of more or less diffusely affected glomeruli.

If we apply these criteria to this patient, it seems most likely to me that he had a diffuse form of nephritis, because his urine consistently contained RBC casts, and once he developed hypertension and nitrogen retention, his condition rapidly deteriorated.

One might well argue that the 20 year period of relatively good health this patient enjoyed despite renal changes favors the presence of some sort of focal disease. The history we are given of the repeated episodes of gross bleeding from the kidneys, and the onset of hypertension and renal failure at age 40, should make one think of polycystic kidneys. On the other hand, the persistent presence of RBC casts must be unusual in polycystic disease, although I understand it can occur, and so also would be the five year period of hypertension without nitrogen retention, and the abrupt onset of uremia.

In reviewing intrarenal factors, it is imperative that one dwell on those for which some sort of specific therapy may be available. Included in this category are: milk-alkali syndrome, collagen-vascular disease, hyperparathyroidism, myeloma, some infectious process, and gout. In reviewing these, the only one at all supported by available clinical evidence is *hyperparathyroidism,* for his calcium level was consistently maintained at a normal range despite a markedly elevated serum phosphorus.

But, peculiar things can happen to calcium and phosphorus relationships in chronic renal failure, because of compensatory responses of the parathyroid glands, and weird changes in serum calcium and phosphorus levels can be enormously hard to interpret correctly. Certainly, other features of hyperparathyroidism were never present during his prolonged illness, such as dyspeptic complaints, evidences of osteoporosis, renal calculi, excessive neuromuscular weakness, and psychological changes.

The most reasonable explanation for the renal parenchymal changes seems to be active chronic glomerulonephritis, in view of the history of sore throat followed by episodes of hematuria, associated with persistent showering of RBC and RBC casts in the urine.

If this patient had active chronic glomular disease, why did he handle it so well and so long, then abruptly fall into a progressive, irreversible state, with hypertension and uremia? We have already suggested the possibility of some complicating development such as renal vascular occlusion or an obstruction to urinary out-flow.

On the other hand, this kind of behavior is sometimes just the nature of the disorder. Whereas, as pointed out by Thomas Addis, patients with chronic glomerulonephritis who fail to recover generally progress so slowly and gradually into renal failure that they are often unaware of what has happened, in a small number of instances, renal decompensation can begin precipitously in patients who apparently have handled their disease admirably for years, as did this patient. Also, as we have perhaps only recently appreciated, although it was recognized by others for years, re-exacerbations of acute nephritis may occur, sometimes late in life, and not infrequently in guises which do not at all suggest an acute process, even to the extent of there being no dramatic changes in the urine.

We must not overlook the fact that five years before death the patient developed pronounced elevation of the blood pressure, and, of course, hypertension may take over the "driver's seat" in chronic nephritis, and, in association with vascular alterations, dominate subsequent happenings. But this patient's eye grounds were not described as showing the changes that generally accompany malignant hypertension, and when he was admitted to the hospital, his diastolic pressure was only mildly elevated. I don't think the facts incriminate a diffuse, progressive arteritis or a pheochromocytoma, for he had not lost weight.

We turn now to a consideration of this patient's sudden death. As you well know, sudden death generally results from some sort of a cardiovascular incident which abruptly renders the heart incapable of maintaining a forward circulation. Included are an acute arrhythmia, myocardial infarction, rupture of the heart or a major vessel, pulmonary embolus, and cardiac tamponade.

Do we have any data favoring the likelihood of any of these? Yes, we do:

1. He had a very sensitive myocardium, moving from one rhythm to another. Several factors could have played a role in this. He was being dialyzed, and shifts in water and electrolyte levels occasioned by this process may lead to arrhythmias. He had an enlarged heart, and there was a history of some chest pain. Myocardial ischemia may have supervened. An acute myocarditis may accompany flare-ups of acute nephritis. Certainly, it is not hard to find reasons why he may have died as the result of a sudden dysrhythmia.

2. He had had two hypotensive episodes and a seizure. Although seizures are not rare in renal dialysis, we have learned that both of these phenomena are very often the sole presentations of a pulmonary embolus. Also, he was described as being very restless and apprehensive, and he developed discomfort in his chest, which had not been present before. Of course, a patient with chronic uremia and heart failure is a sitting duck for pulmonary embolization.

3. These same events point to an acute myocardial infarction, but the ECG hadn't indicated any change, the quality of the heart sounds had remained good, and his cardiac failure had not worsened.

4. When this patient was admitted, he was described as having distended neck veins, dullness at the left base, distant heart sounds, and a pericardial friction rub which subsequently vanished. He had a pulsus paradoxus. He described a tight feeling in his chest. He also had intractable hiccups, which, while they are exceedingly common in uremia, are also observed in pericardial disease. Could his seizure and hypotension have been the result of cardiac tamponade accompanying massive pericardial effusion? We have recognized for years the frequency with which pericardial effusions accompany uremia, but only rather recently have we become aware of the fact that at times these effusions reach such large proportions that cardiac tamponade and death ensue. Such effusions are frequently overlooked in these circumstances. Against this eventuality in this instance is the fact that the patient did not develop a significant tachycardia, a usual accompaniment of tamponade, and the physician who saw the patient terminally observed that the neck veins were not distended.

5. Finally, because this patient was chronically ill and was being dialyzed, the possibility of overwhelming sepsis should be given consideration, but for this we have no evidence whatever.

I believe the clinical data we are given best support the presence of some sort of diffuse renal disease, most likely active chronic glomerulonephritis. For the reasons already presented, a focal process such as polycystic disease deserves notation, but seems much less likely. The changes in the calcium and phosphorus should make one think of hyperparathyroidism, but I suspect these were secondary and not primary phenomena. The abrupt worsening of this patient's well handled chronic renal disorder should make one ask if some new elements were not now at work, in particular, a renovascular obstruction or an obstruction to urinary out-flow. Because of therapeutic potentials, these all should have been thoroughly investigated, and perhaps they were. Not being provided with any impelling evidence for the existence of any of these complicating mechanisms, it seems most reasonable to conclude that his active chronic process abruptly re-exacerbated.

The patient's sudden death was most likely the result of pulmonary embolus, although from an immediate and highly effective therapeutic standpoint, a cardiac tamponade could have been present, and should have been most vigorously excluded. But for the assurance, by the assistant resident who saw this patient before death, that the neck veins were flat, massive, pericardial effusion with tamponade would be my first diagnostic choice.

POST MORTEM FINDINGS

Severe, acute, and organizing fibrinous pericarditis. Pericardial hemorrhage and effusion. Chronic edema of lungs. Bronchopneumonia. Chronic glomerulonephritis, post-streptococcal (?). Renal cell carcinoma, left kidney. Generalized arterio- and arteriolosclerosis, coronary sclerosis. Left ventricular hypertrophy. Chronic congestion of the liver. Secondary hyperplasia of parathyroids. Focal osteitis cystica.

REFERENCES

General

Clark, J. E., and Bluemle, C. W., Jr.: Symposium on diseases of the kidney. Med. Clin. N. Amer. 47:837, 1963.
Franklin, J. S.: Uremia; newer concepts in pathogenesis and diagnosis. Med. Clin. N. Amer. 54:411, 1970.
Franklin, S. S., and Merrill, J. P.: Cause of death in acute renal failure. New Eng. J. Med. 262:711, 761; 1960.
Heptinstall, R. H.: Pathology of end-stage kidney disease. Amer. J. Med. 44:656, 1968.
Merrill, J. P., and Hampers, C. L.: Uremia. New Eng. J. Med. 282:953, 1014; 1970.
Schreiner, G. E., and Maher, J. F.: Uremia: The Biochemistry, Pathogenesis and Treatment. Springfield, Ill., Charles C Thomas, 1961.
Welt, L. G., et al.: Symposium on uremic toxins. Arch. Intern. Med. 126:773, 1970.

Glomerulonephritis

Addis, T.: Glomerulonephritis. New York, The Macmillan Company, 1948.
Addis, T.: Haemorrhagic Bright's disease: natural history. Bull. Johns Hopkins Hosp. 49:203, 1931.
Cameron, J. S.: Bright's disease today: the pathogenesis and treatment of glomerulonephritis, Brit. Med. J. 1:87, 1972.
Cohen, J. A., and Levitt, M. F.: Acute glomerulonephritis with few urinary abnormalities. New Eng. J. Med. 268:749, 1963.
Dixon, F. J.: The pathogenesis of glomerulonephritis. Amer. J. Med. 44:493, 1968.
Ellis, A.: Natural history of Bright's disease: clinical, histological and experimental observations. Lancet 1:1, 1942.
Schwartz, W. B., and Kassirer, J. P.: Clinical aspects of acute glomerulonephritis. In Diseases of the Kidney. M. B. Strauss and L. G. Welt (Eds.). Boston, Little, Brown & Co., 1963, p. 285.

Water and Electrolytes

Schwartz, W. B., and Relman, A. S.: Effects of electrolyte disorders on renal structure and function. New Eng. J. Med. 276:383, 452; 1967.
Windhager, E. E.: Kidney, water and electrolytes. Ann. Rev. Physiol. 31:117, 1969.

Drugs and Toxins

Bauer, J., and Freyberg, R. H.: Vitamin D intoxication with metastatic calcification. JAMA 130:1208, 1946.
DeLuca, H. F.: Vitamin D. New Eng. J. Med. 281:1103, 1969.
Gault, M. H., et al.: Syndromes associated with the abuse of analgesics. Ann. Intern. Med. 68:906, 1968.
Kessler, E.: Hypercalcemia and renal insufficiency secondary to excessive milk and alkali intake. Ann. Intern. Med. 42:324, 1955.
McMillan, D. E., and Freeman, R. B.: The milk-alkali syndrome—study of acute disorder with comments on chronic condition. Medicine 44:485, 1965.
Schreiner, G. E., and Maher, J. F.: Toxic nephropathy. Amer. J. Med. 38:409, 1965.
Tumulty, P. A., and Howard, J. E.: Irradiated ergosterol poisoning. JAMA 119:233, 1942.

Ureteral Obstruction

Alpert, L. I.: Retroperitoneal fibrosis associated with reticulum cell carcinoma. Gastroenterology 62:111, 1972.
Gelford, G. J., et al.: Retroperitoneal fibrosis and methysergide. Radiology 88:976, 1967.
Harbrecht, P. J.: Variants of retroperitoneal fibrosis. Ann. Surg. 165:388, 1967.
Jones, J. H., et al.: Retroperitoneal fibrosis. Amer. J. Med. 48:203, 1970.

Longmire, W. P., et al.: Management of sclerosing fibrosis of the mediastinal and retroperitoneal areas. Ann. Surg. *165:*1013, 1967.

Ormond, J. K.: Bilateral ureteral obstruction due to envelopment and compression by an inflammatory process. J. Urol. *59:*1072, 1948.

Utz, D. C., and Henry, J. D.: Retroperitoneal fibrosis. Med. Clin. N. Amer. *50:*1091, 1966.

Renal Vein Thrombosis

Hamilton, C. R., and Tumulty, P. A.: Renal vein thrombosis in systemic lupus. JAMA *206:*2315, 1968.

McCarthy, L. J., et al.: Bilateral renal vein thrombosis and the nephrotic syndrome in adults. Ann Intern. Med. *58:*837, 1963.

Rosenmann, G., Pollack, V. E., and Pirani, C. L.: Renal vein thrombosis: clinical and pathologic study based on renal biopsies. Medicine *47:*269, 1968.

Renal Ischemia

Eliot, R. S., Kanjuh, V. I., and Edwards, J. E.: Atheromatous embolism. Circulation *30:*611, 1964.

Florez, C. M.: Arterial occlusions produced by emboli from eroded aortic atheromatous plaques. Amer. J. Path. *21:*549, 1945.

Glenn, J. F., and Anderson, E. E.: Reversible renovascular hypertension. Ann. Rev. Med. *18:*219, 1967.

Howard, J. E.: Hypertension as related to renal ischemia. Circulation *29:*657, 1964.

Non-bacterial thrombotic endocarditis (marantic). Brit. Med. J. *3:*5, 1971.

Stamey, T. A., et al.: Functional characteristics of renovascular hypertension. Medicine *40:*347, 1961.

Wooley, C. F., et al.: Nonbacterial thrombotic endocarditis. Arch. Intern. Med. *125:*126, 1970.

Hypernephroma

Berger, L., and Sinkoh, M. W.: Systemic manifestations of hypernephroma: a review of 273 cases. Amer. J. Med. *22:*791, 1957.

Kiely, J. M.: Hypernephroma: the internist's tumor. Med. Clin. N. Amer. *50:*1067, 1966.

Pinals, R. S., and Krane, S. M.: Medical aspects of renal carcinoma. Postgrad. Med. J. *38:*507, 1962.

Polycystic Disease

Dalgaard, O. Z.: Bilateral polycystic disease of the kidneys: a follow-up of 284 patients. Acta Med. Scand. *158:*1, 1957.

Higgins, C. C.: Bilateral polycystic kidney disease: review of 94 cases. Arch. Surg. *65:*318, 1953.

Osteoporosis

Anderson, W. W., et al.: Subtotal parathyroidectomy in azotemic renal osteodystrophy. New Eng. J. Med. *268:*575, 1963.

Howard, J. E., et al.: Clinical disorders of calcium homeostasis. Medicine *42:*25, 1963.

Stanburg, S. W.: Bone disease in uremia. Amer. J. Med. *44:*714, 1968.

Uremic Pericarditis

Alfrey, A. C., et al.: Uremic hemopericardium. Amer. J. Med. *45:*391, 1968.

Beaudry, C., et al.: Uremic pericarditis and cardiac tamponade in chronic renal failure. Ann. Intern. Med. *64:*990, 1966.

Connty, C. M., et al.: Pericarditis in chronic uremia and its sequelae. Ann. Intern. Med. *75:*173, 1971.

Hager, E. B.: Clinical observations on five patients with uremic pericardial tamponade. New Eng. J. Med. *273:*304, 1965.

Pulmonary Embolism

McDonald, J. G., et al.: Major pulmonary embolism, a correlation of clinical findings, haemodynamics, pulmonary arteriography and pathological physiology. Brit. Heart J. *34:*356, 1972.

Q A PATIENT WITH SYSTEMIC LUPUS AND COMPLICATIONS

THE CLINICAL PROBLEM

This was the eighth admission for this 54 year old Cuban divorcee who had a 24 hour history of headache, nausea, vomiting, and general malaise. An aunt had had kidney disease, one sister had rheumatoid arthritis, and another had some type of severe anemia. Several female relatives had deformities of the distal interphalangeal joints of the hands. The patient had had frequent sore throats and occasional pains in her knee joints as a child. She was allergic to penicillin. The patient developed the nephrotic syndrome in 1958. A renal biopsy was compatible with SLE and strongly positive LE cell test results were obtained. In 1964, because of pleuritic chest pain, polyarthritis, and a malar skin rash, she was admitted to The Johns Hopkins Hospital and was followed here subsequently. These features, in association with continued proteinuria, dominated her clinical course from that time on, with an additional problem emerging in 1967 in terms of hypertension and congestive heart failure. In the spring of 1969, she presented with pericarditis and an increase in the urinary abnormalities thought to be associated with an exacerbation of her SLE. Prednisone therapy was increased to 30 mg. daily. She complained of irregular night sweats and of a 35 pound weight loss over the past year. For two months, she had a rash about her neck and increasing blurring of vision. One week prior to admission, she developed pain and swelling in her metacarpophalangeal and proximal interphalangeal joints. Frontal and occipital headaches plagued her. Increasing shortness of breath on exertion and some orthopnea and paroxysmal nocturnal dyspnea were noted. Temperature, 102.6 degrees; pulse, 93 regular; blood pressure, 240/100; weight, 125 pounds. She appeared chronically ill, with Cushing-like changes. Eyes showed marked periorbital edema, dense central cataracts, and questionably elevated disc margins. Skin revealed a maculopapular rash over the posterior neck. Chest was dull to percussion over both posterior basilar lung fields, and rales were heard over both lower lobes. Heart showed a left ventricular heave at the apex, and a right ventricular lift along the left sternal border. Point of maximal intensity: 12 cm. to the left of the midline in the fifth left intercostal space. A systolic ejection murmur was heard along the lower sternal border. The abdomen was nontender. The spleen was palpated a few centimeters below the costal margin. The fingers showed malformed distal interphalangeal joints. There was 4+ pitting edema of the lower legs and presacrum. Neurological examination: normal. Hematocrit, 26 ml./100 ml.; WBCs, 8300/cu. mm., with shift to the left; erythrocyte sedimentation rate, 54 mm. in 1 hr.; platelets, 112,000/cu. mm. Urine: protein, 4+; negative sugar and acetone; RBCs, 8 to 10/24 hr., 2 to 4 WBCs/24 hr., and numerous hyaline casts. Sodium, 133 mEq./liter; potassium, 4.8 mEq./liter; carbon dioxide content, 20 mEq./liter; serum urea nitrogen, 38 mg./100 ml.; glucose, 72 mg./100 ml. Lumbar puncture: clear, colorless, no cells, normal sugar and protein. An ECG showed changes of the Wolff-Parkinson-White syndrome. Initial treatment consisted of prednisone, chlorthiazide, digoxin, guanethidine, and ampicillin, which was soon discontinued, when initial urine culture was found to be negative. Bronchial breath sounds were noted over both lower lobes, with spotty egophony. She continued to have watery diarrhea. An erythematous rash extended over the shoulders and neck, and she developed nasal bridge erythema. On October 12, though febrile, with a temperature of 100.2 degrees, she appeared better. All blood cultures were negative. There were 2+ protein, numerous large granular casts, and many RBCs and WBCs noted in the urine. Hematocrit, 23.5 ml./100 ml.; WBCs, 3300/cu. mm.; platelets, 82,000/cu. mm. Bone marrow aspirate on October 23 contained many cells, with normal erythrocyte and leukocyte maturation and megakaryocytes present. Peripheral smear showed burr cells, helmet cells, and teardrop forms. Creatinine clearance was 10 ml/min. Barium enema on October 24 demonstrated a few diverticula, and an upper GI series showed a small hiatus hernia. On October 28, hematocrit readings were still in between 20 and 25 ml./100 ml., with 2 percent reticulocytes, and the serum was Coomb's negative. Serum urea nitrogen had risen to 59 mg./100 ml., potassium to 6.3 mEq./liter. By October 30, prednisone was increased to 80 mg./day. Further therapy included a low-sodium, 30 gm. protein, 1500 cc. fluid diet, but on November 5, serum urea nitrogen was 95 mg./100 ml., and the patient remained edematous. Diarrhea recurred. Urine culture showed greater than 100,000 *E. coli*, which was treated with tetracycline. On November 10, three days after digoxin had been withheld, there was a sudden onset of precordial pain, which radiated to both shoulders and down the left arm, and the patient developed marked dyspnea and orthopnea. X-ray showed a right middle lobe infiltrate. On November 21, prednisone was increased to 150 mg. daily. Serum urea nitrogen was 240 mg./100 ml. She developed Kussmaul's respirations and bled from multiple mucous membrane sites. Serum urea nitrogen rose to 320 mg./100 ml. On November 27, she suddenly developed severe abdominal pain. The abdomen showed both direct and rebound tenderness and no bowel sounds. A nasogastric tube returned "dark blood." She died quietly the next evening after having apparently gone to sleep.

DISCUSSION OF THE PROBLEM

Beyond any doubt, this patient had SLE, for the course of her illness was altogether typical of this disorder in that it was chronic, occurred in episodes, and involved a variety of organ systems, sometimes singly and sometimes in confusing combinations.

There are, of course, other disorders which are chronic and episodic, and which may involve multiorgan systems. Included are the other so-called collagen disorders, sarcoidosis, lymphomas, granulomatous infections, Whipple's disease, amyloidosis, Crohn's disease, dysproteinemic states, and Mediterranean fever, to name but a few.

But here we get help from the serological tests which were done: LE cells were found, there was a significant elevation of antinuclear titer, and at times the serum complement was reduced. This combination of changes is unique for lupus.

Also, in deriving the diagnosis of SLE, it is helpful to search the family history, for there is some evidence that lupus may be an inherited disorder of peculiar immune reactivity, which expresses itself, in different members of a family, in various clinical guises and in response to different antigenic triggers. In some instances, the trigger appears to be an infection, and in others it is the administration of some drug or serum product, an elective operation, pregnancy, a traumatic accident, or even a stressful psychological disturbance. It is interesting to note that this patient's aunt had kidney disease, a sister had rheumatoid arthritis, and another sister had a severe unexplained anemia.

Sadly, while this patient's long-drawn-out illness allowed her to have some periods of relatively good health, its relentless progression eventually led to her death. Our task is to determine the precise nature of her death. In this regard, it is helpful to categorize the several ways in which death may terminate the course of SLE. These are 10 in number:

1. Fulminant, uncontrolled exacerbations of the disease, marked by high fever, excessive tachycardia, and profound prostration and toxicity, a so-called "lupus crisis." Interestingly, when such patients come to post mortem examination, there may be surprisingly little seen in the way of structural changes. As Dr. Morgan Berthrong once said in discussing such a patient, "It is as if this patient died not of detectable structural damage, but rather of some poorly understood biologic alterations."

2. The second mode of death is that resulting from irreversible structural injury to essential organs, such as the brain, the heart, the kidneys, or the lungs, either singly or in combination.

3. Occasionally, the disease may assume the clinical and histological features of a fulminant polyarteritis, the larger arteries undergoing necrosis, thrombosis, aneurysm formation, or rupture, in a more or less generalized fashion.

4. The various elements of the blood may be profoundly and irreversibly affected, with progressive anemia, thrombocytopenia, and depression of the white blood cell count, alone or in combination.

5. It is essential to realize that a very large percentage of patients with lupus do not die as a direct result of lupus at all, but rather succumb to some type of uncontrolled infectious process. For example, of 40 patients with lupus whom I studied several years ago, autopsies revealed that 30 percent died not primarily of lupus, but of some complicating infection. The importance of remembering this cannot be overestimated. Such infections may be either focal or generalized in nature. While many types of organisms may cause them,

so-called "opportunistic" infections are particularly common, especially if the patient is receiving long-term steroid therapy or anti-immune agents.

6. Some deaths result from complications of therapy, such as a ruptured peptic ulcer, recognition of which may be obscure by the anti-inflammatory effects of the steroids.

7. Failure to manage the patient properly. For example, a precipitous reduction in the dosage of steroids may cause a sudden flare-up of the disease, perhaps an uncontrollable one, or some agent such as an antibiotic may be given needlessly, causing the subsequent development of a drug hypersensitivity state which may precipitate a serious exacerbation of the disorder.

8. Amyloidosis may become a complicating feature, although this is not common.

9. Pulmonary embolism may terminate the illness, as it does so commonly in any kind of chronic, debilitating disorder, especially when associated with fever, anemia, alterations in the serum proteins, fluid retention, heart failure, and uremia. Years ago, Dr. William Osler referred to lobar pneumonia as "the old man's friend." Today, the "friend" more often than not is a pulmonary embolus.

10. Finally, we learned long ago, and in the usual hard way, that every event in the health of a patient with lupus is not necessarily related directly to lupus. As in any long-drawn-out illness, the patient with lupus is heir to any of the disorders which may plague man. The clinician has to constantly remember this and challenge each new event with the question—is this new happening due to lupus, or is it due to some other process?

For example, we once followed the clinical course of a young woman with lupus who began to have convulsive seizures, a not uncommon event in SLE. We concluded this new development was part of the parent disorder. Subsequently, at post mortem, a meningioma was found.

Now, as our next step in diagnosis, let's examine this patient's total course, and see which of these 10 modes of death seems to offer the most reasonable explanation for her death.

While the presence of a fever, rash and joint pains during the last chapter of her illness indicate continued activity of the lupus process, I don't believe her terminal illness could be classified as a so-called "lupus crisis." The fever was only transient, there was no excessive tachycardia, and the degree of toxicity was not marked. She did seem to improve temporarily when the steroid dosage was increased.

Not so readily excluded is the diffuse development of polyarteritic lesions. The rapid progression of her renal insufficiency, associated with cardiac failure, the terminal episode of abdominal pain, preceded by persistent diarrhea, and the migratory nature of her pneumonitis, would all be well explained by such a development. Also, it will be recalled that helmet cells and spherocytes appeared in the patient's blood. These peculiar red cell forms are, of course, seen in so-called angiopathic hemolytic anemia, one of the several causes of which is a diffuse arteritis.

But, on the other hand, when the patient was seen in the clinic, just a week prior to admission, there was no indication of such an accelerating process. The urinary sediment showed no alteration. The diarrhea and the abdominal pain appeared in a setting of severe advancing uremia, of which they are common accompaniments, there was no blood in the stools, and the abdomen remained soft. The patient had no evident myositis or peripheral neuropathy, common features of an acute arteritis. The fever was low-grade and transient, and there was no tachycardia, although these could well have been modified by the larger dosage of steroids she was then receiving. Finally, the type of RBC changes she showed are common in any sort of uremic process.

Surely, there was ample evidence of advancing injury to essential organs, in particular to the kidneys, lungs, and heart. Let us quickly review these. Her illness was introduced by an episode of typical nephrosis. It terminated in progressive uremia. But was everything that affected her kidneys directly related to the lupus? Let us not make the mistake here we just warned against. I don't think it was, and for these reasons: It will be recalled that long before this patient developed renal insufficiency, she had significant systemic hypertension. It has been my own clinical impression that significant systemic hypertension does not usually appear in patients with uncomplicated lupus nephritis until some degree of renal insufficiency has appeared. Therefore, what factors, in addition to lupus, could have affected this patient's kidneys and have led to the early appearance of hypertension? I can think of three.

A few years ago, Dr. Carlos Hamilton and I described the occurrence of renal vein thrombosis in SLE, and, since then, several other cases have been seen in this Clinic. It is interesting to note in this regard that this patient's urine always contained large amounts of protein, even when other alterations in the urinary sediment weren't striking.

Again, not infrequently, a urinary tract infection complicates lupus. We have followed several patients with presumed lupus nephritis who were found at post mortem examination to have pyelonephritis, either instead of or in addition to lupus nephritis. It will be recalled that on several occasions bacteria were cultured from this patient's urine, and she had costovertebral angle tenderness at her last admission.

Amyloidosis is sometimes associated with lupus, but I have never been impressed by the role it plays in renal failure in this disease.

Because of the therapeutic opportunities entailed, an occurrence which is important not to overlook is the acute inception of unilateral renovascular disease leading to hypertension and renal insufficiency in a patient with chronic lupus nephritis. We recall a patient with low-grade, chronic lupus nephritis who abruptly developed marked hypertension and uremia. Appropriate studies revealed an acute vascular lesion of one kidney, which was amenable to surgical therapy, with resulting improvement.

To me, of all of these possibilities, the most appealing is that, in addition to diffuse lupus nephritis, the patient probably had renal vein thrombosis.

This patient had multiple episodes of pleurisy, pleural effusion, and pneumonitis, and increasing shortness of breath. There were signs of consolidation at the lung bases, which came and went. X-rays showed patches of infiltration, now here, now there, with plate-like atelectasis at the lung bases.

Also, it is important to note that there were progressive signs of congestive heart failure. The pulmonic second sound was described as louder than the aortic second sound. A right ventricular heave, indicative of pulmonary hypertension, was said to be present, and, at times, the ECG showed a right axis deviation.

How can we combine these cardiac and pulmonary findings? What could have occurred in the lungs which would have led to pulmonary hypertension and secondary heart failure? There are two likely explanations. In his classic description of the natural course of SLE, Dr. Osler pointed out that the pneumonitis of lupus frequently is a chronic process, the affected alveoli becoming solidly organized by whirls of connective tissue. These fibrotic areas make themselves evident by the sort of plate-like areas of atelectasis seen at this patient's lung bases. In some instances, the organization of the lungs becomes so extensive that pulmonary hypertension results, eventuating ultimately in cor pulmonale. Commonly, there is a disproportion between the mild degree of fibrosis evident in the x-rays and that found at post mortem. That such changes could have developed in this patient is clearly evident.

Second, it is quite likely that some of this patient's episodes of so-called pneumonia with pleurisy were not that at all, but actually resulted from pulmonary emboli. This chronically ill, edematous, anemic, febrile lady clearly was a sitting duck for embolism. It will be remembered that she had several episodes of sudden, severe dyspnea and pain, regarded as being due to myocardial ischemia, although the typical chemical and ECG changes of myocardial infarction never evolved.

It is highly likely, therefore, that this patient will be found to have the diffuse fibrotic changes of pulmonary lupus, as well as multiple pulmonary emboli, leading to cor pulmonale. One can imagine the effects of such a process on the perfusion of the kidneys, already damaged by lupus, and on the obliterated renal veins. Surely one would expect increasing uremia, a dominant feature of this patient's final chapter.

The patient's heart was enlarged, and she was in cardiac failure. There was a murmur of mitral insufficiency. We have already stressed the likelihood of pulmonary changes leading to pulmonary hypertension. In addition, she had had systemic hypertension for a long time. There is good reason to suppose she might have had coronary ischemia secondary to the systemic hypertension, or even resulting from involvement of the coronary arteries by the lupus process, although the latter is not a frequent occurrence. In addition, she may have had lupus myocarditis, and mitral insufficiency owing to lupus is infrequently seen. Frequently, in SLE, there are several quite different factors participating in the onset of congestive heart failure. In this instance, I would feel confident that systemic and pulmonary hypertension played major roles, and that mitral insufficiency with perhaps coronary insufficiency were contributing factors.

Finally, so far as the heart is concerned, this patient had "peculiarly shaped fingers," and so did several members of her family. She is said to have had the Wolff-Parkinson-White conduction abnormality. Now, peculiarly formed fingers are sometimes an accompaniment of congenital cardiac defects of various sorts, as is the Wolff-Parkinson-White syndrome. Could she have had a congenital septal defect in addition to all of her acquired difficulties? The loud systolic murmur and the right ventricular heave would fit such an abnormality. This is an intriguing speculation, but unfortunately we are not given enough information about the appearance of the fingers to estimate their real significance.

Preceding her death, this patient complained of a 35 pound weight loss, with night sweats. Perhaps, like so many other individuals with lupus, this patient succumbed to some complicating infection, and not primarily to lupus at all. What might its nature have been? This question is best considered under two headings—focal infections and generalized infections.

In this chronically ill person, who was receiving steroids and was suffering from an illness in which there were basic peculiarities of immune reactivity, the most likely generalized infection would be that resulting from tuberculosis or some fungus. I know of no way of firmly excluding this possibility with the information at hand. It is true she did not have a sustained fever, but she was being given large amounts of steroids. It is also true there were no suggestive lung changes, but there often are not. The liver is the place to search for such granulomatous infections, and it was never biopsied with a needle. The fact the spinal fluid was clear has only limited significance. One can only point out that this was a perfect setting for the appearance of a disseminated granulomatous infection. It might have been wise to treat her accordingly.

So far as focal infections are concerned, she was admitted with severe occipital headaches and vomiting. A brain abscess was considered, but the spinal fluid was clear, and there were no focal neurological changes. These, of course, by no means exclude such an abscess, but the headaches subsided, and she became more cheerful.

Several clinical features point to infectious endocarditis as the most likely focal infection. These include the loud systolic murmur, the progressive anemia and uremia, the suspected pulmonary embolic occurrences, and the acute abdominal pain with which her illness terminated, representing, perhaps, a mesenteric artery occlusion resulting from an embolus. All one can say is that several blood cultures were sterile, although the patient could well have been infected by some difficult-to-culture organisms, such as a fungus. After all, 15 percent of patients with infectious endocarditis have repeatedly negative blood cultures.

Most observers who saw this patient thought she was having episodes of pneumonia to account for her pulmonary alterations. However, the signs were evanescent and moved from area to area. No organisms were ever cultured from her blood, and those from her sputum were never impressive. It is, of course, possible that her lungs were infected by some unusual organism, such as the *Pneumocystis*, but I prefer to conclude that the changes in her lungs were largely due to the lupus process itself, and to pulmonary emboli.

We have already referred to the likelihood of a renal infection, but cultures of her urine were more often negative than positive. The appearance of spherocytes and helmet cells, of course, brings to mind the possibility of a gram-negative sepsis, but cultures of the blood were sterile. The persistent vomiting and diarrhea suggest a *Salmonella* infection, but again, the stools were guaiac negative, and cultures were sterile.

She had acute abdominal pain, and her stomach contents were grossly bloody shortly before death. Could she have succumbed to a complication of therapy, specifically, a bleeding and ruptured peptic ulcer? This seems unlikely, for it was a terminal event at a time at which she was profoundly uremic, and bleeding from stomach and gut is common at such times. The abdomen was soft, and there was no free air observed on the abdominal x-rays.

Lastly, could this chronically ill woman with a vascular disease have died of a subdural hematoma? There was a vague history of a fall preceding admission. She had occipital head pains, vomiting and questionable papilledema. Few serious conditions are so often overlooked as a subdural hematoma, for the accompanying clinical alterations may be minimal. However, the spinal fluid was entirely normal, there was general agreement that her eye grounds had not changed, she became more alert in her reactions for a time, not duller, and despite prolonged periods of careful observation, there was no change in the neurological findings. Finally, a subdural hematoma would offer a poor explanation for one of the main features of her terminal course—namely, progressive uremia.

In conclusion, we believe that this patient died in some measure as a result of the persistent effects of lupus, which was active to the very end. These effects showed themselves most prominently in altered function of the heart, the lungs, and the kidneys. In addition to the direct effects of the lupus process upon these organ systems, we conclude that other factors were also at play. In the case of the lungs, we believe that there were multiple pulmonary emboli, in addition to pulmonary fibrosis. Where the kidneys were concerned, we suspect that there was renal vein thrombosis in addition to chronic, active lupus nephritis. In the case of the heart, pulmonary as well as systemic hypertension were, no doubt, significant factors, and both coronary and mitral insufficiency may have been contributory factors. An underlying congenital septal defect with the Wolff-Parkinson-White syndrome, in association with distorted fingers, is an intriguing consideration.

While we were not supplied with enough information to enable us to assume a positive position, we strongly suspect that she also developed, toward the last, some type of an infection. If it was generalized in nature, the most likely factor would be tuberculosis or a fungus infection. If localized, endocarditis would be the most likely cause. The rapid deterioration of the patient's renal status and the coup de grâce, suggesting a mesenteric occlusion, cause us to conclude that she did in fact have an infectious endocarditis, perhaps fungal in nature.

POST MORTEM FINDINGS

Chronic proliferative and membranous nephritis (SLE), with advanced renal atrophy. Hypertrophy and dilatation of both ventricles. Hemorrhagic pericarditis. Organizing pneumonia in the left lower lobe. Marked fatty liver. Onionskin changes in spleen (as in SLE). Chronic cholecystitis. Small infarcts in the femoral heads. Diffuse cerebral atrophy.

REFERENCES

General

DuBois, E. L.: Clinical manifestations of SLE. Computer analysis of 512 cases. JAMA 182:513, 1964.

DuBois, E. L.: SLE: A review of the current status of discoid and systemic lupus and their variants. New York, Blakiston Division, McGraw-Hill Book Co., 1966.

DuBois, E. L., and Tufanelli, D. L.: Clinical manifestations of SLE. Computer analysis of 512 cases. JAMA 190:104, 1964.

Estes, D., and Christian, C. L.: Natural history of SLE by perspective analysis. Medicine 50:85, 1971.

Harvey, A. M., et al.: Systemic lupus erythematosus. Medicine 33:291, 1954.

Larson, D. L.: Systemic Lupus Erythematosus. Boston, Little, Brown & Co., 1961.

McDuffie, F. C.: Twenty years of the lupus erythematosus cell. Ann. Intern. Med. 70:413, 1969.

Ropes, M. W.: Observations on the natural course of lupus. Medicine 43:387, 1964.

Tumulty, P. A., and Harvey, A. M.: The clinical course of disseminated lupus erythematosus, an evaluation of Osler's contributions. Bull. Johns Hopkins Hosp. 85:47, 1949.

Familial Lupus

Bringes, S., Zike, K., and Julian, R.: Familial systemic lupus, review of literature. Amer. J. Med. 30:529, 1961.

Joseph, R. R., and Zarafonetis, C. Z. D.: Fatal systemic lupus erythematosus in identical twins: case reports and review of the literature. Amer. J. Med. Sci. 249:190, 1965.

Serological Abnormalities

Christian, C. L.: Immune complex disease. New Eng. J. Med. 280:878, 1969.

Holborow, J., and Johnson, G. D.: Antinuclear factors in systemic lupus erythematosus. Arthritis Rheum. 7:119, 1964.

Shulman, L. E.: Serologic abnormalities in systemic lupus erythematosus. J. Chronic Dis. 16:889, 1963.

Townes, A. S.: Complement levels in disease. Johns Hopkins Med. J. 5:337, 1967.

Drugs and Lupus

Alarcon-Segovia, D., Wakin, K. G., Worthington, J. W., and Ward, L. E.: Clinical and experimental studies on the hydralazine syndrome and its relationship of SLE. Medicine 46:1, 1967.

Blomgren, S. E., Condemi, J. J., Bignall, M. C., and Vaughn, J. H.: Antinuclear antibody induced by procainamide: a prospective study. New Eng. J. Med. 281:64, 1969.

Holley, H. L.: Drugs and the lupus diathesis. J. Chronic Dis. 17:1, 1964.

Specific Organ Involvement

Comerford, F. R., and Cohen, A. S.: The nephropathy of SLE. Medicine 46:425, 1967.

Gold, W. M., and Jennings, D. B.: Pulmonary function in patients with SLE. Amer. Rev. Resp. Dis. 93:556, 1966.

Hejtmancik, M. R., et al.: Cardiovascular manifestations of systemic lupus. Amer. Heart J. 68:119, 1964.

Johnson, R. T., and Richardson, E. D.: Neurological manifestations of systemic lupus erythematosus. Medicine 47:337, 1968.

Koffler, D., and Kunkel, H. G.: Mechanisms of renal injury in SLE. Ann. J. Med. 45:165, 1968.

Labowitz, R., and Schumacher, H. R., Jr.: Articular manifestations of systemic lupus. Ann. Intern. Med. 74:911, 1971.

Shearn, M. A.: Normocholesterolemic nephrotic syndrome. Amer. J. Med. 36:250, 1964.

Infections

Cherubin, C. E., and Nev, H. C.: Infective endocarditis at the Presbyterian Hospital in New York City from 1938–1967. Amer. J. Med. 51:83, 1971.

Kaye, D., McCormack, R., and Hooke, E.: Bacterial endocarditis, changing patterns. Antimicrobiol. Agents and Chemotherapy 37:1961.

Lerner, P. I., and Weinstein, L.: Infective endocarditis in the antibiotic era. New Eng. J. Med. 274:199, 259, 323, 388; 1966.

Utz, J. P.: The spectrum of opportunistic fungus infections. Laboratory Investigation 2:1018, 1962.

R A PATIENT WITH RHEUMATOID ARTHRITIS AND COMPLICATIONS

THE CLINICAL PROBLEM

In 1959, this 55 year old black male developed exertional dyspnea and was found to be hypertensive. After study, the hypertension was considered to be essential in nature, and he was treated with guanethidine. In 1966, he developed severe rheumatoid arthritis, treated with acetylsalicylic acid initially, and then with a course of chloroquine and butazolidine, without obtaining relief. In 1967, he developed chronic renal disease, regarded as secondary to hypertensive arteriosclerotic carviovascular disease. Serum urea nitrogen was 34 mg./100 ml. at that time. In June 1967, he first complained of intermittent periumbilical pain of one week's standing. This was most marked about 20 minutes after eating and lasted one hour, being "helped some" by amphogel. This apparently remitted. However, for six months prior to admission, he noted a similar burning mid-epigastric, nonradiating pain. Three months before admission, this pain worsened and became associated with weakness, tarry stools, and diarrhea, with guaiac positive stools. Hematocrit value was 20 ml./100 ml., and UGI series showed duodenal deformity and an ulcer crater in the duodenum. He was treated with antacids and placed on an ulcer diet. On the night before admission, he noted the sudden onset of a similar pain, associated with dizziness, weakness, and fatigue. He denied having melena or hematemesis. Later he vomited and noted "two tablespoons" of blood. He then came to the Accident Room. Blood pressure was 210/130; respirations, 18; pulse, 94; temperature, 99.4 degrees; weight 118¼ lbs.

He was a chronically wasted black male in no acute distress who was very apathetic. There was a rheumatoid nodule on ventral surface of left wrist, and an early nodule on the exterior surface of left forearm. Marked arteriovenous nicking was present, without hemorrhages, exudates, or papilledema. Chest: Left posterior effusion. Heart: Enlarged to left. There was a grade 3/6 systolic murmur, early, low-pitched, and harsh, with radiation to axilla. Abdomen: Mild epigastric tenderness. Aorta pulsatile and tortuous, and palpable in left flank. No bruit. Rectum: Stools guaiac positive. Extremities: Effusion in knees, elbows, metacarpophalangeal and proximal interphalangeal joints and left ankle. Mild muscular weakness. No edema, clubbing, or cyanosis. Neurological examination: Normal.

Hct was 29 ml./100 ml. Smear showed microcytosis poikilocytosis, and anisocytosis, with an occasional target cell. WBC count 8000/cu. mm., with 75 percent polymorphonuclear leukocytes, and 2 percent monocytes. Platelets adequate. Clotting and bleeding times normal. Urine: trace protein; specific gravity, 1.013; pH 5.0; 5 to 10 WBCs per high power field; 0 casts. Nasogastric aspirate: guaiac positive, no free acid. Electrocardiogram: left ventricular hypertrophy. Chest x-ray: biventricular enlargement, lungs clear. Serum glutamic oxaloacetic transaminase, 18 Karmen units ml.; alkaline phosphatase, 9.3 King-Armstrong units; bilirubin, 0.3 mg./100 ml; bromsulphalein, 8 percent; serum urea nitrogen, 28 mg./100 ml.; creatinine, 1.8 mg./100 ml.; uric acid, 7.6 mg./100 ml.; amylase, 110 Somogyi units/100 ml.; STS, negative. Latex fixation test reactive at 1:5120 and weakly reactive at 1:40,960. Sedimentation rate $^{53}/_{23}$. All bleeding ceased on admission. An UGI series failed to reveal an ulcer. Gastroscopy results were within normal limits. The patient's temperature suddenly spiked to 101.6 degrees, and symptoms of arthritis exacerbated. The next day, he complained of abdominal pain, and he was given an enema. Twenty minutes later, he was heard to cry out and was found lying out of his bed, clutching his bed rail staring out into space, without pulse or respirations. Resuscitative attempts failed.

DISCUSSION OF THE PROBLEM

This patient had three commonly occurring disorders:

1. Hypertension, associated with renal impairment and heart failure.
2. A duodenal ulcer.
3. Chronic arthritis, with rheumatoid-like joint changes.

Our quest is to discover if these three maladies were unrelated incidents, or whether some kind of continuum bound all of them together. In addition, we want to learn what role these processes played at length in his precipitous death.

To begin with, there are a number of disorders which, over a span of time, may become associated with hypertension, renal and cardiac impairment, ulceration of the gut with bleeding, and rheumatoid-like changes in the joints. Included among these are systemic lupus, polyarteritis, scleroderma, enterocolitis, Felty's syndrome, Whipple's disease, Waldenström's macroglobulinemia, and sarcoidosis. Incidentally, it is interesting to note that all of these varied processes are prominently associated with alterations in immune reactivity.

Most of these disorders we can quickly eliminate because their characteristic clinical features were not present, but could he have had SLE, or polyarteritis, or rheumatoid disease, and could the hypertension, renal insufficiency, heart failure, arthritis, and ulcerative gut lesions all have been different manifestations of such an underlying process? Surely the kind of sequential, episodic involvement of multiorgan systems over a long period of time evidenced by this patient is characteristic of members of this so-called collagen disease family.

Let us briefly investigate this consideration. While patients with SLE may acquire alterations in their joints exactly like those of rheumatoid disease, severe distortion of the joints as described here is not usual, nor is the presence of rheumatoid nodules. Late onset of such deforming arthritis in an elderly Negro male would be highly unlikely, statistically, for lupus. From the serological standpoint, he did not have LE cells, although the rheumatoid factor was greatly elevated, which is not customary in SLE. Finally, he had severe hypertension for a number of years, without evidence of renal impairment. When significant diastolic hypertension is maintained in a patient with SLE, renal failure usually is already present or supervenes shortly.

Again, it seems unlikely that all of the disorders which plagued this unfortunate man's health for many years could have been the result of an underlying polyarteritis, even though arteritis may have played a dominant role in the final chapter of his illness, as we shall relate. While rheumatoid-like arthritis may be seen in polyarteritis, it occurs even less commonly than in SLE. A long history of hypertension without significant alterations in renal function and in the urine would diverge from the course of classical polyarteritis. Also, until the final chapter of his illness, there was no history of weight loss, fever, muscle wasting, neuropathy, or abdominal pain, so typical of the life story of classical idiopathic polyarteritis. Therefore, it seems that one must conclude that if he did have an arteritis, and there is surely reason to suspect that at the end of his course he did, such a process must have been part and parcel of the rheumatoid disease, not the other way around.

It seems certain, then, that he did indeed have rheumatoid arthritis, of the late onset type, and of a severe, rapidly progressive sort, with rheumatoid nodules. We will see shortly why these particular characteristics may be of significance in terms of what ensued.

The next question is, to what extent could this rheumatoid process have been responsible for all of the several ills that beset this man, not only in the joints, but also in his heart, kidneys, gut, and blood vessels, and involving hypertension as well.

It might be argued that the rheumatoid process could not have had anything at all to do with either the hypertension or the renal or cardiovascular changes, since all of these preceded by several years the appearance of the rheumatoid joints. But this may be too simplistic a point of view, for it implies that rheumatoid disease is a disorder only of the joints. This would be like assuming that systemic lupus has not begun until it has involved a patient's joints or skin, which of course would be nonsense. The inflamed joints in rheumatoid arthritis are but one manifestation of a generalized disturbance, and it seems only reasonable to assume that other structures may be involved prior to the appearance of "hot" joints.

It has been recognized for over 20 years that varying degrees and types of arteritis may accompany rheumatoid disease. Such arteritic lesions have been divided into (1) those which are necrotizing, and hence resemble those of classical polyarteritis nodosa, and (2) those which are non-necrotizing. The latter may involve very small arteries. Either type of process may be localized or diffuse. A very wide variety of changes may result from such vascular lesions, including pericarditis, myocarditis, coronary occlusion with infarction, mesenteric thrombosis, gangrene, neuropathy, skin ulcers, purpura, scleritis, and visceral infarcts. These and other sequelae of vasculitis may lead to a fatal course of rheumatoid disease, although these vascular lesions have the capacity to heal spontaneously. They often recur, however, sometimes in an episodic, crop-like manner.

The pathogenesis of such vascular lesions is not known, and while some observers attribute a causative role to steroid therapy, 43 of the 78 patients studied in one series have never been given steroids. There is a general agreement that severe vascular lesions are more often associated with the presence of rheumatoid nodules, particularly if the degree of arthritis is severe, and begins abruptly. All of these clinical features, were, of course, present in this patient.

Is it possible that this patient's hypertension and renal disease could have been induced by such rheumatoid vasculitis? Though it is possible, it is unlikely. Several studies have demonstrated a lower incidence of hypertensive cardiovascular disease in patients with rheumatoid arthritis than in groups of matched controls.

While glomerulitis and small granulomas have been described in the kidneys of patients with rheumatoid arthritis, Dr. C. Robert Cooke has told me that when patients with rheumatoid arthritis and hypertensive renal disease come to post mortem examination, their kidneys often fail to show any alterations specific for the rheumatoid process, the changes being those of "garden variety" arteriosclerosis or arteriolosclerosis.

Therefore, I believe we must conclude that those who followed this patient in our clinics were correct, that his hypertension was essential in nature, and that the subsequent renal changes were a sequel to this.

On the other hand, what about his heart, which was very large, in cardiac failure, producing an intense mitral systolic murmur, and which may have been affected by coronary insufficiency, for he complained of angina-like pain?

Were all of these only sequellae of essential hypertension and associated degenerative vascular disease? Or could the rheumatoid process have interjected itself here in a specific role?

We know, of course, that rheumatoid disease may affect all three layers of the heart, and it is quite possible that the murmur of mitral insufficiency described here was due, at least in part, to alterations induced by the rheumatoid process, in addition to the effects of hypertension, anemia, and heart failure.

We must also always remember that sepsis may complicate and terminate the course of severe rheumatoid disease. Let us not forget that this patient was febrile. The acute episode of abdominal pain with which he presented could have come from a vascular lesion originating in a mycotic aneurysm, or an embolism resulting from an acute endocarditis superimposed upon a mitral valve distorted by rheumatoid disease.

Recent studies have indicated a higher incidence of coronary artery disease in patients with rheumatoid arthritis than in matched controls, and there is evidence favoring the conclusion that this may be the result of involvement of the coronary vessels by rheumatoid vasculitis, rather than ordinary degenerative changes. Such could have occurred here, eventuating in the abrupt death of this patient, as a result of either an acute myocardial infarction or an acute arrhythmia.

The history of episodic epigastric distress, relieved by food and the taking of antacids, together with the changes noted in the GI series, is so typical of a peptic duodenal ulcer that it seems to me unquestionable that the patient in fact had such an ulcer.

While a variety of factors may play a role in the onset of peptic ulcer in patients who have the rheumatoid process—including several of the drugs employed to treat the condition, and the frustration and anxiety which must accompany the stress of finding oneself captured by this miserable process—it is a fact that there is an increased incidence of peptic ulcer in patients who have rheumatoid arthritis, even in its untreated state. Why, I do not know. Perhaps it is related to the peculiar small vascular lesions we have alluded to.

We come then, finally, to a consideration of the last, dramatically abbreviated chapter of this patient's chronic illness. What happened to him at the end?

The three cardinal clinical features of the final phase of his illness appear to be these:

1. There was acute upper gastrointestinal bleeding.

2. He had para-umbilical pain, similar to that which he had had before, but this pain was more severe, lasted longer, and did not respond to simple measures, as had his distress in the past.

3. He died suddenly and unexpectedly, crying out after completion of an enema.

A number of the common causes of upper gastrointestinal bleeding we can rapidly eliminate. For example, although he was taking several agents which might have produced a gastritis, gastroscopy was normal. The normal bromsulphalein test excludes varices. The patient vomited and retched several times before producing blood, and one should consider the Mallory-Weiss syndrome, but gastroscopy failed to show a gastroesophageal tear.

Peptic ulcer is, of course, the most common cause of upper gastrointestinal tract bleeding, and this patient's recent past history strongly indicates that he had had a bleeding duodenal ulcer. This could certainly have been a recurrent episode, perhaps with perforation. But, as already stressed, from the description the patient gave of his pain this final time, it seemed to be quantitatively and qualitatively different from that suffered in the past. Furthermore, the GI series failed to show an active ulcer, and there was no clinical or radiological evidence of a perforated ulcer, the abdomen remaining soft, and peristalsis continuing.

Again, pancreatitis does not often present with upper gastrointestinal bleeding, and the serum amylase test gave negative results.

A new growth originating within the esophagus, stomach, or duodenum seems excluded by both the gastroscopy results and the x-rays.

Bleeding phenomena of various sorts are among the major clinical features of amyloidosis, which, as you know, may become an accompaniment of rheumatoid disease. However, there was nothing to suggest the presence of this infiltrative process in other tissues; in particular, there was no neuropathy or purpuric lesions about the eyes, the hair follicles, or around the neck, and the liver and spleen were not enlarged.

It seems most likely, therefore, that the triad of manifestations which ushered in this patient's demise, namely, GI bleeding, mid-abdominal pain and sudden death, were occasioned by some type of an acute vascular incident. What was its nature? Three mechanisms immediately come to mind:

1. A dissecting or rupturing aortic aneurysm.
2. Mesenteric artery thrombosis.
3. Acute bacterial endarteritis, with mycotic aneurysm and rupture.

As we have already emphasized, an arteritis is part of the life story of rheumatoid disease, and necrotizing arteritis with mesenteric infarction has complicated—and unfortunately, terminated—the course of a number of patients such as this. The sudden onset and unremitting nature of this patient's mid-abdominal pain would be typical of a mesenteric infarction. Blood is frequently found in the stomach and stools of such patients. Early in the course, the abdominal findings may be deceptively benign. Fever is an accompaniment, as occurred here.

Obviously, it is not easy to set aside the inviting possibility of necrotizing arteritis, with mesenteric artery thrombosis, in a patient with nodular rheumatoid disease. However, there are features which don't fit. He was not the usual type of patient with rheumatoid arthritis who would be expected to develop necrotizing arteritis. This complication of rheumatoid disease is generally encountered in patients who, in addition to nodules, have peripheral neuritis, scleritis, skin ulcers, purpura, pericarditis, or other evidences of an on-going, progressive, acute arteritis. Such were not present here. On the other hand, such additional features may not always be present, and we cannot fully exclude the presence of a necrotizing arteritis because of their absence. However, the fact that this patient never developed evidences of "dead gut," such as abdominal tenderness and signs of peritoneal irritation, even after the passage of several days, further militates against this possibility.

This patient had considerable diastolic hypertension, and a very dilated, tortuous aorta. He died suddenly, after a period of unremitting, poorly understood pain, associated with unexplained upper gastrointestinal bleeding. Furthermore, he had a disease—rheumatoid arthritis—which could lead to injury to the walls of the aorta and play a causative role in the development of an aortic aneurysm and its subsequent acute dissection or rupture. Such incidents have been described in a number of patients with polyarteritis, giant cell arteritis, and, less often, rheumatoid disease.

While aneurysms most often rupture into the pericardial, pleural, or peritoneal cavities, they sometimes rupture into the third portion of the duodenum, and in doing so, may exactly mimic a bleeding duodenal ulcer. I once followed the disease course of such an unfortunate patient. He was a rugged, elderly Texan who called long distance to say that he had never considered himself the type, but had just been told that he had a bleeding duodenal ulcer. He had experienced epigastric distress and episodes of hematemesis, and a GI series had been interpreted as showing a duodenal ulcer. Knowing he had an abdominal aneurysm, we suggested he fly here. Shortly after arrival, he exsanguinated while being examined in the X-ray Department. The abdominal aneurysm had been bleeding intermittently into his duodenum.

Could this present patient's "bleeding ulcer" of some three months ago have been a similar incident? One might argue that there was no murmur heard, but this is not unusual, nor is the absence of altered peripheral pulses. Stronger arguments against rupturing aneurysm are the facts that the bleeding appeared modest in amount, and special films taken to demonstrate an abdominal aneurysm were interpreted by experts as being negative. Nevertheless, a ruptured abdominal aneurysm is a possibility which cannot be completely excluded.

I am impressed by this patient's febrile course, and the story of a chill at the onset of his pain. Also, some of his joints flared and developed effusions.

All patients with so-called collagen disorders are prone to infections, which they may handle poorly, and which may present in unusual, easily overlooked guises. In rheumatoid disease, for example, the development of a complicating staphylococcal arthritis has been seen several times in this clinic, and generally in settings in which its presence was not appreciated.

Could this patient's chronic rheumatoid disease have been complicated by the onset of a staphylococcal sepsis, with the development of pyogenic arthritis and endarteritis of the aorta or of one of its mesenteric branches, with the formation of a mycotic aneurysm and its subsequent rupture, causing sudden death of the patient? An acute bacterial endocarditis could also have accompanied this process.

This suggestion may sound somewhat far-fetched, but we have, on several occasions, been amazed to find staphylococci growing luxuriantly in joints which we thought were merely undergoing a flare-up of rheumatoid arthritis, and acute bacterial endarteritis of the aorta or its branches has been described in elderly males whose aortae were distorted by the changes of rheumatoid and degenerative processes. Sometimes *Staphylococcus* has been the invading organism, but a number of other organisms have been responsible, including *Salmonella*.

The circumstances of this patient's sudden death suggest several mechanisms for it. It was related in time to the giving of the enema, and, of course, the stress of undergoing an enema, just as straining at stool in the use of the bedpan, may sometimes cause pulmonary embolism. This patient's chronic illness certainly made him a candidate for such an event. His hypertension and coronary artery disease clearly set the stage for an acute myocardial infarction or dysrthymia.

If we are correct in our supposition that his abdominal pain and bleeding are best explained by some type of acute vascular accident, then the coup de grâce may well have been a dramatic rupture of the aorta, or one of its major branches, although immediate death generally does not follow such incidents.

If this patient had represented more typically the sort of patient with rheumatoid disease who ultimately develops necrotizing arteritis, I would be satisfied to indict this process as being the sole villain in the story. But, this patient was not typical, for the reasons given. I suspect that in addition to rheumatoid disease, essential hypertension, coronary artery disease, and peptic ulcer—all of the latter possibly intimately related to the rheumatoid process —his chronic illness was terminated by the inception of a septicemia, with septic joints and endarteritis of the abdominal aorta or one of its mesenteric branches, followed by mycotic aneurysm and terminal rupture. The mitral valve may also have been affected by this process. The organism could have been a *Staphylococcus* or one with similar invasive qualities.

POST MORTEM FINDINGS

Acute healing and healed arteritis, generalized, with marked involvement of gallbladder and gastrointestinal tract, and occasional lesions demonstrated in skeletal muscle, spleen, and renal pelvis. Focal areas of destruction of aortic wall, aortic arch, and at level of diaphragm, with early aneurysm formation. Focal aortic dissectional perforation at level of diaphragm. Retroperitoneal and mediastinal hematomas. Massive left hemothorax. Marked chronic synovitis. Generalized arteriosclerosis. Left ventricular hypertrophy. Focal tubular atrophy and chronic inflammation of the renal cortices. Focal mucosal hemorrhages of the small intestine, colon, and tracheobronchial tree.

REFERENCES

General

Christian, C. L.: Immune-complex disease. New Eng. J. Med. 280:878, 1969.
Conference on the immunologic aspects of rheumatoid arthritis and systemic lupus. Arthritis Rheum. 6:409, 1963.
Hollander, J. L.: Arthritis and Allied Conditions: A Textbook of Rheumatology. 7th ed. Philadelphia, Lea & Febiger, 1966.
Kulka, J. P.: The pathogenesis of rheumatoid arthritis. J. Chronic Dis. 10:388, 1959.
Sharp, J. T., et al.: Observations on the clinical, chemical and serological manifestations of rheumatoid arthritis based on 154 cases. Medicine 43:41, 1964.

Systemic Rheumatoid Disease

Baggenstoss, A. H., and Rosenberg, E. F.: Visceral lesions associated with chronic rheumatoid arthritis. Arch. Path. 35:503, 1943.
Bevans, M., et al.: Systemic lesions of malignant rheumatoid arthritis. Amer. J. Med. 16:197, 1954.
Cruickshank, B.: Heart lesions in rheumatoid disease. J. Path. Bacteriol. 76:223, 1958.
Fingerman, D. L., and Andrus, E. C.: Visceral lesions associated with rheumatoid arthritis. Ann. Rheum. Dis. 3:168, 1943.
Hart, F. D., and Golding, J. R.: Rheumatoid neuropathy. Brit. Med. J. 1:1594, 1960.
Hollingsworth, J. W.: Local and Systemic Complications of Rheumatoid Arthritis. Philadelphia, W. B. Saunders Company, 1968.
Labowitz, W. B.: The heart in rheumatoid disease. Geriatrics 21:194, 1966.
Mays, E. E.: Rheumatoid pleuritis. Dis. Chest 53:202, 1968.
Petty, T. L., and Wilkins, M.: The five manifestations of rheumatoid disease of the lung. Dis. Chest 49:75, 1966.
Rheumatoid neuropathy. Brit. Med. J. 1:516, 1971.

Arteritis in Rheumatoid Disease

Bienenstock, H., Minick, R., and Rogoff, B.: Mesenteric arteritis and intestinal infarction in rheumatoid arthritis. Arch. Intern. Med. 119:359, 1967.
Bywaters, E. G.: Peripheral vascular obstruction in rheumatoid arthritis and its relationship to other vascular lesions. Ann. Rheum. Dis. 16:84, 1957.
Bywaters, E. G. L., and Scott, J. T.: The natural history of vascular lesions in rheumatoid arthritis. J. Chronic Dis. 16:905, 1963.
Johnson, R. L., et al.: Steroid therapy and vascular disease in rheumatoid arthritis. Arthritis Rheum. 2:224, 1959.
Meriwether, J. H., Jr., et al.: The renal vascular lesion in rheumatoid disease. Arthritis Rheum. 10:298, 1967.
Schmid, R. F., Cooper, N. S., Ziff, M., and McEwen, C.: Arteritis in rheumatoid arthritis. Amer. J. Med. 30:56, 1961.
Sokoloff, L., and Bunim, J. J.: Vascular lesions in rheumatoid arthritis. J. Chronic Dis. 5:668, 1957.

Infection in Rheumatoid Disease

Argen, R. J., et al.: Suppurative arthritis. Arch. Intern. Med. 117:661, 1966.
Karten, I.: Septic arthritis complicating rheumatoid arthritis. Ann. Intern. Med. 70:1147, 1969.
Kass, E. H., and Finland, M.: Corticosteroids and infections. Adv. Intern. Med. 9:45, 1958.
Myers, A. R., et al.: Pyoarthrosis complicating rheumatoid arthritis. Lancet 2:714, 1969.
Wilkerson, J. T., et al.: Septic arthritis: the unexpected complication. Postgrad. Med. 45:127, 1969.

Amyloidosis in Rheumatoid Disease

Gedda, P. O.: Amyloidosis and other causes of death in rheumatoid arthritis. Acta Med. Scan. 150:443, 1955.

Pettersson, T., and Wegelius, O.: Biopsy diagnosis of amyloidosis in rheumatoid arthritis. Gastroenterology 62:22, 1972.

Other Forms of Arteritis

Ball, J.: Rheumatoid arthritis and polyarteritis nodosa. Ann. Rheum. Dis. 13:277, 1954.
Davson, J., Ball, J., and Platt, R.: Kidney in periarteritis nodosa. Quart. J. Med. 17:175, 1948.
Harvey, A. M., Shulman, L., Tumulty, P. A., and Conley, C. L.: Systemic lupus erythematosus. Medicine 33:291, 1954.
Muehrcke, R. C., et al.: Lupus nephritis: a clinical and pathologic study based on renal biopsies. Medicine 36:1, 1954.
Ralston, D. E., and Kvale, W. F.: The renal lesions of periarteritis nodosa. Mayo Clin. Proc. 24:18, 1949.
Slocumb, C. H.: Arthralgia and arthritis of lupus erythematosus. Proc. Staff Mayo Clin. 15:638, 1940.
Soffer, L. J., et al.: Renal manifestations of systemic lupus erythematosus. Ann. Intern. Med. 54:215, 1961.
Winkelmann, R. K., and Spencer, H.: Polyarteritis nodosa. Quart. J. Med. 26:43, 1957.
Winkelmann, R. K., and Winkelmann, W. B.: Cutaneous and visceral syndromes of necrotizing or "allergic" angiitis. Medicine 43:59, 1964.

Abdominal Pain and Bleeding

Anagmostopoulos, C. E., et al.: Aortic dissections and dissecting aneurysms. Amer. J. Cardiol. 30:263, 1972.
Beebe, R. T., et al.: The early diagnosis of ruptured abdominal aneurysm. Ann. Intern. Med. 48:834, 1958.
Cabal, E. C., and Holtz, S.: Polyarteritis as cause of intestinal hemorrhage. Gastroenterology 61:99, 1971.
Holmes, K. D.: Mallory-Weiss syndrome: review of 20 cases and literature review. Ann. Surg. 164:89, 1966.
Lawrence, M. S., et al.: Ruptured abdominal aortic aneurysm. Ann. Thoracic Surg. 2:159, 1966.
Offinger, L. W., and Austen, W. G.: A study of 136 patients with mesenteric infarction. Surg. Gynec. Obstet. 124:251, 1967.
Patterson, M.: Fatal gastrointestinal bleeding. JAMA 175:19, 1961.

S A PATIENT WITH A HEMOGLOBINOPATHY

THE CLINICAL PROBLEM

The patient was a 27 year old black mother of two children who was admitted because of high fever, coma, and profound anemia.

Three years previously, she had had a severe, acute illness said to be similar to the present illness, during which she had "pneumonia" and anemia. She recovered well and afterwards she was told she had a "rare blood type."

She was well until three days before admission, when she began to complain of generalized aching, malaise, and vomiting following ingestion of a cabbage meal. Her private doctor examined her and gave her Donnatal, aspirin, and codeine. Her condition continued to deteriorate, and she complained of severe pain in the abdomen, back, and down the left leg. These pains were described as resembling indigestion. The day before admission she had difficulty in walking; she was unable to remain still, was agitated, irritable, and dizzy, and the pains were described now as being more like labor pains. Late in the evening she was more somnolent and slept well. Early the next morning she spoke to her husband when he left for work; however, two hours later she was not arousable, and an ambulance was called. There was no history of chest pain, fever, chills, sweats, passage of blood, abortion, severe heat exposure, dysuria, or other symptoms of acute illness.

Blood pressure was 140/80; pulse 120; respirations, 22; temperature, 106 degrees rectally. She was an obese, acutely ill, disoriented, but occasionally communicative patient. Her skin was generally hot, and there was a hyper-pigmented, thickened, raised chronic dermatitis of the lower legs and feet. No cyanosis or petechial hemorrhages were noted. The neck was slightly stiff. There was no lymphadenopathy. She complained of pain in the right hip when the leg was flexed, but there was no local tenderness. Her lungs and heart were normal, as were the abdominal and pelvic examinations. The second pulmonic sound was greater than the second aortic sound. No abnormal neurological signs were present except for her mental status.

Hematocrit was 18 ml./100 ml.; reticulocyte count, 0.95 percent, WBC count, 32,000/cu. mm., with 21 percent juvenile neutrophils, 41 percent neutrophils, and 32 percent lymphocytes. The only comments regarding the blood smear were that the platelets were adequate, and there was slight anisocytosis, poikilocytosis, and hypochromia. Urine examination revealed 1+ proteinuria; no bile; urobilinogen positive, 1:4; and a negative sediment. Stool guaiac test was 1+ on the stool obtained during the rectal examination. Electrocardiogram showed sinus tachycardia. X-rays of her chest, skull, and abdomen were normal. Lumbar puncture was performed; the opening pressure was 350 mm. water, and the closing pressure was 250 mm. water. There was only one cell; Pandy test, negative; protein, 10 mg./100 ml.; glucose, 110 mg./100 ml. (blood sugar, 150 mg./100 ml.). Prothrombin, 50 percent. Electrolyte and amylase levels were not remarkable. Bilirubin, 1.2 mg./100 ml., with 0.8 mg. being direct reacting.

The patient was sponged with ice water, and given intravenous fluids containing large doses of vitamins, penicillin, and chloramphenicol. She received one unit of whole blood, aspirin suppositories, and, on her second day, staphcillin intravenously. Her temperature dropped to 103 degrees shortly after admission and remained at about that level. Her pulse was 110 to 130, respirations 28 to 40, and blood pressure normal. Her mental status fluctuated—at times she was lucid but at other times barely responsive to pain.

On the second hospital day, the lumbar puncture was repeated and an opening pressure of greater than 600 mm. water was recorded; 2 cc. of fluid were removed, and a closing pressure of 300 mm. water was recorded. The fluid was slightly bloody and there were 11,000 RBCs and 130 WBCs per milliliter. A bone marrow specimen was obtained, which showed "poorly stained, dark nucleated cells." About noon on the second day her respirations became more labored and she expired.

DISCUSSION OF THE PROBLEM

Fundamentally, this patient's illness was composed of three elements:

1. An episode of acute abdominal pain.
2. An episode of acute cerebral dysfunction.
3. Profound anemia and marked leukocytosis.

It seems profitable to analyze the clinical features of each, with the hope that a thread of continuity binding them together becomes evident.

We shall start with the acute episode of cerebral dysfunction, because the clinical data supplied about it are more complete than the somewhat scanty information given about the others.

The cerebral episode began abruptly. She kissed her husband farewell, and two hours later could not be aroused. Thereafter, her state of consciousness waxed and waned, but was never fully regained. She threw herself about restlessly, was incontinent of urine, and breathed rapidly and noisily. And yet, no focal neurological abnormalities were seen, nor were signs of meningeal irritation. Although the spinal fluid pressure was distinctly elevated, no cellular elements were seen on the first tap, and on the second, there were 11,000 RBCs but only 130 WBCs. Chemical tests revealed no increased protein or other abnormality.

Now, not too many kinds of disorders could produce such changes. Certainly, meningitis and encephalitis are excluded by the dearth of protein and cells in the spinal fluid. A brain abscess is unlikely, for the same reason, and furthermore, most brain abscesses are associated with at least some focal neurological signs. There were no pupillary or other focal abnormalities to suggest a subdural hematoma, which is usually associated with a progressive cerebral dysfunction, not with a precipitious change of consciousness as noted here. Similarily, a solid tumor can be excluded, although hemorrhage into a tumor or cyst sometimes results in the dramatic appearance of signs and symptoms. But, if this had transpired here and produced the degree of elevation of the spinal fluid pressure observed in this patient, focal signs would certainly be anticipated. Exposure to a toxic substance could do this, but there was none. Also possible is a metabolic disorder, such as porphyria, but marked elevation of spinal fluid pressure and presence of RBCs in the fluid do not occur in this condition. A diffuse cerebritis, seen in a variety of disseminated infections, comes to mind in this setting, but significant amounts of protein and cells should have appeared in the spinal fluid.

We are left, then, with the conclusion that her cerebral dysfunction must have been circulatory in origin. What was its nature? A hemorrhage or occlusion of a single vessel, large enough to elevate the spinal fluid pressure appreciably, should have led to some focal neurological signs, but there were none. Therefore, she must have suffered multiple, very small vascular occlusions, perhaps associated with occlusion of the dural sinuses. Only in this way could high spinal fluid pressure have been associated with relatively clear spinal fluid in the absence of focal neurologic abnormalities.

Now, let us advance to the second element of this unfortunate woman's illness, the acute episode of abdominal pain. By all odds, the single most helpful factor in ferreting out the cause of any abdominal pain is an adequate history and, in particular, a detailed description of the character of the pain. We are seriously handicapped in this case by its lack.

We are able to garner only the following information:
1. The pain was generalized in the abdomen.
2. There was radiation to the back and down the left leg.
3. There was pain in the right hip on flexion.
4. It was very severe pain, and seemed to wax and wane.
5. It was described "like indigestion," and also "like labor pains."
6. It was associated with malaise and vomiting after the ingestion of cabbage, and also with generalized aching and some pain in the joints. Fever and chills were denied, but her temperature was 106 degrees.

The following findings from the physical examination seem pertinent:
1. Although she was critically ill, she was never in shock.
2. Temperature, pulse, and respiration were all increased.
3. Her abdomen was soft, and remained so.
4. No masses or enlargements of organs was felt.
5. She was pale but not jaundiced.
6. The bowel sounds were diminished.

Clearly, this information could be applied to many different processes. We shall attempt to winnow these out briefly.

Could the high fever have been caused by cholangitis and sepsis, secondary to gallbladder disease and gallstones? She was not jaundiced, the abdomen was soft, and there was no mass. The liver was neither enlarged nor tender. It should be pointed out, however, that the usual acute abdominal signs may be absent in a woman as sick as this. Finally, gallbladder disease would not account for the patient's striking anemia, unless she had an associated blood dyscrasia, such as a hemoglobinopathy. As you know, gallstones are common in these disorders, and abdominal crises may be confused with gall colic, and vice versa.

Acute pancreatitis is sometimes associated with abscess formation and subsequent sepsis. But the abdomen was soft, and the serum amylase level did not rise.

Perforation of a peptic ulcer must always be considered when there is pain in the back, but once again the softness of the abdomen raises an objection as does a normal flat abdominal film.

A ruptured appendix, Meckel's diverticulum, or colonic diverticulum might lead to pylephlebitis and sepsis, but there were no focal signs or symptoms whatever to indicate such a lesion.

Some mechanical obstruction is brought to mind by the description of pain resembling labor, with radiation to the back, but there was but little vomiting, no distention, and a "quiet" abdomen, in addition to an unremarkable flat plate.

A renal stone or papillary necrosis is excluded by the clear urine, normal serum urea nitrogen, negative flat plate, and absence of tenderness in the region of the kidneys.

She had never been known to have gastrointestinal symptoms before, and this, together with the soft abdomen, eliminates regional enteritis or ulcerative colitis.

She was too young for a gastrointestinal carcinoma, although she could have had a lymphoma, but, as already indicated, there were no signs of a perforation or of an obstruction which might have been the result of such a process.

The back pain and, in particular, its radiation down the left leg, should make one think about some intrapelvic disorder, for the sciatic nerve can be irritated by ovarian and other pelvic abnormalities, but nothing abnormal was palpated in the pelvic cavity.

There are but two structures within the abdominal cavity not yet scrutinized, namely, the lymph nodes and the blood vessels.

The very diffuseness and vagueness of the pain, and its radiation into the back, as well as its severity and the absence of muscle spasm, focal tenderness, and peritoneal irritation, all suggest an inflammatory or neoplastic process in the retroperitoneal structures. The profound anemia and the leukocytosis obviously complement this possibility, as does the description of the bone marrow findings.

In opposition, one might ask why such a process should precipitously flare up in a female previously regarded as well, and whose weight had increased in one year to 220 pounds? Furthermore, there was no evidence of a tumor or inflammatory mass in the abdominal cavity or elsewhere, and the chest film was clear. But this possibility cannot be completely eliminated, since all the information we have about the patient's antecedent health is purely hearsay.

A number of features point to the pain's vascular origin: its severity, the restlessness and agitation of the patient, the radiation into the back and down the left leg, the silent abdomen, and the absence of masses of palpable organs. Such a process might have implicated the large, or the small vessels, and might have been widespread, affecting the gut, the soft tissues, and even the bones themselves.

The profound anemia suggests a dissecting aneurysm, but this patient was not the type of a person to have such a disorder. She was young, there was no history of trauma, she had none of the characteristics of Marfan's syndrome, and she did not have diabetes or hypertension. All the peripheral pulses were present, no bruits were described, and she was not in shock, Massive intraabdominal bleeding seems unlikely in view of the normal serum urea nitrogen and bilirubin levels.

But could there not have occurred elsewhere in this patient vascular changes similar to those we have postulated to have taken place in her head, with occlusion of multiple small vessels by some embolic or thrombotic process? A similar change could have led to the pain in the right hip and in the spine and pelvic bones. The finding of blood in the stool and the marked leukocytosis would be compatible. The abdominal findings were indeed benign, but we have seen patients with massive mesenteric occlusion and a disarmingly soft abdomen. The only physical alteration may be the absence of peristaltic sounds, which was noted here. Furthermore, these alterations may have involved retroperitoneal and other vessels, and not solely the mesenteric vessels, as already indicated.

Before concluding this portion of our discussion, we should mention a cause of acute abdominal pain frequently overlooked until the patient has been operated on at least once (and usually several times) without benefit. This is porphyria. Porphyria deserves thoughtful consideration in these particular circumstances because of the following:

1. The severe, cramping nature of the pain, which often mimics such things as gallstones, mesenteric occlusion, appendicitis, and so forth.
2. The paradoxical benignity of the abdominal physical signs.
3. The sudden appearance of the changes in the central nervous system.
4. The worsening of the patient's condition after taking a drug.
5. The appearance of some kind of pigmented, vesicular lesions on the legs.
6. Failure to respond to treatment, and rapid conclusion in death. However, the excessively high fever, the very pronounced leukocytosis, the severe anemia, the pronounced degree of elevation of the spinal fluid pressure, and the absence of any focal neurological alterations exclude porphyria.

We come then to the last element of this patient's illness, the profound anemia and marked leukocytosis.

The salient features of the hematologic alterations were these:
1. Extreme anemia.
2. A normal number of platelets.
3. Marked leukocytosis, with brisk shift to the left.
4. A reticulocyte count of only 0.9 percent.
5. A degree of hypochromia, poikilocytosis, and anisocytosis.
6. A bone marrow showing large numbers of poorly staining, dark nucleated cells.

Unfortunately, for the clinician, a great many different types of conditions could have induced these same changes, and we shall have to examine several.

Could she have hemorrhaged? This seems unlikely. Except for the weakly positive guaiac stool, there was no visible or historical evidence of bleeding. Returns from the Levine tube were clear, and there was nothing to indicate bleeding into any of the body cavities. The serum urea nitrogen level was normal, and the bilirubin was but slightly elevated. Arguing against more chronic bleeding was failure of the reticulocyte count to be even slightly elevated.

Could this have been primarily an active hemolytic process? The diagnosis of a hemolytic anemia requires demonstration of the presence of two factors: (1) increased blood destruction, and (2) increased blood formation. We have little of either here. The reticulocyte count was only 0.9 percent, the bilirubin only 0.2 mg./100 ml., the urobilinogen only 1 Erlich unit/4 hrs. While there was some anisocytosis, no nucleated RBCs were described. The changes in the white blood cells and perhaps also the bone marrow would, of course, fit a hemolytic process. We conclude that if there was a hemolytic process, it was low grade and not accountable for the entire course of events.

Was this process a bone marrow failure? It was certainly not aplasia, in view of the adequate platelets and WBCs. She was obese and there is no need to question the adequacy of her diet. The cells were not macrocytic, and both the nature of the neurological changes and the appearance of the bone marrow exclude pernicious anemia. There was nothing indicative of an endocrine disorder, and she did not have uremia. Her cells were not microcytic as in pyridoxine dificiency. So-called auto-immune disorders like SLE, in my experience, rarely if ever produce an anemia of this degree in the absence of very brisk hemolysis, which was not noted here.

Acute, overwhelming infection is suggested by this patient's course, but in the absence of massive hemolysis, how could suppression of the bone marrow by an infection have possibly induced such a marked degree of anemia in three days? The marked leukocytosis and normal platelet count are additional arguments against such suppression.

Invasion of the bone marrow by some neoplasm, including myeloma, lymphoma, or leukemia, or by a widespread granulomatous infection, such as tuberculosis or a fungus, is not so readily excluded, particularly in view of the cryptic description of the bone marrow as being "invaded by masses of nucleated cells." On the other hand, there are certainly features of typical myelophthisic or myelo-invasive disease which were not mentioned here, including increased numbers of platelets, nucleated RBCs, and marked variations in size, shape, and color of the cells. Furthermore, this patient was told some three years before this acute illness that she was anemic and, despite this fact, she continued to become obese. So far as we know, she was generally well. There was no history of antecedent weight loss, weakness, sweating, fever, and so forth, although, unfortunately, patients frequently fail to tell the physician about these early telltale details.

Could this patient have had some type of congenital anemia? Several bits of evidence suggest this. First, the history of an episode of pneumonia some three years prior to admission, in a setting, incidentally, said to be similar to the present illness. Episodes of pneumonitis are not uncommon, for example, in sickle cell disease, sometimes stemming from infection, other times from vascular occlusion. Following recovery from the pneumonia, the patient was told of some abnormality in her blood, her husband and children were called in for a check-up and she was advised to visit the clinic. She did not do this, and apparently felt well. To feel well despite a significant degree of anemia is, of course, a hallmark of congenital anemia. The lesions on her legs could conceivably have been associated with a chronic anemia.

What kind of a congenital anemia might she have had? Not the spherocytic hemolytic variety, obviously, and probably not sickle cell anemia of the S-S type, for she had none of the other structural hallmarks of this disorder, and it would be unusual for a patient with S-S disease to have had two children and to have reached the age of this patient, weighing 220 pounds, although it *could* happen. However, she could have had one of the other kinds of sickle hemoglobinopathy, as, for example, the S-C variant.

It might be argued that no sickle cells were seen, but this is entirely consonant with this disorder. A more cogent argument is the fact, already emphasized, that there was but little evidence of hemolysis, despite the profound anemia. However, it is well known that two different mechanisms may play a role in the anemia of sickle cell disease. One is hemolysis, and the other is bone marrow failure. A patient with sickle disease may experience a marked worsening of his anemia owing to bone marrow failure, in the absence of any exacerbation of the hemolytic process. This phenomenon is said to be associated sometimes with a variety of infectious processes. Such could have taken place here. The bone marrow could be suffused with erythroid hyperplasia at such times, as might have been the case here. It is true that in S-C disease the liver and spleen are usually enlarged, and they were not felt here, but this can happen. A stronger point against the diagnosis is absence of target cells in the smears.

And so we have completed our analysis of the three elemental components of this patient's illness. What has evolved? The best explanation for the central nervous system changes appears to be multiple small vascular occlusions. Likewise, the abdominal pain would seem to be most reasonably understood on the basis of multiple vascular occlusions involving mesenteric or retroperitoneal structures (or both), and perhaps bone as well. The blood changes are most compatible with some sort of congenital abnormality of the hemoglobin and bone marrow failure, or less likely, with involvement of the marrow by a malignant or infectious process.

If we tie these three sets of phenomena together in the most logical way, we should have the correct diagnosis inevitably—almost!

Multiple small vascular occlusions, such as postulated here, would have to be the product of some embolic or thrombotic process, or both. Disorders leading to these are best categorized as follows:

1. Some collagen-vascular disorder.
2. A disseminated infection.
3. Thrombotic thrombocytopenic purpura.
4. A blood dyscrasia—anemia, leukemia, polycythemia.
5. A new growth, including lymphoma and myeloma.
6. A dysproteinemia, macroglobulinemia.
7. Fat embolism.

As already indicated, the blood picture would be unusual for systemic lupus erythematosus. Furthermore, there was nothing in the past health to suggest a chronic, episodic polyorgan system disorder.

For some of these same reasons, and in addition because she was a young female, we can exclude polyarteritis nodosa (PAN). Also, PAN usually involves medium-sized vessels, and the complete absence of focal neurological signs or renal changes would be unlikely for PAN.

Thrombotic thrombocytopenic purpura might indeed behave like this, but it seems there was nothing peculiar about the number or character of the platelets, nor were the characteristic alterations seen in the RBCs—although they might have been overlooked, of course. Again, in thrombotic thrombocytopenic purpura, one would have expected to find definite evidence of a hemolytic anemia, and the spleen was not enlarged.

The abrupt onset, the very high fever, and the greatly elevated WBC count suggests a widely disseminated or overwhelming infection, such as a staphylococcic or gram-negative sepsis or miliary tuberculosis. Against a staphylococcic or other sepsis is the fact that, despite the critical state she was in, her blood pressure was always well maintained. No petechial spots were seen, the spleen was not felt, and the urine was clear. There was no evidence of a focus of infection in the heart or elsewhere. We have already stressed the incompatibility of such an acute infection with the blood changes noted here.

A widespread granulomatous infection such as tuberculosis is less easily eliminated, perhaps, from a hematological standpoint, and we must not forget that disseminated tuberculosis can exactly reproduce the blood picture of leukemia. But this would have been an exceedingly fulminant course for tuberculosis, if it is true that, as we were told, she was entirely well only a few days before admission. Also, her chest x-ray was clear. One might have expected tubercles in the meninges, and the spinal fluid examination failed to indicate their presence.

A neoplasm, and in particular a lymphosarcoma or reticulum cell sarcoma, or even a myeloma, is suggested by the report of the bone marrow being crowded with dark nucleated cells. As for myeloma, I don't believe we have ever seen this disorder in a female only 27 years old.

Occlusion of multiple small vessels could be induced by such neoplasms in several different ways, including:
1. Infiltration of the vessel walls.
2. As a secondary process to cachexia and dehydration.
3. Through the laying down of amyloid.
4. Concurring with a septicemia.
5. Through sludging of the blood by the appearance of macroglobulins or cold agglutinins, in association with the tumor.

Widespread, sudden infiltration of the walls of many small blood vessels, causing occlusion, must be an unusual phenomenon in tumors. There was no cachexia or dehydration. Amyloid does not suddenly spread itself throughout the lumens of widely dispersed vessels. Nothing pointed to the presence of macroglobulins. The patient's blood showed no peculiarities when drawn into a syringe, nor did it form rouleaux. There was no bleeding tendency. The characteristic tortuosity and sausage-like dilatations of the fundic vessels, and the hemorrhages and exudates of macroglobulinemia, were not described.

Arguing against the possibility of a tumor with secondary infection is the fact that we are assured that the patient was not ill in any way, and had reached her greatest lifetime weight of 220 pounds just three days prior to her death. Again, there was no evidence of tumor tissue in the chest, abdominal cavity, pelvic organs, or lymph glands. We should mention, however, that the type of skin abnormality described could be the sort seen in lymphomatous disorders, and we find it difficult to exclude positively a process such as lymphosarcoma, in view of the limitations of this history.

We come then, to the final consideration, that this patient must have had some sort of a primary blood disorder. While leukemia is suggested by the description of the infiltrative changes in the bone marrow, the character of the peripheral blood did not suggest leukemia, although in these circumstances one has to consider aleukemic leukemia. However, the normal platelet count would not fit, nor would the lack of enlargement of the lymph nodes, liver, or spleen.

It seems most reasonable, therefore, to conclude that the abnormality resided in the RBCs and, as already suggested, to conclude that the patient must have had a hemoglobinopathy, probably of the S-C variety. This appears to offer the most logical explanation for the illness suffered some three years prior to admission, during which the patient had a pneumonia, and was found to have "some kind of a blood disease," which occasioned the family to be called in and examined. It explains a history of "good health" despite anemia, which may well have been chronic, although we can't be certain. It accounts for the sudden onset of the severe abdominal pain and of the subsequent neurological developments, with rapid progression to death. It also offers a solution to the pain in the right hip and perhaps in other bones as well. It also fits, although perhaps not as comfortably as one would wish, the changes in the peripheral blood and bone marrow.

Some final thoughts need to be added. On admission, the patient's temperature was 106 degrees. This is higher than is usually observed in vascular crises, and higher than usually results from central nervous system damage alone in adults. This raises the possibility of an associated infection, which I think is quite likely. Not infrequently, crises in sickle disease are precipitated by a variety of infections.

For example, *Salmonella* infections have a penchant for doing this, producing, in particular, a *Salmonella* osteomyelitis, and such an infection may have been the trigger here. It is even possible that some acute intraabdominal incident, such as acute cholecystitis, may have been the source of infection.

In vascular crises, fat emboli and even shreds of bone marrow have been found obliterating the lumens of capillaries and small vessels, as have conglomerations of sickled RBCs. Such emboli are thought to be the result of bone marrow infarction. It is possible that this patient's marked respiratory distress and loud pulmonic second sound may have been produced by such fat and sickle cell embolic and thrombotic events.

In summary, the most likely explanation for this unfortunate course of events would seem to be congenital hemoglobinopathy, probably of the S-C type, with vascular crises resulting in obstruction of multiple small vessels in the brain, lungs, abdominal cavity, and bones, perhaps complicated by secondary infection, questionably a salmonellosis.

POST MORTEM FINDINGS

Electrophoretic studies revealed that the patient had sickle cell hemoglobulin-C disease. The terminal event was the result of massive multifocal infarction of bone marrow, with subsequent bone marrow and fat embolism. Sections of the bone marrow showed sinusoidal engorgement of masses of sickled erythrocytes and widespread areas of necrosis. There were abundant fat emboli in the pulmonary capillaries, renal glomeruli, and brain. The difficulty in interpretation of the bone marrow aspirates arose from the fact that they were taken from areas of necrosis or partial necrosis, with resultant alterations in the appearance of the cells.

REFERENCES

Amorosi, E., and Ultman, J.: TTP—report of 16 cases and review of the literature. Medicine 45:139, 1966.
Beutler, E. (Ed.): Hereditary Disorders of Erythrocyte Metabolism. New York, Grune & Stratton, 1968.
Bone marrow failure. Seminars Hematol. 4:175, 1967.
Charache, S., and Page, D. L.: Infarction of bone marrow in sickle cell disorders. Ann. Intern. Med. 67:1195, 1967.
Connor, E. B.: Sickle cell anemia and infection. Medicine 50:97, 1971.
Dacie, J. V.: The Hemolytic Anemias. 2nd ed. New York, Grune & Stratton, 1960.
Desforges, J. F., and Wang, Y. F. W.: Sickle cell anemia. Med. Clin. N. Amer. 50:1519, 1966.
Jandl, J. H. (Ed.): Symposium on disorders of the red cell. Amer. J. Med. 41:657, 1966.
Motulsky, A. G.: Frequency of sickling disorders in U. S. blacks. New Eng. J. Med. 288:31, 1973.
Murayama, M.: Molecular mechanisms of red cell "sickling." Science 153:145, 1966.
Perutz, M. F., and Lehmann, H.: Molecular pathology of human haemoglobin. Nature 219:902, 1968.
River, G. L., Robbins, A. B., and Schwartz, S. O.: S-C hemoglobin—a clinical study. Blood 18:305, 1961.
Umlas, J., and Kaiser, J.: Thrombohemolytic purpura (TTP): a disease or a syndrome? Amer. J. Med. 49:783, 1970.

A PATIENT WITH SYSTEMIC LUPUS ERYTHEMATOSUS (SLE) AND EXTENSIVE, PROFUSE BLEEDING

THE CLINICAL PROBLEM

This 59 year old woman was admitted for the eleventh time on March 12, 1965, because of melena and anemia. She died six weeks later. The patient's family history was positive for vague rheumatic complaints and acute nephritis. In 1932, at age 26, the patient was seen in the outpatient department, complaining of fatigue. No explanation could be found for this and it was thought to have an emotional basis. In 1935, she developed diplopia and increased fatigability and was admitted to the hospital for the first time. The muscle weakness appeared to respond somewhat to neostigmine, and she was thought to have myasthenia gravis. Shortly after discharge she stopped taking neostigmine because her weakness had considerably decreased, and her diplopia and ptosis had disappeared. Subsequently, however, she developed a malar rash, and in 1936 a diagnosis of discoid lupus was made in the dermatology outpatient clinic.

The patient was relatively well until the next year, when she first developed vague arthralgias, and at this time she was found to have a biologic false positive test for syphilis. Subsequently she complained of vague aches and pains, and in 1951 she developed a clear-cut polyarthritis. In 1952, she became extremely ill and was again admitted to the hospital, with chills, fever, malar rash, pleurisy, arthritis, and pneumonia. At this admission, there was found the first of numerous positive LE preparations.

The patient responded satisfactorily to ACTH therapy until 1953, when she was readmitted with fever, chills, arthritis, and acute nephritis. In 1954, she developed a duodenal ulcer which responded to medical therapy. In 1955, she once more had an episode of arthritis, this time associated with marked conjunctivitis. In 1960, she was again admitted with an episode of severe polyarthritis, and in 1961 with an episode of pleurisy, cough, and hemoptysis. In 1962, the clinical features of Sjögren's syndrome were noted. In 1963, she again had arthritis and pneumonia with pleurisy, and in 1964, she was seen on several occasions with vague gastrointestinal complaints.

In January of 1965, the patient developed arthritis, pleurisy, and a cramping epigastric pain, which occurred one to two hours after meals and was aggravated by spices and partially relieved by antacids. An upper gastrointestinal series showed a duodenal ulcer. One week prior to admission, she noted black, tarry stools and came to the outpatient department, where it was discovered that her hematocrit value, which had been 35 ml./100 ml. in January, had fallen to 22 ml./100 ml., and she was admitted to the hospital.

On admission, her blood pressure was 140/84; pulse, 76; rectal temperature, 100 degrees. She was described as a slightly obese, well developed, chronically ill Caucasian woman. The mucous membranes were pale and the patient appeared to be very anxious and tense, but in no acute distress. The skin over the nose and malar areas was atrophic and hyperpigmented. There was alopecia with atrophic skin over the left frontal area, and an erythematous papular eruption was present bilaterally over the pretibial areas. There were a few moist rales over the left lung base posteriorly. The heart was moderately enlarged, with a harsh grade II/VI apical systolic murmur. The liver was palpated 6 cm. below the right costal margin in the midclavicular line, and the spleen tip 4 cm. below the left costal margin. The neurologic examination was normal.

The patient's hematocrit value was 23 ml./100 ml., and the WBC count was 2400/cu. mm., with a slight shift to the left. Platelet numbers were adequate or slightly increased on smear. Urinalysis showed 3+ proteinuria, numerous RBCs and three to five WBCs cells per high power field, and occasional granular casts. Stool guaiac tests were negative on nine occasions. Serum alkaline phosphatase, 2.3 Bodansky units; total serum proteins, 6.2 gm./100 ml.; albumin, 2.4 gm./100 ml.; globulin, 3.8 gm./100 ml. Serum glutamic oxaloacetic transaminase, 26 Karmen units/ml.; serum glutamic pyruvic transaminase, 14 Karmen units/ml.; serum bilirubin, less than 0.8 mg./100 ml.; prothrombin time, greater than 50 percent of normal; creatinine clearance, 9.6 cc. per min.; VDRL (Venereal Disease Research Laboratories) test, weakly reactive. Clotting time was 9 min.; bleeding time, 2.5 min.; and tourniquet test was 1 to 2+ positive. A urine culture was negative, as were five blood cultures.

On admission to the hospital the patient was treated with an ulcer diet plus antacids. She did well except for continued microscopic hematuria until the sixth hospital day, when she developed small hemorrhagic lesions on her right thumb and left forefinger, and her hematocrit reading fell to 19.5 ml./100 ml. On her seventh hospital day she was noted to have a disturbed affect, and she was started on prednisone therapy, 60 mg. per day. She thereafter developed an agitated depression, and on her ninth hospital day she was started on chlorpromazine, 25 mg. three times a day. On her eleventh hospital day, she complained of paralysis and hypesthesia of her legs, urinary frequency, and abdominal pain. She was also noted to have numerous ecchymotic and purpuric areas over her body. Bladder catheterization yielded 800 cc. of dark brown urine, and abdominal x-rays revealed many air fluid levels in the left lower quadrant, dilatation of the ascending and transverse colon, and obscured retroperitoneal structures. Prothrombin time, clotting time, plasma fibrinogen, and circulating anticoagulant studies were all normal or negative. Her platelet count was 129,000/cu. mm. By her fourteenth hospital day, her serum urea nitrogen had risen to 128 mg./100 ml., and her hematocrit had fallen to 25 ml./100 ml. On the seventeenth hospital day, a left ankle abscess was drained, and methicillin therapy was begun. *Staphylococcus aureus*, resistant to penicillin, was cultured. A biopsy specimen of the skin adjacent to the abscess showed an acute vasculitis. On the twenty-second hospital day, circulating anticoagulants were first demonstrated. The hematocrit value continued to fall. For a short period of time she improved, but then suddenly went into shock.

Over the next four hours she complained of both chest and abdominal pain, and passed several grossly bloody stools. Bowel sounds were initially present, but, as her abdomen became progressively distended and rigid, the bowel sounds decreased and then disappeared. Paracentesis produced bloody fluid from the right upper quadrant, and a small amount of bloody fluid was aspirated from the stomach. She died despite vigorous treatment with vasopressors, whole blood, and plasma expanders.

DISCUSSION OF THE PROBLEM

When analyzing any complex clinical problem, which this most certainly is, it is hazardous to begin with any assumptions; however, I do believe that it is sound to assume that this patient did, in fact, have systemic lupus erythematosus (SLE), just as she was thought to have during the 23 years she visited the various clinics of this hospital. Indeed, the story of her 23 years of sickness is actually a classic biography of the natural history of SLE. Among other features, the course of her illness illustrates so vividly the three dominant characteristics of the life story of SLE:

1. Chronicity: in this instance, a span of 23 years.
2. Episodicity: periods of varying degrees of ill health interspersed with periods of remission of varying duration.
3. Multiplicity of organ system involvement.

Therefore, we shall confine our attention to the final chapter of her saga of lupus, and attempt to answer the question, "What was the nature of the coup de grâce which finally freed this patient from this all-encompassing illness, the occasion to her of so much misery, both mental and physical, for so long a period of time?"

The clinical features of this final episode which strike us as most pertinent are as follows:

1. It occurred at a time when she was receiving no specific therapy.
2. It occurred in circumstances which indicated that the lupus process was active, as manifested my malaise, weight loss, pneumonitis, pleurisy, and generalized arthralgias.
3. There was extensive and profuse bleeding: from the GI tract, into the skin and subcutaneous tissues, from the kidneys, and ultimately into the abdominal cavity.
4. The patient complained of epigastric pain, and there was a previous history of a demonstrated duodenal ulcer and of melena.
5. There was progressive nitrogen retention, associated with hematuria and proteinuria.
6. Widespread neurological deficits suddenly appeared, including psy-

chosis, weakness and paresthesia of the lower extremities, and an atonic urinary bladder.

7. After a period of transient improvement, the patient suddenly went into severe shock (from which she could not be withdrawn), associated with increased abdominal pain, an initially soft abdomen giving place to rigidity and adynamic ileus, bright red blood passing per rectum and aspirated preterminally from the right upper quadrant of the abdomen.

These seem to us to be the basic items of this clinical puzzle. What is the most reasonable manner in which to make these pieces fit together?

Since bleeding was the most vivid manifestation of her final illness, perhaps we should consider this phenomenon first.

Bleeding, whether in the form of mild purpura or as a massive hemorrhage, is a common occurrence in patients with SLE. As a matter of fact, unexplained bleeding in any female between the ages of 20 and 40 is of itself reason to give thought to the diagnosis of SLE. Such bleeding may originate from a variety of quite different mechanisms:

1. An acute arteritis.
2. Thrombocytopenia.
3. Presence of an anticoagulant.
4. Secondary infection.
5. Presence of macroglobulins.
6. Deposition of amyloid.
7. Concomitance of thrombotic thrombocytopenic purpura.
8. Liver injury.
9. Uremia.
10. Drugs used in therapy: (a) Cushing's syndrome; (b) allergy.
11. Pancreatitis.

It should be emphasized that in any particular incident of bleeding, one or several of these factors acting in consort may be responsible for the bleeding, and the observer must winnow out the factor or factors which seem most likely to be active.

Let us attempt to do this here. Several can be dismissed quickly. The platelet count and bleeding time were normal. There was no indication of important liver injury. The bleeding began at a time when she was not receiving any specific therapy, and steroids had not been given for some time past. Although she was, indeed, uremic when the bleeding commenced, her serum urea nitrogen was not at a level which is generally associated with the kind and degree of bleeding noted here. During the early period of her bleeding, the serum amylase level was repeatedly normal. The same can be said of the circulating anticoagulant which was ultimately discovered, but which was absent in the first phases of her bleeding.

A significant concentration of macroglobulin in her blood can be excluded because of the absence of the characteristic changes in her eye grounds, and also because of the absence of rouleau formation of the red blood cells, of a history of Raynaud's phenomenon, or of bleeding from the nose and mouth, the latter so typical of macroglobulinemia. In other words, there was no clinical evidence of sludged blood.

Purpura and other bleeding phenomena are a part of the changes which are commonly induced by amyloidosis, and, of course, SLE is one of the disorders which may be complicated by the deposition of the peculiar material of this condition. However, unless I am mistaken, the instances within this hospital in which significant deposition of amyloid has occurred in SLE have been very few indeed. It is true that the patient's liver and spleen were enlarged and she had proteinuria, but such changes are commonly seen in straightforward SLE. There was nothing to indicate the laying down of amyloid elsewhere. The kind of central nervous system deficits this patient developed would be most unusual in amyloidosis, which characteristically affects the peripheral nerves, and only rarely the spinal cord or the brain. Finally, a typical feature of the purpura of amyloid is its presence about the eyes and about hair follicles, neither of which was described here.

The concomitance of SLE and the peculiar disorder thrombotic thrombocytopenic purpura is, of course, suggested by the type of generalized bleeding this patient endured, and by the strikingly sudden onset of the widespread neurological abnormalities, as well as by the renal alterations. It is not easy to lay this possibility aside. However, the relatively normal platelet count, and also the absence of schizocytes and burr cells in the peripheral blood, seem to me to lessen the likelihood that this strange process could have been present.

Secondary infections of all sorts plague the clinical course of patients with SLE, and as a matter of fact, often cause their death. So frequently do such complicating infections appear in patients with SLE, and so readily do they imitate the parent disease, that it is a wise rule never to accept a new change in a patient with SLE as necessarily a part of SLE until one has first carefully excluded infectious complications.

Septicemias of any sort, and in particular gram-negative septicemias, may be associated with widespread hemorrhagic phenomena owing to occlusion of multiple small vessels. Such occlusions sometimes mimic those produced by thrombotic thrombocytopenic purpura or by forms of arteritis.

Could this patient have had such an infection? She was suspected at one time of having tuberculosis, but I am not aware of tuberculosis producing such changes. Cultures of her urine showed nothing significant. Her lungs were clear. Could she have had an intra-abdominal abscess, the result of perforation of her long-standing peptic ulcer? Of course this is possible, and we will discuss this point later.

There are features of this patient's course which very strongly point to bacterial endocarditis, namely:
  1. A loud apical systolic murmur.
  2. Progressive anemia.
  3. The development of a nephritis with uremia.

4. The sudden appearance of neurological changes, which could have been the result of embolism.

5. Terminally, sudden onset of intra-abdominal bleeding, which could have been the result of a mycotic aneurysm.

Finally, she did have a staphylococcal abscess drained over her left ankle. We are loath to lay aside this possibility. However, a strong point against this or any other infection was the fact that repeated blood cultures were negative, and these were obtained at the height of her hemorrhagic tendencies, in addition at a time when she was not receiving antibiotics.

We must conclude, therefore, that the primal cause of her bleeding must have been an active vasculitis, which was part and parcel of her on-going SLE. This impression receives weight from the fact that a skin biopsy showed an active arteritis.

In thinking about the arteritis of SLE, it is well to recall that while this disorder characteristically affects small vessels, larger vessels may be injured by virtue of involvement of their vasa vasorum. Also, changes exactly similar to those of polyarteritis nodosa are seen in SLE occasionally, with perhaps a smaller number of eosinophils being present in the lesions. Such arteritic lesions can become extensive and massive in SLE, leading to widespread hemorrhage and even to gangrene of the extremities. There is surely enough reason to speculate about such changes taking place here.

Next, let us ask ourselves what is the most reasonable way in which to relate the diffuse arteritic alterations just postulated to the terminal episode, characterized as it was by (a) a period of seeming improvement, followed by (b) sudden appearance of shock, transiently responding to blood replacement, (c) the development of a rigid, tender abdomen with adynamic ileus, and (d) brisk hemorrhage per rectum, and bleeding into the abdominal cavity. A wide variety of possibilities present themselves. Let us briefly review them.

1. As a result of the rupture of vessels, patients with arteritis may form large hematomas, particularly in the region of the liver, spleen, and kidneys, but actually anywhere within the abdominal cavity. In the past two years we have seen three such patients. These hematomas may be mistaken for solid tumor masses, abscesses, or aneurysms, if they lie adjacent to pulsating vessels. They may rupture, inducing shock. However, in this instance, no such mass had been felt prior to onset of shock, and such a ruptured hematoma would not account for the brisk intestinal hemorrhage which accompanied the onset of shock.

2. Hemoperitoneum may be caused by rupture of the liver or the spleen. While there was no apparent cause for rupture of the liver, her spleen was enlarged, and it is conceivable that a spleen might rupture spontaneously if acutely affected by an arteritic process—although I have never heard of such happening in SLE. However, there was no tenderness or fullness about the spleen after this incident occurred and, furthermore, how could a ruptured spleen produce *intestinal* bleeding?

3. We have already spoken of our concern that this patient might have

acquired some infection, perhaps an intra-abdominal abscess resulting from a ruptured peptic ulcer. Rarely, such abscesses may erode a vessel and produce hemoperitoneum and shock. The fact that this patient was on steroids could have set the stage for the development of such an abscess, and at the same time it could have masked all the usual clinical appearances of such a lesion. On the other hand, this patient's abdomen was repeatedly examined, both clinically and radiologically, and not even a hint of the presence of such an inflammatory lesion was ever found. Furthermore, one would be hard put to understand how such an abscess could cause hemorrhage intraluminally into the gut, such as marked this patient's final hours.

4. The likelihood that this patient may have had an active peptic ulcer seems excessively high, what with the past history of duodenal deformity and tarry stools. When ulcers bleed, they may also perforate; could not the simultaneous occurrence of these two catastrophes have produced the changes noted here?

Obviously this possibility is not lightly discarded, but there are some facts in the history which do not quite fit this explanation.

  a. Initially, her abdomen was remarkably free of local spasm and tenderness. However, we must again emphasize the masking potentialities of adrenal steroids, for we have examined several patients with fecal peritonitis whose abdomens felt quite "benign," thanks to the steroids they were taking.
  b. A significant collection of blood in the abdominal cavity is certainly not a usual accompaniment of a ruptured and bleeding ulcer. Generally, chronic ulcers of the sort this patient probably had are buried deeply in the pancreas, or are surrounded by so much inflammatory tissue that gross bleeding into the free abdominal cavity does not take place. In a study of 100 patients with hemoperitoneum by Battersby, only 5 percent were found to be associated with a ruptured ulcer.

5. There are two good reasons to speculate about an acute hemorrhagic pancreatitis.

  a. Pancreatitis is said to occur with increased incidence in patients who are taking adrenal steroids over a prolonged period of time.
  b. The pancreas is not uncommonly involved in an acute arteritis.

Moreover, pancreatitis is one of the relatively small group of abdominal disorders in which severe shock makes its appearance early, whereas in ruptured peptic ulcer, it is more often a delayed phenomenon. Again, intraabdominal and intraperitoneal bleeding, as well as retroperitoneal bleeding, can occur in acute pancreatitis, the result of the effect of digestive enzymes on tissues and vessels. Obviously, this is a possibility to be taken most seriously here.

But, again, there is evidence which does not suit such a diagnosis. The patient had no pain in her back. There was no nausea, vomiting, or retching. The abdomen was initially quite soft. Once more, however, we have to remember the possible masking effects of steroids. Also—and this is most important—the stress laid on the acuteness of abdominal signs in pancreatitis in the older literature is no longer regarded as being realistic, for not infrequently, even without steroids, abdominal tenderness and spasm are of only mild or moderate degree, particularly in early stages. Nevertheless, in a fulminant pancreatitis, such as would be anticipated here, one surely would have expected more provocative changes in the upper abdomen than were described here. Also, massive bleeding from the GI tract is not a very common accompaniment of acute pancreatitis. Further, the appearance of gross blood in the abdominal cavity so early in the course of pancreatitis would seem to be an unusual result of pancreatic enzymes, and one might have expected fat particles in the fluid to have been removed. No fat particles were described. It is too bad a serum amylase test was not performed at this time. However, on several previous occasions when the patient had abdominal pain, the amylase level was determined. On one occasion it was 400 Somogyi units/100 ml., but on all others it was low.

6. Occlusion of mesenteric vessels, owing to thrombi or to emboli (the latter perhaps arising from myocarditis) is a not unlikely happening in the setting of acute arteritis we have described, and it may be associated with hemoperitoneum and shock. In addition, emboli could account for neurological and renal alterations. The latent period which transpired here between the onset of shock and the subsequent disappearance of bowel sounds and development of distention, rigidity, and adynamic ileus is typical of a mesenteric occlusion. Bleeding into the gut also occurs, as you well know. However, such bleeding is generally of a mild degree, presenting as melena, and the brisk hemorrhaging from the upper and lower ends of the GI tract described here would be out of character for mesenteric occlusion by thrombi or emboli.

7. Malignant tumors are among the more common causes of a hemoperitoneum. This patient was 59, and we must not forget that patients with SLE can also acquire other kinds of disease processes. In this regard, I recall a woman with recognized SLE, followed here for several years, who began to have convulsive seizures. It was concluded these must be a part of her SLE process, and she died soon afterward. At post mortem examination, an operable meningioma was discovered. All symptoms and signs in the patient with SLE are not necessarily a result of SLE. This axiom is worth remembering. In this particular setting, in the absence of localizing signs and symptoms pointing to a specific type of neoplasm, and in view of the description of an enlarged spleen and liver, we should place lymphoma high on the list of potential invaders, especially since in recent times there have been several reports of the concomitance of SLE and lymphomata. This has occasioned some excitement among the ranks of the auto-immunologists—who sometimes appear to be somewhat overexcitable! But enlargement of this patient's liver and spleen had been noted for a long time, no other masses were palpable within the abdomen, a G.I. series had failed to disclose any infiltrating lesion and, finally, lymphoma does not explain the renal or neurological changes very well.

8. We come, then to our final consideration, which is that the hemoperitoneum could have resulted from a ruptured dissecting aneurysm. Such aneurysms accounted for blood in the abdominal cavity in 14 percent of the patients Battersby studied, although bleeding from aneurysms more frequently occurs in the retroperitoneal tissues than directly into the abdominal cavity. Better than anything else, an aneurysm fits these aspects of the total course of events of this patient's catastrophic termination:
   a. The sudden development of paralysis of the legs, and an atonic urinary bladder.
   b. The sudden onset of shock.
   c. The terminal pain in the chest as well as in the abdomen.
   d. The latent period, before adynamic ileus and distention and rigidity of the abdomen became evident.
   e. The bleeding into the gut, as well as into the cavity of the abdomen.

It might be argued that no murmurs or alterations in the peripheral pulses were described, but these physical changes either may not be present at all, or are present only inconstantly, and often are unfortunately overlooked, particularly if a very ill patient is being examined under emergency circumstances, as was the case here.

But why should this patient have developed an aneurysm, and why did it rupture? The most plausible explanation is that it was the result of acute arteritic changes in the vasa vasorum, leading to necrosis of the tunica media. I have never seen or heard of such a complication occurring in a patient with SLE, but it has been described in rare instances in polyarteritis nodosa.

In conclusion, then, I believe that this patient with long-standing SLE entered a phase of her disease in which widespread acute arteritis was a predominant alteration. As a part of this process, and of its effects upon the walls of large and small vessels alike, she developed a dissecting aneurysm of the aorta, which ultimately ruptured into the abdominal cavity and gut. She possibly also had a peptic ulcer.

POST MORTEM FINDINGS

Disseminated lupus erythematosus with widespread arteritis. Multiple aneurysms of the superior mesenteric artery, with terminal rupture into mesentery and peritoneal cavity. Subdural hematoma of the spinal cord.

REFERENCES

DuBois, E. L.: Clinical manifestations of SLE. Computer analysis of 512 cases. JAMA *182*:513, 1964.

DuBois, E. L.: SLE: a review of the current status of discoid and systemic lupus and their variants. New York, Blakiston Division, McGraw-Hill Book Co., 1966.

DuBois, E. L., and Tufanelli, D. L.: Clinical manifestations of SLE. Computer analysis of 512 cases. JAMA *190*:104, 1964.
Estes, D., and Christian, C. L.: Natural history of SLE by perspective analysis. Medicine *50*:85, 1971.
Harvey, A. M., Shulman, L. E., Tumulty, P. A., Conley, C. L., and Schoenrich, E. H.: Systemic lupus—review of literature and analysis of 138 cases. Medicine *33*:291, 1954.
Ropes, M. W.: Observations on the natural course of lupus. Medicine *43*:387, 1964.

Index

Abdomen, fluid in, delineation of, 85
  in physical examination, 82
  pain in, causes of, 85, 86
Abdominal aneurysms, clinical
  presentations of, 81
Abscess, intrahepatic, diagnosis of, 86
  liver, patient with, diagnostic
    discussion of, 229–233
  perinephric, diagnosis of, 87
  subdiaphragmatic, diagnosis of, 87
Acropachy, diagnostic significance of,
  64
Alcoholic patient, counseling of, 33
Amyloidosis, patient with, diagnostic
  discussion of, 315–321
Aneurysms, abdominal, clinical
  presentations, of, 81
Aortic insufficiency, congestive heart
  failure and, patient with,
  diagnostic discussion of, 296–303
Arteries, peripheral, in physical
  examination, 79
Arteritis, giant cell, as cause of fever
  of unknown origin, 152
Arthritis, rheumatoid, complications
  and, patient with, diagnostic
  discussion of, 342–349
Ascites, patient with, diagnostic
  discussion of, 268–277
Attitude, of patient, effect of illness
    on, 12
  toward physician, 11
  of physician, toward patient, 14
  toward patient's family, 42

Bacteroides, as cause of fever of
  unknown origin, 146
Biopsies, surgeon-internist
  communication in, 117

Bleeding, profuse, systemic lupus
  erythematosus and, patient with,
  diagnostic discussion of, 362–370
Blood pressure, determination of, 54
Body temperature, 137–138. See also
  Temperature.
Breath, shortness of, significance of,
  74
Breathing capacity, gross assessment
  of, 75
Brucellosis, as cause of fever of
  unknown origin, 146

Carcinoma, pancreatic, diagnosis of,
  87
  physical examination and, 84
Cardiac surgery, persistent fever and
  malaise after, diagnostic
  discussion of, 214–219
Cardiac tamponade, 79
Charcot's fever, 148
Chest, in physical examination, 72
  pain in, severe venous in-flow
    block, coronary artery disease
    and, patient with, diagnostic
    discussion of, 258–266
Circulation, in physical examination,
  76
Clinical management, biopsies in, 117
  briefing of patient in, 116–117
  conservatism vs. action in, 119
  consultants in, selection of, 103
  diagnostic studies in, selection of,
    104–108
  diet in, 116
  differential diagnosis in, listing of,
    103–104
  drugs in, 111–115
    cost of, 112

373

Clinical management (*Continued*)
  drugs in, development of
      dependencies upon, 114
    failures in, 115
    instructions to patient in, 113
    proper administration of,
      113–114
    reactions to, 114–115
    tranquilizing, 115
  general considerations in, 101–123
  hospitalization in, decision on, 110
  knowledge of facts in, 118
  "minor" patient complaints in, 115
  observation in, 108
  operations in, planning of, 117–118
  orders in, writing of, 110–111
  plan of, presentation of, sense of
      timing in, 102
  progress notes in, 122–123
  progress visits in, 120–122
  stability in, value of, 119–120
  worksheet in, 104
Clinician. See also *Physician*.
  definition of, 1
  function of, 3
Clubbing, of fingers and toes,
    diagnostic significance of, 64
Collagen-vascular disorders, as cause
    of fever of unknown origin,
    151–152
Coloration, of hair, in physical
    examination, 56
Communication, with consultant,
    45–48
  with family of patient, 39–42
  with family of patient with
    incurable illness, 179, 180–
    183
    at time of death, 183–185
  with patient, 4, 11–15
    practical guidelines for, 6
  with patient with incurable illness,
    172–176
Congestive heart failure, aortic
    insufficiency and, patient with,
    diagnostic discussion of, 296–
    303
Congestive hepatomegaly, 77
Conjunctivitis, diagnostic implications
    of, 68
Constrictive pericarditis, 79
Consultant, examination by, 46
  primary physician and, 45
    disagreement between, 47, 48
  role of, 45–48
  selection of, in clinical
      management, 103
Contractures, Dupuytren's,
    significance of, 63

Coronary artery disease, chest pain,
    severe venous in-flow block and,
    patient with, diagnostic
    discussion of, 258–266
Coxsackie virus, abdominal pain
    caused by, diagnosis of, 86
Crohn's disease, as cause of fever of
    unknown origin, 152–153
Cryptococcal meningitis, patient
    with, diagnostic discussion of,
    278–284
Cyanosis, 54, 55

Death, of patient with incurable
    illness, 183–185
  sudden, patient suffering,
    diagnostic discussion of,
    234–240
Deposits in integument, significance
    of, 59
Diabetic patient, counseling of, 33
Diagnosis. See also names of specific
    ailments to be diagnosed.
  differential, clinical evidence in,
      detailed analysis of, 192–193
    gathering of, 189–190
    organization of, 190–192
    provisional diagnosis from, 195
  common errors in, 196–197
  illustrative example of, 197–199
  listing of disorders in, 193–195
  in clinical management,
    103–104
  systematic approach to, 189–199
  explanation of, to patient, 32
  problem-oriented, 201–371
  vs. management, 1
Diagnostic studies, cessation of,
    decision for, 107–108
  in functional disorders, 128
    avoidance of, 129
    discussion of, with patient, 130,
      131
  order of performance of, 106
  selection of, 104–108
  tempo of, 106–107
  troublesome, 108–109
Diaphragms, examination of, 73
Diet, in clinical management, 116
Differential diagnosis. See *Diagnosis,
    differential*.
Drug fever, 148–149
Drugs, functional disorders and, 129,
    130
  in clinical management, cost of,
    112
  development of dependencies
      upon, 114
  failures in, 115

INDEX

Drugs (*Continued*)
  in clinical management,
    instructions to patient in, 113
  prescription of, 111–115
  proper administration of,
    113–114
  reactions to, 114–115
  tranquilizing, 115
Dupuytren's contractures, significance
    of, 63

Edema, significance of, 57
Effusion, pericardial, 78
Emboli, pulmonary, multiple, patient
    with, diagnostic discussion of,
    207–213
Embolism, pulmonary, as cause of
    fever of unknown origin, 152
  clinical presentations of, 80
Episodic polyorgan system disease,
    chronic, patient with, diagnostic
    discussion of, 305–314
Examination, physical, 51–91. See
    also *Physical examination*.
Exophthalmos, 67
Exploratory laparotomy, in fever of
    unknown origin, 156–161
Extremities, in physical examination,
    63
  skin of, examination of, 65
Eyes, in physical examination, 67

Face, in physical examination, 67
Factitious fever, 154
Family, patient's, attitude of, during
    physical examination, 52
  communication with, 39–42
    in incurable illness, 179,
      180–183
      at times of death, 183–185
  consultant's relations with, 46,
    47
  discussions with, 40
  effect of illness on, 39
  hostile, protections against, 41
  in incurable illness, 179, 180–183
    counseling at time of death,
      183–185
  physician's attitude toward, 42
Fat, subcutaneous, in physical
    examination, 61
Fatal illness, patient with, 171–185.
    See also *Illness, incurable*.
Feet, structure of, diagnostic
    significance of, 63
Fever, Charcot's, 148
  drug, 148–149

Fever (*Continued*)
  factitious, 154
    vs. true, 53
  of unknown origin, 137–164
    Bacteroides as cause of, 146
    brucellosis as cause of, 146
    causes of, 138–139
    collagen-vascular disorders as
      cause of, 151–152
    course of, 142–143
    Crohn's disease as cause of,
      152–153
    diagnosis of, difficulties of,
      138–140
    drugs as cause of, 148–149
    exploratory laparotomy in,
      156–161
    eye examination in, 68
    giant cell arteritis as cause of,
      152
    histoplasmosis as cause of, 145
    infectious mononucleosis as cause
      of, 147
    leptospiral infections as cause of,
      147
    meningococcal infections as
      cause of, 147
    patient's history in, 140–141
    physical examination in, 142
    pulmonary embolism as cause of,
      152
    Salmonella as cause of, 146
    sarcoidosis as cause of, 146
    therapeutic trial in, 154–156
    tuberculosis as cause of, 143–145
    tularemia as cause of, 146
    tumors as cause of, 150–151
    vs. factitious fever, 154
    Whipple's disease as cause of,
      153
  pattern of, 138
  persistent, malaise and, patient
    with, after cardiac surgery,
    diagnostic discussion of,
    214–219
Finger(s), clubbing of, diagnostic
    significance of, 64
  structure of, diagnostic significance
    of, 63
Fingernails, changes in, observation
    of, 65
Fluid, abdominal, delineation of, 85
Focal infections, as cause of fever of
    unknown origin, 147–148
Functional disorders, 125–135
  diagnostic studies in, 128
    avoidance of, 129
  discussion of, with patient, 130,
    131

Functional disorders (*Continued*)
  drugs and, 129, 130
  treatment of, 132
  vs. organic disease, 128
Fundic vessels of eye, examination of, 68, 69
FUO, 137–164. See also *Fever, of unknown origin.*

Gastrointestinal hemorrhage, obscure, patient with, diagnostic discussion of, 249–256
Genitalia, in physical examination, 88
Giant cell arteritis, as cause of fever of unknown origin, 152
Gland(s), parotid, in physical examination, 66
  thyroid, examination of, 71
Granulomatous processes, significance of, 59
Gums, examination of, 70

Hair, in physical examination, 56
Hamman-Rich syndrome, patient with, diagnostic discussion of, 286–294
Hands, appearance of, diagnostic significance of, 63
Head, in physical examination, 67
Heart, in physical examination, 76
Heart failure, congestive, aortic insufficiency and, patient with, diagnostic discussion of, 296–303
Hemoglobinopathy, patient with, diagnostic discussion of, 351–361
Hemorrhage, gastrointestinal, obscure, patient with, diagnostic discussion of, 249–256
"splinter," significance of, 58
Hepatomegaly, congestive, 77
Histoplasmosis, as cause of fever of unknown origin, 145
History-taking, 17–27. See also *Interview.*
  analysis of earlier diagnoses in, 21
  detecting clues in, 17
  explanation to patient in, 18
  importance of, 7
  in fever of unknown origin, 140–142
  methodology of, 18
  personal and social, 25
  recording of, 26
  review of past illness in, 19
  review of present illness in, 19
Hypercalcemia, patient with, diagnostic discussion of, 201–205

Icterus, detection of, 54, 55
Illness, effect of, on patient's attitude, 12
  fatal, patient with, 171–185. See also *Illness, incurable.*
  incurable, patient's family in, 179, 180–183
    patient with, 171–185
      communicating with, 172–176
      management of, 172, 176–180
  management of, vs. diagnosis, 1
  progressive, patient with, 171–185. See also *Illness, incurable.*
  severity of, estimation of, 89
    general evidence for, 89
    specific evidence for, 90
  total impact of, 3
Incurable illness, patient with, 171–185. See also *Illness, incurable.*
Infections, as cause of fever of unknown origin, 143–148
Infectious mononucleosis, as cause of fever of unknown origin, 147
Infiltrates in integument, significance of, 59
Integument, deposits and infiltrates in, 59
Interstitial pneumonitis of Hamman-Rich, patient with, diagnostic discussion of, 186–194
Interview, "final" or summarizing, 29–36
  response of patient in, 35
  significance of, 29
  structuring of, 30
  terms used in, 31
Intrahepatic abscess, diagnosis of, 86

Joint, affected, examination of, 64

Kidney. See also *Perinephric abscess* and *Uremia.*
  systolic bruits around, detection of, 82

Laparotomy, exploratory, in fever of unknown origin, 156–161
Leptospiral infections, as cause of fever of unknown origin, 147
Lips, in physical examination, 70
Liver, abscess of, patient with, diagnostic discussion of, 229–233
  palpation of, 83

Lupus erythematosus, systemic, complications and, patient with, diagnostic discussion of, 333–341
   family history in, 140, 141
   profuse bleeding and, patient with, diagnostic discussion of, 362–370
Lymph nodes, in physical examination, 66

Malaise, persistent fever and, patient with, after cardiac surgery, diagnostic discussion of, 214–219
Malignant tumors, early cutaneous and subcutaneous metastases of, 60
Malocclusion of teeth, 70
Management, clinical, general considerations in, 101–123. See also *Clinical management.*
   outlining program of, to patient, 34
   vs. diagnosis, 1
Mediastinal mass, patient with, diagnostic discussion of, 241–248
Mediastinum, in physical examination, 75
Meningitis, cryptococcal, patient with, diagnostic discussion of, 278–284
Meningococcal infections, as cause of fever of unknown origin, 147
Mononucleosis, infectious, as cause of fever of unknown origin, 147
Mouth, in physical examination, 70
Murmurs, extracardiac, 81
Muscles, in physical examination, 61
Myositis, significance of, 61

Nails, changes in, observation of, 65
Nasopharynx, in physical examination, 69
Neck, in physical examination, 71
   venous engorgement of, significance of, 77
Neoplasms, as cause of fever of unknown origin, 150–151
Nodules, rheumatoid, 60

Obese patient, counseling of, 33
Operations, surgical, planning in, 117–118
Oral cavity, in physical examination, 70

Organic disease, vs. functional disorder, 128

Pain, abdominal, causes of, 85, 86
   as symptom, 22
   associated phenomena of, 24
   cause of, 23
   character of, 23
   chest, severe venous in-flow block, coronary artery disease and, patient with, diagnostic discussion of, 258–266
   decrease in, 24
   increase in, 23
   location of, 22
   radiation of, 22
   time relationships of, 24
Pallor, detection of, 54
Pancreas, carcinoma of, diagnosis of, 87
   physical examination and, 84
Papilledema, recognition of, 68
Parotid glands, in physical examination, 66
Patient, alcoholic, counseling of, 33
   attitude of, effect of illness on, 12
      toward physician, 11
   attitude of physician toward, 14
   body structure of, 53
   briefing of, concerning clinical management, 116–117
   clinical management of, general considerations in, 101–123. See also *Clinical Management.*
   coloration of, in physical examination, 54
   communication with, 4, 11–15
      practical guidelines for, 6
   consultant's relations with, 46
   diabetic, counseling of, 33
   explanation of diagnosis to, 32
   family of, communication with, 39–42. See also *Family, patient's.*
   general appearances of, during physical examination, 52
   hospitalized, progress visits to, 120–122
   instructions to, concerning prescribed drugs, 113
   "minor" complaints of, 116
   obese, counseling of, 33
   outlining management program to, 35
   personality of, analysis of, 13
      during physical examination, 52
   physical examination of, 50–91. See also *Physical examination.*

Patient (*Continued*)
  response of, to "final" or summarizing interview, 35
  responsiveness of, during physical examination, 52
  with functional disorder, 125–135
  with incurable illness, 171–185
Pelvis, inflammatory disease in, diagnosis of, 88
Pericardial disease, physical examination and, 78
Perinephric abscess, diagnosis of, 87
Peripheral arteries, in physical examination, 79
Peripheral veins, in physical examination, 80
Personality of patient, analysis of, 13
  during physical examination, 52
Petechiae, significance of, 58
Physical examination, 51–91
  abdomen in, 82
  chest in, 72
  deposits, infiltrates and nodules in, 59
  edema in, 57
  extremities in, 63
  eyes in, 67
  family members' attitude during, 52
  general appearance of patient during, 52
  general observations in, 51
  general setting of, 52
  genitalia in, 88
  hair in, 56
  head and face in, 67
  heart and circulation in, 76
  importance of, 7
  in fever of unknown origin, 142
  lips and oral cavity in, 70
  lymph nodes in, 66
  mediastinum in, 75
  muscles in, 61
  nasopharynx in, 69
  neck in, 71
  parotid glands in, 66
  particular observations during, 54
  patient's personality during, 52
  patient's response during, character of, 52
  pericardial disease and, 78
  peripheral arteries in, 79
  peripheral veins in, 80
  scars and tattoos in, 56
  severity of illness and, estimation of, 89
  skeleton in, 88
  skin eruptions in, 58
  skin in, observation of, 54

Patient (*Continued*)
  sternum in, 76
  subcutaneous fat in, 61
  superior vena cava in, 76
  trachea in, 72
  vascular lesions in, 57
  vital signs in, 53
Physician. See also *Clinician*.
  attitude of, toward patient, 14
    toward patient's family, 42
  attitude of patient toward, 11
  primary, consultant and, 45
    disagreement between, 47, 48
Pigmentation, increased or decreased, 55
Pneumonia, pneumococcal, fulminant, patient with, diagnostic discussion of, 221–228
Pneumonitis, interstitial, of Hamman-Rich, patient with, diagnostic discussion of, 186–194
Polyorgan system disease, episodic, chronic, patient with, diagnostic discussion of, 305–314
Progress notes, writing of, 122–123
Pulmonary emboli, multiple, patient with, diagnostic discussion of, 207–213
Pulmonary embolism, as cause of fever of unknown origin, 152
  clinical presentations of, 80
Pulse rate, significance of, 53
Purpura, distribution of, significance of, 58

Rales, post-tussic, 74
Respiratory rate, importance of, 53
Rheumatoid arthritis, complications and, patient with, diagnostic discussion of, 342–349
Rheumatoid nodules, 60
Ribs, examination of, 73
Rubs, pericardial, 78

Salmonella, as cause of fever of unknown origin, 146
Sarcoidosis, as cause of fever of unknown origin, 146
Scalp, in physical examination, 67
Scars, diagnostic pertinence of, 56
Skeleton, in physical examination, 88

INDEX

Skin, adherence of, to subcutaneous tissues, 56
  coloration of, examination of, 54
  deposits, infiltrates and nodules upon, 59
  eruptions of, significance of, 58
  of extremities, examination of, 65
  pigmentation of, increased or decreased, 55
  texture of, examination of, 55
  thickening of, 56
Skull, auscultation of, in physical examination, 67
Spiders, vascular, 57
Spleen, palpation of, 84
"Splinter hemorrhages," significance of, 58
Sternum, in physical examination, 76
Subcutaneous fat, in physical examination, 61
Subdiaphragmatic abscess, diagnosis of, 87
Superior vena cava, in physical examination, 76
Systemic lupus erythematosus, complications and, patient with, diagnostic discussion, 333–341
  family history in, 140, 141
  profuse bleeding and, patient with, diagnostic discussion of, 362–370

Tamponade, cardiac, 79
Tattoos, diagnostic pertinence of, 57
Teeth, malocclusion of, 70
Telangiectases, 57
Temperature, 137–138
  elevated, 53. See also *Fever*.
  factors affecting, 137
  normal, 137
Thoracic cage, examination of, 72
Thyroid gland, examination of, 71

Toes, clubbing of, diagnostic significance of, 64
Tongue, examination of, 71
Trachea, in physical examination, 72
Tuberculosis, as cause of fever of unknown origin, 143–145
Tularemia, as cause of fever of unknown origin, 146
Tumors, as cause of fever of unknown origin, 150–151
  malignant, early cutaneous and subcutaneous metastases of, 60

Uremia, chronic, patient with, diagnostic discussion of, 323–331
Uveal tract, alterations in, 68

Vascular lesions, on extremities, significance of, 64
  significance of, 57
Vascular spiders, 57
Veins, peripheral, in physical examination, 80
Vena cava, superior, in physical examination, 76
Venous engorgement of neck, significance of, 77
Venous in-flow block, severe, chest pain, coronary artery disease and, patient with, diagnostic discussion of, 258–266
Vital signs, 53

Wheezing, significance of, 73, 74
Whipple's disease, as cause of fever of unknown origin, 153
Worksheet, in clinical management, 104